Culture and PTSD

THE ETHNOGRAPHY OF POLITICAL VIOLENCE

Tobias Kelly, *Series Editor*

A complete list of books in the series
is available from the publisher.

CULTURE AND PTSD

Trauma in Global
and Historical Perspective

Edited by

Devon E. Hinton

and

Byron J. Good

PENN

UNIVERSITY OF PENNSYLVANIA PRESS

PHILADELPHIA

Published by
University of Pennsylvania Press
Philadelphia, Pennsylvania 19104-4112
www.upenn.edu/pennpress

Printed in the United States of America on acid-free paper

1 3 5 7 9 10 8 6 4 2

Library of Congress Cataloging-in-Publication Data
Culture and PTSD : trauma in global and historical perspective /
edited by Devon E. Hinton and Byron J. Good.
     pages cm — (The ethnography of political violence)
   Includes bibliographical references and index.
   ISBN 978-0-8122-4714-5 (alk. paper)
     1. Post-traumatic stress disorder—Case studies.
2. Ethnopsychology—Case studies.   3. Cross-cultural counseling—
Case studies.   4. Transcultural medical care—Case studies.
I. Hinton, Devon E., editor.   II. Good, Byron, editor.   III. Series:
Ethnography of political violence.
   RC552.P67C85 2015
   616.85'210089—dc23
                                                      2015014672

CONTENTS

PART I

Introduction and Theoretical
Background

Introduction: Culture, Trauma, and PTSD

Byron J. Good and Devon E. Hinton

Since the 1970s, the terms "trauma," "posttraumatic stress disorder" (or PTSD), and "trauma treatment" have become so much a part of everyday language in the United States that they seem to most Americans to name natural realities. Although the general public could hardly recite the criteria of the most recent American Psychiatric Association's *Diagnostic and Statistical Manual*—the DSM-5—the image of persons suffering intensive, recurrent memories or flashbacks of traumatic experiences they have suffered is now part of common understandings of human nature. The ideas that reliving such traumatic events through intrusive memories can reproduce the terror associated with events and lead to social withdrawal and impairment, that repressing and re-remembering such memories is possible, and that working through these memories in some form of psychotherapy can lead to improvement are now deeply embedded in popular American understandings of trauma, illness, and recovery. It was therefore provocative when in 1995 Allan Young wrote in the introduction to his classic book *The Harmony of Illusions: Inventing Post-Traumatic Stress Disorder*: "The disorder is not timeless, nor does it possess an intrinsic unity. Rather, it is glued together by the practices, technologies, and narratives with which it is diagnosed, studied, treated, and represented and by the various interests, institutions, and moral arguments that mobilized the efforts and resources" (Young 1995:5).

Among anthropologists and cultural critics of mainstream psychiatry, Young's position is now widely accepted. For many, it is linked to a broader critique of the universality of psychiatric diagnostic categories in general—and of the globalization of psychiatry. The more specific critique of PTSD and trauma treatment as the pathologization of normal forms of suffering—in settings of war and violence, for example—is for many particularly compelling. But while quoting Young on the "invention" of PTSD is common, it is less common to attend to Young's rejection of the suggestion that his saying PTSD is a "historical product" means that it is "not real." "On the contrary," Young writes, "the reality of PTSD is confirmed empirically by its place in people's lives, by their experiences and convictions. . . . My job as an ethnographer of PTSD is not to deny its reality but to explain how it and its traumatic memory have been *made* real, to describe the mechanisms through which these phenomena penetrate people's lifeworlds, acquire facticity, and shape the self-knowledge of patients, clinicians, and researchers" (5–6). The program set forth by Young, of exploring the ways that traumatic memory is made real, penetrating people's lifeworlds and shaping self-knowledge, is in many ways more challenging than engaging in debates over the status of PTSD. And it is the subject of this book.

Culture and PTSD is an examination of the ways that PTSD—and trauma and trauma treatment more broadly—are made real in diverse, cross-cultural settings far from the clinics of the post–Vietnam War Veterans Administration in which Young did his research and twenty years removed from that work. The central chapters are ethnographic and historical, providing rich data about the local experiences of complex forms of violence and the deployment of psychiatric categories and psychosocial treatments in these settings. The chapters raise explicit questions about whether phenomena comparable to the DSM description of PTSD are to be found in other societies and at other times in history. And they raise explicit questions about particular diagnostic criteria. But the book is not organized as a debate over the ontological status of PTSD. The essays do not focus primarily on the question of whether PTSD is a real, universal disease, or whether, as psychiatrist Derek Summerfield (1999) claims, it should be considered a "pseudocondition." This book is rather an examination by anthropologists, psychiatrists, and psychologists about the fit between PTSD, as is represented in the current *Diagnostic and Statistical Manual* (DSM-5) and in clinical research, and local forms of illness experience. And it is an exploration of the deployment of trauma, PTSD, and trauma treatments in settings such as Navajo country in New Mexico and Oaxaca in Mexico, and settings of conflict and violence, including Haiti, Peru, and Aceh, Indonesia. While the book addresses classic questions about the historical and cross-cultural validity of the PTSD construct, its real focus is an examination of how individuals, families, and communities in very diverse cultural settings experience the effects of wars, brutal civil conflicts, and domestic violence, and on how communities, clinicians, and public health specialists respond to individuals who experience prolonged suffering as a consequence.

Debates Framing the Book

This book is framed by two sets of contemporary debates. First, these chapters were written as revision of the American Psychiatric Association's *Diagnostic and Statistical Manual* and the preparation of the new manual, the DSM-5, was under way. The anxiety disorders committee took seriously questions of cultural validity, and critical reviews—such as Hinton and Lewis-Fernández's review (2011) of the cross-cultural validity of PTSD criteria—have played a role in the revision of the manual. Debates about specific symptom clusters and diagnostic criteria will be discussed below.

At the same time, narrow debates about the wording of diagnostic criteria were easier to address in the revision of the DSM than larger debates about the framing of the diagnostic manual. For PTSD, issues of narrowly defined categories versus more pervasive conditions have been long-standing concerns in both clinical work and research. PTSD in the psychiatric diagnostic system is defined as a response to a specific trauma event that produces particular clusters of symptoms. But how is this relevant to the more pervasive trauma, such as that resulting from years of child abuse or living in localities of ongoing insecurity and violence or long-term involvement as combatants or civilians, for clinicians and trauma researchers? For many, broader issues such as these are more important and far more difficult to respond to than the wording of specific criteria for PTSD and acute trauma diagnoses. In the current revision of the DSM, these broader issues were left unresolved—again. As the essays in this book show, the broader view of complex trauma is more relevant in many settings in which anthropologists and global mental health specialists work than the narrower view of PTSD represented in the DSM. This book contributes to an understanding of these more complex forms of trauma, their effects on lives in particular cultural settings, and the implications for trauma treatment and trauma research in cross-cultural settings.

The terms "complex trauma" and "complex PTSD" are used in this book and are part of ongoing debates. Both terms have a variety of meanings (Bryant 2010, 2012; de Jong et al. 2005; Herman 1992, 1993; Resick et al. 2012).

Complex trauma can refer to experiencing a severe trauma or multiple traumas over an extended period of time. Some define complex trauma as resulting from extended periods of child abuse, while others argue that complex PTSD may result from "a range of adult experiences, including war, civil conflict, torture, and other experiences involving pervasive loss of control over aversive consequences" (Bryant 2012:253). Complex trauma can refer to experiencing prolonged trauma while in a state of vulnerability, such as when young or when subject to multiple stresses. The term "complex PTSD" often refers to the clinical picture that may result from complex trauma, with complex trauma, as indicated above, said to result from many causes: the nature and severity of traumatic experience; duration of the trauma; age the trauma occurs and developmental effects; genetic vulnerability; or current levels of stress. The term also may refer specifically to the complexity of the clinical picture, including specific symptoms, in particular, somatization and emotion regulation difficulties, and comorbidity with other diagnosable conditions (major depressive disorder, other anxiety disorders such as panic disorder, and somatoform disorders, as well as personality disorders). Put more broadly, the complexity of the disorder may be related to social response and stigma associated with the traumatizing events (such as those experienced by many Vietnam vets) and to cultural interpretation of particular trauma-related symptoms. For example, as chapters in this book demonstrate, a culture that has catastrophic cognitions about somatic symptoms resulting from traumatic experience or PTSD may amplify the anxiety associated with traumatic memory and associated symptoms, resulting in more comorbidities among other effects.

Many of the chapters in this book address PTSD as understood in a broad perspective. The difference between PTSD as defined by DSM-5 and PTSD in a broader sense, that is, complex PTSD or trauma-related disorder, needs to be kept clear. This chapter and Chapter 1 use the term "posttraumatic stress syndrome" to indicate the wide set of symptoms that actually occur in a locality owing to trauma, from DSM-type PTSD symptoms to depression, generalized anxiety disorder, substance abuse, poor emotion regulation, or hyperreactivity to multiple triggers, among other symptoms in the "trauma symptom pool" (see Chapter 1). We also consider the term "posttraumatic stress syndrome" to include the local meaning of trauma symptoms (e.g., attribution of symptoms to local cultural syndromes), local consequences of having the symptoms (e.g., interpersonal and economic course), and ways of seeking treatment for symptoms. There are local "posttraumatic stress syndromes"—a Cambodian one, a Haitian one—which will overlap but also differ radically. The term "posttraumatic stress syndrome" better conveys the sense of the lived, contextualized experience of trauma than does the narrower term "PTSD"; it better describes the lived experience of illness than does the disease concept PTSD (Eisenberg 1977; Kleinman et al. 1978). At the same time, we recognize that much of the literature that describes PTSD actually refers to conditions or clinical presentations that are more akin to complex forms of posttrauma conditions than to simple PTSD. (When the term "posttraumatic" is used, it must be remembered that often trauma is ongoing and continuing, not just one past event, and in addition, that there are multiple types of ongoing stress. Hence the term "complex trauma" is often used as is discussed in this chapter and in Chapter 1 [Hinton and Good]. We use the term "posttraumatic stress syndrome" with the assumption of this broader frame. Many chapters in this volume discuss these issues, such as that of Jenkins and Haas [Chapter 5] and James [Chapter 11].)

Nosologically oriented researchers seek to find symptoms that are unique to particular disorders in order to create DSM categories that are distinct or heterogeneous, reducing the presence of the same symptoms in multiple diagnostic categories, increasing differentiation of disorders, and improving differential diagnosis (Bryant 2012; Resick et al. 2012). This is true for PTSD and acute trauma diagnoses. But for clinicians, as well as researchers with interests beyond nosology, not only are features of responses to trauma that are unique to PTSD important, but the entire range of symptoms and disorders that result from diverse forms of traumatic experience have great importance for understanding and responding to these conditions, particularly in culturally diverse populations. This book brings special attention to this broader range of phenomena, what we refer to as the posttraumatic stress syndrome, that is, to a broader set of trauma symptoms and how these play out in different cultural and global contexts. Given the eruptions of episodic violence globally, high endemic violence in some societies and in particular settings in nearly every society, widespread sexual and domestic violence, and forms of extreme traumatic experience for which there is universal risk, both PTSD and posttraumatic stress syndrome are important public health issues globally. These are the focus of the studies in this volume.

If the revision of the *Diagnostic and Statistical Manual* served as one context for the essays in this book, debates about the legitimacy of focusing on trauma and trauma treatment in global humanitarian settings serve as a second critical context. Attention to trauma and trauma treatment in settings of complex emergencies (e.g., IASC 2007), as well as debates about the legitimacy of psychosocial and mental health interventions in global humanitarian work, have become far more widespread and urgent than was the case when Young wrote about the making real of PTSD. Many, including anthropologists and cross-cultural psychiatrists, such as Arthur Kleinman, have strongly criticized the labeling of acute responses to traumatic violence as a mental disorder, arguing that this represents a pathologization and professionalization of normal forms of human suffering, a form of globalized medicalization of human responses to disaster and violence. Anthropologists interested in mental illnesses across cultures have also criticized the assumption—without adequate empirical research—that PTSD is a universally valid condition. These arguments have been elaborated by critics of humanitarianism and development, such as Derek Summerfield (1999:1449) who calls PTSD "a pseudocondition, a reframing of the understandable suffering of war as a technical problem to which short-term technical solutions like counseling are applicable." For Summerfield, the extension of notions of trauma and PTSD to non-Western societies may represent a form of psychological imperialism that "risks an unwitting perpetuation of the colonial status of the non-Western mind" (2000:422). Vanessa Pupavac (2001), Mark Duffield (2001), and others have linked the focus on trauma by humanitarian organizations to the pathologization of whole societies. The demand for "psycho-social interventions," they argue, serves as a "new form of international therapeutic governance" (Pupavac 2001:358) that contributes to the "mobile sovereignty" (Pandolfi 2008:263; cf. Fassin and Pandolfi 2010) of international aid organizations more than to the relief of suffering in the communities they intend to help.

These criticisms have been taken up by those who question the increasing role played by humanitarian organizations in settings of complex emergencies over the past several decades (see Good, Good, and Grayman [Chapter 12]). In her remarkable book about violence and reconciliation among the Quechua communities in Peru in the years following the end of the Shining Path era, Kimberly Theidon (2013) describes the significance of the "trauma industry" and its effects on how nongovernmental organizations framed their mental health missions, how the Truth and Reconciliation Commission coded data from the interviews conducted, and how the report described the long-term effects of the violence on those who had experienced and witnessed it. In the coding of interviews, a wide variety of deeply embodied descriptions of pain and suffering—embedded in what

Theidon calls "sensuous psychologies" (24–53)—were simply coded as "trauma." Theidon argues that this represented not only a globalization of trauma and PTSD as categories, shaping how international communities viewed the effects of violence, but that the dismissal of local Quechua terms represented a much deeper and long-standing view by urban, professional Peruvians of the indigenous communities as backward and incapable of abstract thought, a people whose complaints required translation into the modern language of trauma to be comprehensible. A history of colonialism and racism thus shaped the view of indigenous people and the need to code their experience in the reality-based, modern language of trauma and PTSD in order to devise mental health responses.

Many involved in the global mental health movement would agree that mental health and psychosocial interventions focused narrowly on trauma and trauma treatment are misplaced in postdisaster or postconflict settings. There is strong evidence that major disasters, conflicts, and violence increase the prevalence of mental health problems broadly, including the clusters of disorders associated with PTSD. Studies repeatedly show a "dose effect" linking levels of experiences of traumatic violence to risk for depression, anxiety disorders, and acute psychoses, as well as PTSD. And many of the settings in which humanitarian organizations work have extraordinarily limited mental health resources. Advocates for global mental health thus see humanitarian responses to disaster or violence as providing an opportunity to build mental health services more broadly. In this context, the critique of PTSD, trauma treatment, and psychosocial interventions often provide donor organizations with a rationale not only for not building effective responses to trauma-related conditions, but for refusing to invest in capacity building for mental health care more generally. The stakes are thus high in debates about how to think of trauma in settings of complex emergencies and what the most appropriate responses should be.

Given the massive scope of mental health problems in postdisaster and postconflict settings, are there empirically supported clinical and public health interventions that are effective? Is there evidence that providing mental health treatments for PTSD and other trauma-related mental health problems actually "jeopardizes local coping strategies," as suggested by Pupavac (2001)? What is the evidence for the effectiveness of purported "local coping strategies"?[1] And what, on the other hand, is the evidence for long-term effects of medical and psychosocial treatments for acute trauma and chronic, long-term forms of PTSD?

The essays in this book address questions that are central to the study of PTSD in cross-cultural perspectives, questions about what we can learn about PTSD and trauma-related mental health problems from cross-cultural research. But these questions are placed in the context of urgent questions about how to proceed, about whether the deployment of PTSD as a tool of identifying and responding to human trauma-related suffering is effective or actually creates new forms of victims and pernicious demands to demonstrate traumatic experience as a means of determining who is provided compensation and care.

Framing the cross-cultural study of PTSD in these terms—in technical diagnostic terms about the validity of particular symptom clusters across cultures, in relation to humanitarian work in resource limited settings, and in ethnographic terms concerning how PTSD is made real in diverse settings—is a reminder of significant changes since the writing of Young's *Harmony of Illusions*. Concerns about experiences of soldiers remain, but with traumatic brain injury now playing a new—or recurrent, given the similarities to the diagnosis of "shell shock"—role in discussions and treatment. Identifying and responding to PTSD is far more closely related to human rights activities than in the past and are closely linked to the moral imperative of the human rights movement. PTSD and trauma treatment play an important role in advocacy for increased investment in global mental health. Terms such as "historical trauma" (see Ball and O'Nell [Chapter 10]) place PTSD in a broader context of moral claims and the search for social and political forms of restitution. And debates about sexual violence and gender issues have taken an increasingly important place in global settings; these debates are often waged in terms of trauma, PTSD, and trauma treatment. These are all central issues in the essays in this book.

Historical Background

How have the terms "trauma" and "PTSD" come to be used to do such important cultural and moral work in American society and in global debates? Richard McNally argues in his essay in this book (Chapter 2) that although shell shock was commonly observed for soldiers in World War I and World War II, the cluster of symptoms now defined as PTSD are difficult to find in the records of medical treatments of soldiers in the great world wars. If this is the case, how did the current constellation of symptoms, meanings, and practices now associated with PTSD come to be recognized, produced, and made the focus of a wide variety of treatment modalities and the site of an extraordinary body of scientific research, particularly in the neurosciences?

Young and Breslau (Chapter 3) argue that the current conceptualization of PTSD arose in direct response to the Vietnam War. Current ideas about trauma and PTSD emerged, they show, in response to problems suffered by Vietnam veterans. Following the Vietnam War the concept was introduced in the DSM-III and became a diagnostic category to explain the psychological wounds of war, which enabled access to benefits and helped shift the society's view of the soldier presenting with psychological distress from that of shirker or weakling to victim deserving support and remuneration (Fassin and Rechtman 2009). In previous wars, a psychological state was not a condition warranting recompense; rather, one needed to have a true *physical disorder* like "irritable heart" or "soldier's heart" to gain such benefits. Trauma— overexertion in the case of irritable or soldier's heart, or a shell blast in the case of shell shock in World War I—was then understood to have psychological effects, constituting a physiopsychology (Kugelmann 2009; Micale and Lerner 2001). In the Vietnam War, a psychological wound—PTSD—was cast as analogous to the inevitable effects of an overwhelming stressor, like a building that is physically stressed to the point of collapse. But such psychological disorders still carry stigma. This has contributed to the continual emergence of ambiguous, physiopsychological syndromes and promotions of categories such as Gulf War syndrome, a condition in which toxic exposures during war have given rise to multiple unexplained complaints, a kind of "toxic neurasthenia" (Jones and Wessely 2005; Kilshaw 2009).[2]

While exposure to combat and the experiences of Vietnam veterans returning to an America hostile to the war constitute one historical lineage of PTSD, there is a second lineage that has been equally important in determining the meanings trauma, PTSD, and trauma treatment have come to take on, particularly in the United States. It is impossible to discuss trauma treatment in this country without evoking issues of traumatized children, sexual abuse, incest and domestic violence, debates about false memories, and an enormous bureaucratic, therapeutic, and legal apparatus for managing claims of sexual predation. Brown, Scheflin, and Hammond (1998) provide an important history of this lineage of PTSD and the controversies it generated, as well as the empirical evidence associated with the false memory controversy. While the modern era of child abuse concerns can be traced back to the 1950s and the recognition by radiologists that skeletal lesions were parentally inflicted, it was not until 1962 that C. Henry Kempe described the "battered child syndrome" and provided medical data about child abuse (Kempe et al. 1962). The recognition of child abuse led to dramatic change, and by 1966 every state except Hawaii had enacted statutes mandating physician reporting of child abuse (Brown et al. 1998:6). Child sexual abuse was the last frontier of recognition of and response to child abuse, and passage of the federal Child Abuse Prevention and Treatment Act in 1974 mandated reporting and evaluation of suspected child sexual abuse and the investigation and prosecution of offenders. These mandates came without clear guidelines for assessing allegations of sexual abuse, and child abuse investigations were highly idiosyncratic and often highly prejudicial. Brown et al. (1998) describe how the original goals of providing care for children were often subverted, and by the late 1970s and 1980s laws and procedures came increasingly to focus on finding fault and prosecuting offenders rather than providing care for those injured (Conte 1991). Many of the debates about legitimacy of identifying "perpetrators" resulted from an era of excessive and highly suggestive interviewing tactics, and the focus on sex offenders continues to garner far more legal and bureaucratic investment than attention to providing services for those needing care.

Childhood sexual abuse was the domain not only of pediatricians and child protection advocates, but of feminist researchers, scholars, and therapists as well. Armstrong (1994) argues that Western societies went through three eras: an Age of Denial (up to the 1970s), an Age of Validation (1970s to 1990), and an Age of Backlash (after 1990). Writings on father-daughter incest (Herman 1981), on hidden sexual abuse of children, and on rape and rape trauma emerged in the 1970s, with an increasing body of research supporting the recognition of the prevalence of sexual abuse. It was only in the 1980s that the sequelae of incest and sexual violence were recast in terms of PTSD (Brown et al. 1998).

The development of phase-specific trauma treatment played a critical role in bringing together these two cultural histories associated with PTSD—that associated with the Vietnam War and that associated with the recognition of sexual abuse, particularly of children. Mardi Horowitz's *Stress Response Syndromes* (1976) was critical both in framing trauma response in terms of alterations between intrusive reexperiencing and general numbing of responsiveness, and in the development of phase-oriented treatment of PTSD. While the growing consensus about the treatment of PTSD had its historical roots in Pierre Janet, who advocated treatment of trauma and dissociation in stages including stabilization, memory processing, and rehabilitation (Brown et al. 1998:9; van der Kolk and van der Hart 1989), the years following Horowitz's book saw enormous development of the field of trauma treatment as a central modality in psychological services. Although memory processing has been a part of most trauma treatment from the initial days, consensus has developed concerning the dangers of rapid recall and abreaction methods. The early consensus on this issue pointed forward to evidence for the hazards of debriefing approaches, which has shaped guidelines for international psychosocial responses to trauma.

The emergence of a focus on dissociation and dissociative disorders, the fierce controversies about false memories, and the development of an enormous body of empirical research about the nature of traumatic memory are beyond the scope of this introduction. What becomes clear, however, in this brief schematic description of the cultural history of PTSD is that our understanding of trauma, PTSD, and trauma treatment today results from the remarkable convergence of efforts to understand and respond to experiences of war veterans, particularly Vietnam War veterans, and efforts to treat children and adults suffering the effects of childhood trauma and sexual abuse, as well as sexual violence into adulthood. It should be of little surprise that containing these diverse meanings in the DSM diagnoses of acute stress disorder and PTSD requires a remarkable act of simplification. And it should be of little surprise that such simplification would poorly serve clinicians treating a diverse array of trauma-related mental health disorders.

There is today an enormous literature associated with evidence-based practice guidelines for the treatment of PTSD (Foa et al. 2009 and Friedman et al. 2014 present reviews of the literature on the major treatment modalities; cf. Cukor et al. 2010 for a short review), as well as a significant body of work outlining the evidence for diverse modalities of treating complex traumatic stress disorders (see essays in Courtois and Ford 2009). Nearly all point to various forms of cognitive behavioral therapy as demonstrating effectiveness (Cahill et al. 2010), and psychopharmacologic treatment with antidepressant medications, particularly the SSRIs, has been shown to be effective, while the benzodiazepines have not (Friedman et al. 2009, 2014). Few studies have evaluated what forms of treatment are both feasible and effective in low resource settings in which large parts of the population have experienced severe and protracted violence (see Nakimuli-Mpungu et al. 2013 as one example).

Essays in this volume suggest that while phenomena quite similar to PTSD in North America and Europe are widely present across cultures, a narrow focus on the validity of this construct may well obscure the limitations associated with recognizing and responding to PTSD as defined by current diagnostic manuals. They also raise the question of whether evidence-based treatments for PTSD can be effective as public health measures in dealing with trauma-related disorders in postconflict settings for societies or groups attempting to respond to historical trauma, or in locations of ongoing ontological insecurity and endemic violence. Trauma seemingly results in a complex array of effects that vary by cultural context—what we have described as posttraumatic stress syndromes. The PTSD cluster of symptoms is only one subset of symptoms associated with such syndromes. This volume is an exploration of the larger set of phenomena, of which PTSD is a part, a set of studies of how such phenomena are understood and responded to in diverse cultural-historical settings, and an examination of how the PTSD construct has been deployed to make PTSD real in very diverse social settings.

PTSD: Biology and Recovery

Trauma and PTSD have been the focus of an enormous body of research in the neurosciences and neuropsychology, particularly since the establishment of the National Center for PTSD in 1988 (see chapters in Kirmayer et al. 2007 for an important review of this work). Underlying contemporary research are classic studies of the fight-or-flight response to threatening events and classical conditioning models. Some studies continue to focus on embodied responses to fear and processes of fear extinction, with particular interest in fear extinction as a form of new learning rather than the extinction of memory (for summaries, see Barad and Cain 2007; Quirk et al. 2007). A body of research focuses on the processing, storage, and retrieval of traumatic memories, with particular interest in differences between processing of normal versus traumatic memories and between body memory and declarative memory. Traumatic memories are consistently characterized by "fragmentary and intense sensations and affects, often with little or no verbal narrative content" (van der Kolk et al. 2001:9). The amygdala has been shown to be particularly critical in the processing of traumatic memory (Ledoux 1996). Any reminder of the trauma is said to activate the amygdala, which results in a fight-or-flight type of response: palpitations, fear, shortness of breath. This is said to result in reexperiencing (or flashbacks) and in hyperreactivity to any trauma reminder. Other studies argue that trauma results in a hyperreactivity to a range of cues (e.g., to noises, stresses, or worry itself), and that early adversity may even modify genes permanently toward that state (Bohacek et al. 2013; Heim et al. 2000; Mayer 2007).

Although studies of the processing of memory are critical to understanding basic neurobiological processes associated with PTSD, it is often difficult to determine why the majority of persons who suffer traumatic events—at a level meeting DSM criterion A for PTSD—*do not* develop PTSD. Most persons are highly resilient. Meta-analyses of epidemiological studies have found that only approximately 20 percent of persons who experience traumatic events develop PTSD (Yehuda and McFarlane 1995). Breslau and Kessler (2001) showed that while 75 percent of adult Americans suffer traumatic experience fulfilling DSM-IV criteria, only 12 percent actually develop PTSD. Shalev (2007) argues that while most persons suffer initial experiences characteristic of PTSD, most naturally recovery. He suggests, therefore, that PTSD be seen as a disorder of recovery, and that research should be focused on identifying processes that disrupt normal recovery rather than basic processes associated with response to trauma.

Cognitive-behavioral therapists argue that persons who develop chronic PTSD are characterized by particular patterns of dysfunctional cognitions about themselves and the world (Foa et al. 1999). Many have argued PTSD may represent a "pathological block to normal memory consolidation, resulting in trauma memories being retained in short-term storage, thereby allowing rapid and inappropriate triggering of recall" (Silove 2007:247). Van der Kolk (2007) argues that developmental issues are critical to risk for PTSD, and that "PTSD captures only a limited aspect of posttraumatic psychopathology, particularly in children" (226). He argues that when their primary "caregivers are emotionally absent, inconsistent, frustrating, violent, intrusive, or neglectful," individuals are at far greater risk for developing chronic PTSD. This includes children who develop what a task force of the National Child Traumatic Stress Network calls "developmental trauma disorder" in children, as well as what is described as "complex trauma" or "disorders of extreme stress not otherwise specified" (DESNOS) (Luxenberg, Spinazzola, Hidalgo et al. 2001; Luxenberg, Spinazzola, and van der Kolk 2001). But while neurobiological, cognitive, and developmental issues may be important in determining who is at heightened risk for failing to recover from traumatic experiences, current social and cultural factors—such as lack of social support, continued adversity, or inability to make sense of traumatic events—may be even more important (see, e.g., Brewin et al. 2000; Shalev 2007).

This book suggests that these issues need to be placed in social and cross-cultural context. On the one hand, chapters in this book show diverse ways in which traumatic experiences are understood, expressed, and made sense of. On the other hand, they suggest that trauma results in a broad arousal symptom pool—which includes the DSM symptoms but others as well—that forms a key part of the biological effects of severe trauma: hyperreactivity to stimuli and emotions, poor emotion regulation, sleep disorders like severe insomnia and sleep paralysis, multiple somatic complaints. (Those who advocate for complex PTSD as a DSM diagnosis argue in particular that symptoms of "emotion dysregulation" distinguish complex from usual PTSD [Bryant 2012].) These various symptoms may be induced by the nature and severity of the trauma and ongoing vulnerabilities, and the symptoms may be amplified by cultural ideas about the mind and body and about the meanings of particular symptoms. Ethnopsychologies and ethnophysiologies specific to given cultures and local cultural illness syndromes may lead to heightened attention to particular symptoms (hypersemiotized symptoms), as well as to "catastrophic cognitions," leading to bio-attentional looping that produces a certain trauma-based illness reality (cf. Hinton and Good 2009). Ethnopsychologies and ethnophysiologies give rise to certain ideas about redress and cure, to local therapeutic practices, and to certain trauma-based identities and self-narratives. And local religious and ritual traditions may be key in determining whether individuals are able to make sense of and recover from particular traumatic experiences, including both embodied and declarative memories of trauma. These and other analytic frames or contextualizations are discussed by Hinton and Good in Chapter 1 of this volume and are illustrated in all the book chapters.

PTSD in DSM-III, DSM-IV, and DSM-5

The formal definition and diagnostic criteria for PTSD have been debated and have undergone limited but significant changes within the *Diagnostic and Statistical Manual* since being introduced in DSM-III. The PTSD diagnosis was first introduced in 1980 in the *Diagnostic and Statistical Manual of Mental Disorder-III*, or DSM-III (American Psychiatric Association 1980). (On the history of the PTSD concept, see McNally [Chapter 2]; Young and Breslau [Chapter 3]; Ball and O'Nell [Chapter 11].) In DSM-III, PTSD was comprised of three clusters of symptoms (American Psychiatric Association 1980). The first cluster consisted of reexperiencing symptoms, such as recollections and dreams of the event; the second of avoidance and numbing symptoms, such as avoidance of reminders, a sense of blunted emotion (viz., a restricted range of affect), and loss of interest in activities; and the third of hyperarousal symptoms such as startle and hypervigilance. The criteria were minimally changed in the next edition of the manual, DSM-IV (American Psychiatric Association, 1994), or in the DSM-IV-TR (American Psychiatric Association 2000), which is shown in Table I.1.

Table I.1. PTSD: DSM-IV-TR Criteria (309.81)

A. The person has been exposed to a traumatic event in which both of the following were present:

   (1) the person experienced, witnessed, or was confronted with an event or events that involved actual or threatened death or serious injury, or a threat to the physical integrity of self or others

   (2) the person's response involved intense fear, helplessness, or horror. *Note:* In children, this may be expressed instead by disorganized or agitated behavior.

B. The traumatic event is persistently reexperienced in one (or more) of the following ways:

   (1) recurrent and intrusive distressing recollections of the event, including images, thoughts, or perceptions. *Note:* In young children, repetitive play may occur in which themes or aspects of the trauma are expressed.

   (2) recurrent distressing dreams of the event. *Note:* In children, there may be frightening dreams without recognizable content.

   (3) acting or feeling as if the traumatic event were recurring (includes a sense of reliving the experience, illusions, hallucinations, and dissociative flashback episodes, including those that occur on awakening or when intoxicated). *Note:* In young children, trauma-specific reenactment may occur.

   (4) intense psychological distress at exposure to internal or external cues that symbolize or resemble an aspect of the traumatic event

   (5) physiological reactivity on exposure to internal or external cues that symbolize or resemble an aspect of the traumatic event

C. Persistent avoidance of stimuli associated with the trauma and numbing of general responsiveness (not present before the trauma), as indicated by three (or more) of the following:

   (1) efforts to avoid thoughts, feelings, or conversations associated with the trauma

(*continued*)

Table I.1. (continued)

---

(2) efforts to avoid activities, places, or people that arouse recollections of the trauma

(3) inability to recall an important aspect of the trauma

(4) markedly diminished interest or participation in significant activities

(5) feeling of detachment or estrangement from others

(6) restricted range of affect (e.g., unable to have loving feelings)

(7) sense of a foreshortened future (e.g., does not expect to have a career, marriage, children, or a normal life span)

D. Persistent symptoms of increased arousal (not present before the trauma), as indicated by three (or more) of the following:

(1) difficulty falling or staying asleep

(2) irritability or outbursts of anger

(3) difficulty concentrating

(4) hypervigilance

(5) exaggerated startle response

E. Duration of the disturbance (symptoms in criteria B, C, and D) is more than one month.

F. The disturbance causes clinically significant distress or impairment in social, occupational, or other important areas of functioning.

Source: *Diagnostic and Statistical Manual of Mental Disorders*, 4th ed., text revision [DSM-IV-TR], pp. 271–72. Copyright 2000. American Psychiatric Association. Reprinted with permission.

More significant changes were introduced in the criteria for PTSD in the recently published DSM-5 (American Psychiatric Association 2013) (see Table I.2) (for a discussion, see Friedman et al. 2011).[3] There was a narrowing of the numbing and avoidance cluster, making it solely an avoidance cluster, and the creation of a new cluster called "negative alterations in cognitions and mood associated with the traumatic event(s)," which includes the DSM-IV's numbing items[4] and two new items: a self- and other-blame item ("persistent, distorted cognitions about the cause or consequence of the traumatic event[s] that lead the individual to blame himself/herself or others") and an emotion-type item, namely, "persistent negative emotional state (e.g., fear, horror, anger, guilt, or shame)." Also, in DSM-5, the wording of two of the DSM-IV numbing items has been changed (and as was indicated above, the new version of these two items, along with the other DSM-IV "numbing items," have been moved to the "negative alterations" cluster). The "restricted

Table I.2. PTSD: DSM-5 Criteria (309.81)

A. Exposure to actual or threatened death, serious injury, or sexual violation in one (or more) of the following ways:

1. Directly experiencing the traumatic event(s).
2. Witnessing, in person, the event(s) as it occurred to others.
3. Learning that the traumatic event(s) occurred to a close family member or close friend. In cases of actual or threatened death of a family member or friend, the event(s) must have been violent or accidental.
4. Experiencing repeated or extreme exposure to aversive details of the traumatic event(s) (e.g., first responders collecting human remains; police officers repeatedly exposed to details of child abuse).
   Note: Criterion A4 does not apply to exposure through electronic media, television, movies, or pictures, unless this exposure is work related.

B. Presence of one (or more) of the following intrusion symptoms associated with the traumatic event(s), beginning after the traumatic event(s) occurred:

1. Recurrent, involuntary, and intrusive distressing memories of the traumatic event(s).
   Note: In children older than 6 years, repetitive play may occur in which themes or aspects of the traumatic event(s) are expressed.
2. Recurrent distressing dreams in which the content and/or affect of the dream are related to the traumatic event(s).
   Note: In children, there may be frightening dreams without recognizable content.
3. Dissociative reactions (e.g., flashbacks) in which the individual feels or acts as if the traumatic event(s) were recurring. (Such reactions may occur on a continuum, with the most extreme expression being a complete loss of awareness of present surroundings.)
   Note: In children, trauma-specific reenactment may occur in play.
4. Intense or prolonged psychological distress at exposure to internal or external cues that symbolize or resemble an aspect of the traumatic event(s).
5. Marked physiological reactions to internal or external cues that symbolize or resemble an aspect of the traumatic event(s).

C. Persistent avoidance of stimuli associated with the traumatic event(s), beginning after the traumatic event(s) occurred, as evidenced by avoidance of one or both of the following:

1. Avoidance of or efforts to avoid distressing memories, thoughts, or feelings about or closely associated with the traumatic event(s).
2. Avoidance of or efforts to avoid external reminders (people, places, conversations, activities, objects, situations) that arouse distressing memories, thoughts, or feelings about or closely associated with the traumatic event(s).

(continued)

Table I.2. (continued)

D. Negative alterations in cognitions and mood associated with the traumatic event(s), beginning or worsening after the traumatic event(s) occurred, as evidenced by two (or more) of the following:

1. Inability to remember an important aspect of the traumatic event(s) (typically due to dissociative amnesia and not to other factors such as head injury, alcohol, or drugs).
2. Persistent and exaggerated negative beliefs or expectations about oneself, others, or the world (e.g., "I am bad," "No one can be trusted," "The world is completely dangerous," "My whole nervous system is permanently ruined").
3. Persistent, distorted cognitions about the cause or consequence of the traumatic event(s) that lead the individual to blame himself/herself or others.
4. Persistent negative emotional state (e.g., fear, horror, anger, guilt, or shame).
5. Markedly diminished interest or participation in significant activities.
6. Feelings of detachment or estrangement from others.
7. Persistent inability to experience positive emotions (e.g., inability to experience happiness, satisfaction, or loving feelings).

E. Marked alterations in arousal and reactivity associated with the traumatic event(s), beginning or worsening after the traumatic event(s) occurred, as evidenced by two (or more) of the following:

1. Irritable behavior and angry outbursts (with little or no provocation) typically expressed as verbal or physical aggression toward people or objects.
2. Reckless or self-destructive behavior.
3. Hypervigilance.
4. Exaggerated startle response.
5. Problems with concentration.
6. Sleep disturbance (e.g., difficulty falling or staying asleep or restless sleep).

F. Duration of the disturbance (criteria B, C, D, and E) is more than 1 month.

G. The disturbance causes clinically significant distress or impairment in social, occupational, or other important areas of functioning.

H. The disturbance is not attributable to the direct physiological effects of a substance (e.g., medication, alcohol) or another medical condition.

range of affect" item is now a "persistent inability to experience positive emotions," transforming the item from a numbing item to more of a depressive-type item, an anhedonia item. The "foreshortened sense of future" item is now a "persistent and exaggerated negative beliefs or expectations about oneself, others, or the world."[5] Thus, the new cluster that is named "negative alterations in cognitions and mood associated with the traumatic event(s)" contains a heterogeneous mix of items with many being depression-like items: the two reworded items; an amnesia item, which may well be a depressive item in that depression can give rise to a sense of mental slowing and poor memory; and the "pervasive negative state" item, with that negative state possibly being depression.[6]

In DSM-5, the arousal cluster is somewhat changed. In the cluster description, the term "reactivity" has been added to the term "arousal." Also, another criterion has been added: "reckless or self-destructive behavior." Anger is again in the arousal cluster, and anger is more emphasized in the overall DSM–5 criteria because another cluster, namely "negative alterations in cognitions and mood," has a persistent negative mood item, and this may be a state of anger.

There are ongoing debates about the symptom clusters in the PTSD criteria, the putative "dimensions of PTSD," and whether DSM-IV and DSM-5 PTSD leave out key dimensions or key symptoms (Armour et al. 2012; Elhai and Palmieri 2011). For example, some have suggested somatic symptoms to be a core dimension of PTSD, particularly in non-Western cultures, and that somatic symptoms should form another criterion in the arousal cluster or be another PTSD dimension (for a review, see Hinton and Lewis-Fernández 2011). Somatic symptoms, it is argued, may be prominent in certain groups for multiple reasons, including the severity of trauma and the cultural interpretation of symptoms (for a detailed discussion, see Hinton and Good [Chapter 1]). For example, somatic symptoms are caused by the arousal associated with PTSD, and in certain cultures those somatic symptoms are attributed to cultural syndromes: palpitations attributed to "weak heart" in the Cambodian case. Consequently, there is a hypervigilant surveying of the body for the symptoms associated with a syndrome, and catastrophic cognitions upon discovering them, with those catastrophic cognitions increasing arousal. Owing to these reasons, in certain cultures the arousal dimension will have within it many somatic symptoms that are associated with cultural syndromes, that is, there will be an arousal cluster of the typical PTSD arousal symptoms along with somatic symptoms associated with various culture-specific syndromes.

A further cultural critique of DSM criteria holds that there are many trauma-related symptoms that are not in the DSM-IV and DSM-5 criteria that are a key part of the response to trauma (for an overview, see Hinton and Good [Chapter 1]). The current volume shows many examples of symptoms that occur in trauma-related disorders that are not in the DSM-5. For example, among Cambodian refugees, not only are somatic symptoms such as dizziness upon standing (orthostatic dizziness) central complaints, but also are multiple other non-DSM-5 PTSD symptoms such as sleep paralysis. As illustrated by the current volume, PTSD is just one of many disorders that result from trauma (for a review, see Hinton and Lewis-Fernández 2011). The core response to trauma includes not just the currently specified PTSD items and clusters, but also somatic symptoms, depression, bereavement, anxiety, and panic attacks, as well as acting out and substance abuse, raising questions about whether these are comorbid disorders or should be incorporated into a broader posttraumatic stress syndrome. Depending on the cultural group, certain of these other psychopathological dimensions may be more prominent. In addition, cultural syndromes like the Khmer "wind attacks" (*gaeut khyâl*)[7] or "heart weakness" (*khsaoy beh doung*) may be a core aspect of the trauma-related distress in a locality, creating a unique cluster of complaints and inflecting trauma-symptom presentation and meaning, producing a certain profile of DSM comorbidities (e.g., prominent panic attacks), resulting in certain kinds of symptom clustering, and profoundly altering the attempted treatments of symptoms and the course of recovery. Through these means, these syndromes and local understandings pattern trauma-related experiencing profoundly, forming certain sensuous psychologies (Theidon 2013), local embodied ontologies, that are linked to local healing traditions and the local ethnopsychology, ethnophysiology, and ethnospirituality, and these syndromes and local understandings result in a certain social and personal course of trauma-related experiencing.

Finally, as suggested throughout this Introduction, failure of the DSM-5 to address complex PTSD and to distinguish between initial symptoms associated with traumatic experience and long-term or chronic PTSD that results from an inability to recover, limit the value of PTSD as described in the DSM-5 for cross-cultural settings. Chapters in this volume provide evidence for the importance of understanding complex forms of posttrauma disorders, including those associated with pervasive childhood abuse and trauma, and long-term trauma related to wars or civil conflicts. Such trauma creates complex symptom presentations and shapes multiple ontological domains (for an overview, see Hinton and Good [Chapter 1]). Chapters in this book address specific issues of validity of the PTSD construct, and some chapters provide evidence concerning specific symptom clusters. But the larger conversation with the DSM categories in this book concerns the broader issues of the relation between the DSM-5 categories and the larger posttraumatic stress syndromes observed in diverse cultural settings.

Book Themes and Questions

This volume examines the question of how trauma and PTSD come to be constituted and experienced in cross-cultural and historical contexts. These chapters suggest five overall themes critical to understanding trauma, PTSD, and trauma treatment, raising important questions and directions for future research.

First, what is the nature of local phenomenologies of posttrauma experiences and symptoms? Chapters in this volume demonstrate that culture has important influences on local illness vocabularies, understandings of how trauma affects mental and bodily experience (the local ethnopsychology and ethnophysiology), attention to particular symptoms, and practices aimed at reducing these symptoms. Assessing the validity of the PTSD construct and criteria across cultures requires not simply asking whether there are cases in which symptoms co-occur in the way described in the DSM, but how DSM-defined PTSD relates to local forms of illness experience.

Second, running throughout the book is a series of questions about the importance of "ontological security" in the very conceptualization of "post" traumatic stress disorders (cf. Green 1999; Hinton et al. 2009; James 2008). James, in her chapter on Haiti (Chapter 11), makes most explicit the importance of insecurity as a basic feature of social life that shapes experience. The issue of the "post" in PTSD is called into serious question in many of the settings in which anthropologists work. Security pertains to multiple domains that include safety, spiritual, existential, economic, and environment concerns. A key aspect of trauma can be seen as a sense of being under threat following a traumatic event, a feeling that a trauma may occur again. Ongoing or current threats to security will reverberate with this concern. This raises quite fundamental questions about whether it is meaningful to diagnose PTSD in settings of continued insecurity, or whether the very concept assumes that trauma is in the past and individuals are currently living in settings of ontological security. Determining the nature of PTSD and PTSD symptoms in settings of security and settings of continued violence or economic insecurity is a critical issue for research.

Third, we have raised throughout this Introduction the issue of the adequacy of a concept of posttrauma disorders focused on relatively limited traumatic events and the importance of experiences of pervasive and complex trauma—in developmental contexts or in settings of long-term exposure to violence—in cross-cultural settings. The chapters in this book bring this issue into particularly sharp focus. While they do not suggest that phenomena represented by DSM criteria are absent or unimportant in cross-cultural settings, they do raise important questions about the relevance of more pervasive, complex forms of traumatic experience in a conceptualization of posttrauma disorders.

Fourth, although not the explicit focus of the chapters of this book, the authors demonstrate the critical importance of local social, cultural, and religious practices that contribute to recovery from trauma (or resilience or self-remission of symptoms). The chapters describe specific local strategies for making sense of disaster or violence, the failures of sense making, and diverse practices of resilience that contribute to recovery (on these processes, see also Hinton and Kirmayer 2013). They raise important questions about why these processes may be successful for some individuals and not for others, and more general comparative questions about how members of different societies achieve recovery and understand and respond to those who fail to recover.

Fifth, these chapters speak to the debates about the utility of the PTSD concept in humanitarian work and in local therapeutic environments. How has PTSD as a concept been deployed, how have trauma treatments been deployed, and how effective have they been? What therapeutic responses can be effective in settings with widespread experiences of violence and with limited mental health resources? Is the PTSD concept useful in the task of developing local mental health systems in settings with extremely few psychiatrists? Has it been deployed in ways that contribute to the development of mental health services capacity, or does a focus on trauma and PTSD reduce attention to broader strategies for developing mental health services? How does targeting DSM-defined PTSD affect the broader range of symptoms or disorders associated with trauma?

Finally, a number of the chapters provide important data for responding to questions about whether deployment of the concepts of trauma, PTSD, and trauma treatment produces "victims" and contributes to the pathologization of whole societies, or whether it provides mechanisms for effective response to social suffering. Do processes of identifying individuals who have experienced massive trauma and developed prolonged symptoms, advocated by many human rights groups, support the identification of perpetrators and provide effective means of compensation? Are these processes effective in identifying those who need medical and psychosocial interventions? Or does the deployment of concepts of PTSD lead to the struggle to produce "trauma portfolios," as James describes for Haiti (Chapter 11), thus engaging individuals in prolonged bureaucratic procedures requiring demonstration of continued suffering rather than providing genuine support that promotes recovery?

These are the broad issues that are raised by the chapters of this volume. Let us now turn to a close examination of the chapters.

Summary of Chapters

Part I: Introduction and Theoretical Background

This introductory chapter is intended to place the book in the context of the historical emergence of the PTSD concept, to indicate the importance of cross-cultural studies for understanding posttrauma disorders, and to situate the essays in this book in relation to critical debates that have arisen particularly in the past decade.

In Chapter 1, Hinton and Good describe three general models to use to assess the trauma survivor in a culturally sensitive manner: using eleven analytic perspectives, avoiding certain kinds of errors, and employing dynamic, multiplex models of how trauma-related distress is generated. The chapter outlines eleven analytic perspectives from which to examine the existential position of the trauma survivor, providing a framework that brings the chapters in the book into conversation with one another and showing how the chapters aim at a rich contextualization of trauma-related disorder in particular sociocultural and historical contexts. Based on the analysis of the eleven ontological dimensions, Chapter 1 describes some common errors made by clinicians and researchers when examining trauma in cross-cultural perspective. The chapter also discusses multiplex models of the generation of trauma-related disorder, giving emphasis to the notion of complex trauma and the related concept of the "arousal complex" or "reactivity complex" (a much broader concept than "poor emotion regulation").

Part II: Historical Perspectives

The three chapters in this section examine PTSD in historical context. McNally gives an overview of several controversies about the PTSD construct, critiquing both the social constructivist view (that PTSD is the invention of a certain sociocultural group) and the acultural view (that PTSD as described in the DSM is an accurate mapping of trauma-related disorders, free of cultural context). He argues for the importance of open-ended queries about symptoms and notes the problem that when assessing PTSD symptoms in any context, diverse social and cultural factors influence the reporting of symptoms and bodily experience. McNally gives a historical view of PTSD, describing the emergence of PTSD in DSM-III in response to experiences in the Vietnam War: the new diagnosis served to validate the distress of Vietnam veterans and allowed a way of providing benefits. He notes that in the Vietnam War, many "psychiatric casualties" had no combat exposure and many had delayed onset. He points out that it was in this context that the concept of numbing emerged to explain delayed onset of PTSD symptoms: numbing was seemingly the first response followed by the development of PTSD symptoms.

McNally discusses the unique symptoms seen in each war setting. In the narratives collected by physicians in World War I, certain symptoms we call PTSD were not salient whereas others not now prominent took central stage: in the narrative of a WWI veteran with shell shock, flashbacks were not found but rather such symptoms as irritability, depressed mood, dreams about the war, and apparent sleep paralysis. But he notes this absence of flashback in the assessment narrative might have been a result of methods of questioning rather than true absence. Other than these issues of possible overinclusion, McNally points out the problem of category truncation—of trauma-related disorder having a wide range of symptoms not included in the DSM-IV PTSD category. McNally shows that many symptoms, including somatic symptoms, not in the DSM PTSD diagnostic criteria were seemingly common in past wars. And he shows that symptoms that were common in Vietnam veterans are less emphasized in the current conceptualization of trauma's effects: guilt, which was a prominent part of the Vietnam War distress presentation (though now in DSM-5, self-blame is a criterion) and rage at society (though now in DSM-5, persistent negative emotional state is a criterion, which may include such a sense of persistent rage).

McNally examines possible definitions of PTSD, including the abnormal response to trauma no matter what the range of symptoms. He points to the problem of defining what constitutes a "trauma." There is a danger of "bracket creep" if what is considered a trauma is too broad, such as including under the rubric the experience of feeling helpless upon learning of threats: as an example of this kind of bracket creep, he notes that in one study that 4 percent of Americans were classified as having PTSD after 9/11 despite living far away, apparently by watching the event on television. McNally ponders the theoretical implications of considering that pulling a tooth can produce PTSD. For example, he asks whether in the West some cases of PTSD serve as an "idiom of distress" that is taken on for reasons analogous to Charcot's patients in the Salpêtrière enacting the steps of grand hysteria (Didi-Huberman and Charcot 2003; Haskell 2011), that is, a sort of final ethnobehavioral pathway to express distress that is provided by a society (Carr and Vitaliano 1985).

Young and Breslau also examine the historical origins of the PTSD concept and argue that it is a heterogeneous entity because the supposed cause (a trauma) is so variable and at times almost nonexistent, even imagined. They note that the definition of stressor has shifted: from being an objectively verifiable extreme threat in DSM-III to in DSM-IV being simply an event considered as threatening to oneself from the person's perspective or threatening to others when the event is witnessed. DSM-5 has a similar definition, though slightly narrowed (see McNally [Chapter 2]), for example, specifying that learning of a trauma can only qualify as a trauma if the event occurred to a close family member or a friend. Young and Breslau describe DSM's memory logic, in which a traumatic event (A) leads to a bad memory (B), and that memory leads to both of the following: constant arousal (C) and avoidance of anything that reminds the person of the trauma event as well as numbing (D). Young and Breslau review the problem of expanding what is considered causative of PTSD to the point that the presence of symptoms (C and D), leads to a search for any bad memories (B) that may explain the experiencing of those symptoms (C and D)—that is, a process of retrospective attribution. In respect to the heterogeneity issue, Young and Breslau point out that the symptoms of major depression and generalized anxiety disorder (GAD) are similar to many of the symptoms in the PTSD criteria, and that often the person with PTSD will be given those two diagnoses.[8] It would also suggest that a person with GAD or major depression may notice that they have many of the PTSD symptoms and this then may give rise to the search for the cause in some trauma.

Young and Breslau note the potential large increase of PTSD diagnoses and hence the rate of meting out of disability benefits to veterans if the liberal definition of a stressor (criterion A) is used. They review cases from Charcot and discuss one that demonstrates the invention of memory. The man in question did not have trauma but vividly conjured it in mind in anticipatory fear to the point of insisting on having passed through the trauma; the case shows how conjuring to mind an imagined and feared event (a carriage rolling over the leg, a nearby bomb explosion) comes to be viewed as a true memory. In addition, Young and Breslau argue that someone reviewing past life events may come to view one of them as traumatic not only by such distortion but simply through emotion inflation—reconfiguring a past event as pathogen. Experiencing distress leads to a review of past events in search of those that caused current distress, and through *Nachträglichkeit*, the "pathogenic event" is found and imbued with a sense of harrowing power, of dark significance. A further mechanism encouraging retrospective discovery of a "pathogenic trauma" is self-narrative making. If finding the pathogen allows the person to cast current distress such as anger, depression, anxiety, or substance abuse as part of the narrative of a "hero," of a combat survivor, with invisible psychic wounds, then this process may be accelerated; in such a way, the person creates a new and preferable identity—and this choice may have important economic consequences. Private memory is central to self-fashioning and the narration of the self; through the PTSD diagnosis, the person is not a failure but a survivor, a war hero. Even in cases of true severe trauma, the master narratives of trauma's effect will strongly shape the experiencing of those with trauma.

Young and Breslau show the continual dance between textual definitions of disorder (DSM), prototypical cases (i.e., pure cases such as those that result from a severe trauma that seem to exemplify the illness characteristics and may serve as pure representatives of the kind[9]), and actual clinical populations. They refer to prototypes as cases where a severe traumatic event seemed to result in PTSD symptoms, and they state that clinical cases are much more complex entities. There is also the problem of autosuggestion and

malleable memory. Young and Breslau describe how each war seems to result in certain "assemblages" that constitute new forms of war-related distress and how those forms may enter society as the prototypical image of
trauma. These assemblages will be influenced by current medical knowledge,
institutional cultures, and popular attitudes. These assemblages result in
unique trauma subjectivities. As they point out, somatic syndromes often
took central place in such assemblages, in the associated trauma subjectivities: the prominence of gastrointestinal concerns and fears of peptic ulcers
among soldiers in World War II. Or in the Gulf War, the fear of deadly chemical agents and contamination led to prominent somatic complaints. And
following 9/11, the effect of viewing those events constituted a seeming new
trauma assemblage that is referred to as "distant PTSD," as described by
Young and Breslau.

Boehnlein and Hinton's chapter investigates the overlap of traumatic
brain injury (TBI) and PTSD in historical perspective. They situate in historical context the present debates about whether the complaint of having TBI
may sometimes serve as the new guise of a PTSD, what might be called "mimicked TBI"; this occurs when TBI is not present but TBI-like symptoms are
enminded and embodied as a distress form, when TBI is not present but
trauma-related symptoms lead to the diagnosis of TBI. Trauma-related symptoms such as PTSD overlap greatly with TBI symptoms: TBI symptoms include headache, dizziness, fatigue, insomnia, vision problems, sensitivity to
light and sound, memory problems, difficulties with focus and concentration,
impulsivity, depression, irritability, anxiety, and personality changes. As
Boehnlein and Hinton discuss, several previous war syndromes and their
symptoms—irritable heart in the Civil War, railroad spine in the late nineteenth century, and shell shock in WWI—were attributed to physical damage but were usually psychological in origin. For example, shell shock was
thought to result from a concussive injury (from a blast); and shell shock
was thought to bring about many of the symptoms that we now classify as
PTSD symptoms, as well other symptoms. In the current episteme of war
syndromes, TBI inflects the understanding of psychological trauma because
it leads to a special scrutinizing for the presence of symptoms like headache,
memory loss, and poor concentration among those with a history of head
trauma (which includes being present in the zone of a bomb explosion)—soon
these TBI-type symptoms may be more salient in all psychological trauma
presentations. In the current episteme of war syndromes, there are several
types of overlap between TBI and PTSD, creating a complex typology: pure

TBI, which act as paradigmatic cases in Young and Breslau's terminology, in which PTSD is not present and the person does not think him- or herself to have PTSD; pure PTSD, in which TBI is not present and the person does not think him- or herself to have TBI; co-occuring TBI and PTSD, in which the person self-labels trauma-related symptoms such as PTSD symptoms as TBI, with the presence of PTSD being ignored; and mimicked TBI in the absence of PTSD or any trauma-related psychological symptoms, in which the person has anxiety and/or depressive symptoms (e.g., anxiety, irritability, headache, poor concentration) from non-trauma-related causes and attributes those symptoms to TBI though TBI is not present.

Part III: Cross-Cultural Perspectives

Part III consists of eight chapters describing studies of trauma, trauma-related conditions, and trauma treatment in distinctive social and cultural contexts.

Jenkins and Haas detail how trauma plays out in a particular American subculture: the life experiences of adolescents in a community in New Mexico. They use the term "psychic trauma" rather than "PTSD"; the term "PTSD" conjures a certain circumscribed set of symptoms—such as trauma recall or anger—whereas the group they studied experienced adverse advents that have a far broader range of negative effects. And as they note, the PTSD criteria include certain symptoms that may not apply to other cultures—for example, numbing and avoidance in certain Latin American contexts—and do not include others that may be central in a locality. The authors call for an ethnography of traumas and stresses, and the effects on the local social world. They show how local traumas interact with local stressors to create a specific trauma ontology. The youth they studied in residential care grew up in situations marked by frequent traumas, by high levels of poverty, and by drug culture: the highest per capita rate of death by heroin overdose in America is found in rural New Mexico. Intergenerational legacies of structural violence are pervasive: parents often have psychological and substance abuse problems, making it difficult for them to provide protective parenting. Trauma by someone in the home shatters the bonds of social trust in profound and distinct ways. Rape is common. Self-cutting is frequent, seemingly used as a way to cope with negative affect or as a way to express a desperate need for help, a kind of idiom of distress and final ethnobehavioral pathway. Worsening matters, government services are being withdrawn.

The actions of those in these social worlds, according to Jenkins and Haas, are best viewed from the perspective of a "sociology of psychic trauma," analyzing how state structures and local realities combine to create crushing structural violence on the level of the family and the individual. There is the social course of trauma, the social embeddedness of trauma, in which trauma itself shapes social structures and interactions: ongoing stresses combine with frequent traumas to impact local life, and in turn, lead to more trauma—so go the vicious cycles. When seen through this optic, the illusion of human agency seems to dissolve. What becomes visible are crushing lines of structural violence, and how those forces play out on the national, state, local, and family level. As Jenkins and Haas's analysis highlights, there are various types of structural violence. There is the structural violence that a person experiences from living in contexts where violence is rampant, ranging from gang violence, crime, family-level violence (e.g., owing to anger generated by PTSD), to exposure to drug culture and all that it entails. Also, there is violence that comes to be perpetrated for structural reasons, such as when intergenerational problems and local stresses (e.g., economic issues) result in persons' perpetrating actual violence and abuses; that is, violence is seemingly generated by economic, social, and other conditions. And there is "structural violence" in the metaphoric sense: stresses (e.g., poverty) and deprivations (e.g., lack of education) that constitute a key aspect of endemic adversity. All these types of structural violence are present in the locality described by Jenkins and Haas, and the authors try to delineate all these lines of force that are the vectors of structural violence. Whereas Lewis (1959, 1966) describes a "culture of poverty," Jenkins and Haas detail a "culture of violence and stresses" ("culture of trauma and stresses") and they illustrate how these forces infiltrate and permeate the local social world. This is not to deny human agency but rather to point out the endemic structures that shape personhood, biology, and life experiences, to trace the lines of structural violence—and consider questions of agency. (The theme of structural violence is addressed in many chapters of the volume: see Hinton and Good [Chapter 1].)

In the next chapter, Duncan shows how the definition of the traumatic varies across cultures: in Oaxaca, whereas migration and other events are professionally framed as traumatic, not so domestic violence—it is just a "part of life." It is considered a man's right to hit his wife, and that his doing so in jealousy means he cares for her. Events that would elsewhere be seen as traumatic are not viewed as so in this context. But the conceptualization of the traumatic and its effects are in flux. Duncan describes a location of high levels of trauma, and of high levels of stress, such as poverty and lack of potable water, and a location where campaigns about trauma and its effects have begun in the form of billboards and by other means and where therapeutic groups have become increasingly common in clinics. In one case that she describes, which involves a therapy group in a clinic, each woman is asked to describe a trauma and is told that not expressing it will lead to the trauma operating inside her like a pathogen, producing emotional distress. Campaigns against violence such as gender-based violence, high rates of such violence, and campaigns urging women to seek services for the effects of such violence: these all combine to lead many women to seek mental health services.

Through these campaigns and receiving services, a certain "trauma assemblage" results, to build on Young and Breslau's phrasing, the emergence of a new trauma subjectivity. Women are told that trauma results in certain symptoms, and they learn about the role of mental health professionals and about the supposed need for self-esteem and empowerment to recover from trauma's blow. Multiple means aim to educate women about psychological violence such as humiliations and insults, and about the need to get mental health care for sequelae of these events. Western-type PTSD and related ideas are taught in various ways in the goal of "sensitizing" (*sensibilización*). In this trauma assemblage, domestic abuse is not thought by local professional treaters to cause PTSD, but rather to result in anxiety and depression. As Duncan points out, this view is in contrast to surveys that show that as many as 20 percent of the women in Oaxaca have PTSD, and that intimate partner violence is a risk factor for PTSD. Though domestic violence does seemingly produce PTSD symptoms, Duncan hypothesizes that so diagnosing women might have negative consequences, in particular the medicalization of the problem: giving a pill to the woman who has suffered such violence rather than addressing the violence itself. But she argues that the expansion of the Euroamerican understanding of mental health in these settings is generative of novel social practices and self-understandings that are indeed empowering and that shine light on structural and routinized abuse and violence.

Pedersen and Kienzler put forward a general bio-psycho-social model of how distress and psychological disorders are produced among Quechua speakers in Peru. They advocate a model in which causality can occur at any of various levels, emphasizing current life problems and stresses. The authors review the literature showing that structural violence and disadvantage—poverty, low socioeconomic class, lack of support—create particular vulnerabilities. And they review the literature on the impact of current stress and daily stressors on mental health as compared to the impact of traumatic events. In addition, the authors examine local meaning systems, analyzing the narratives of highland Quechua about their experience of violence and adversity to determine the local idioms of distress and ethnopsychology. The local ethnopsychology emphasizes how traumatic events along with current stress and worry worsen mental health. The authors present a semantic map of this local ethnopsychology's conceptualization of the effects of trauma and adversity (for a semantic map of this kind among Cambodian refugees, see Hinton and Good [Chapter 1]). For example, "worrying thoughts" (*pinsamientuwan*) are considered to possibly lead to insanity, and those persons who have passed through chronic adversity are thought to be highly vulnerable and are compared to a tattered cloth that rips easily or a friable piece of wood. The informants also speak of sadness (*llaki*) characterized by multiple somatic symptoms such as headache and stomach pain. *Llaki* are thought to be caused by *pinsamientuwan*. The authors present the results of a study showing how these idioms relate to DSM-type diagnoses and to functioning. In this way, the authors show how DSM disorders relate to local diagnostic labels (syndromes, idioms of distress, metaphors depicting vulnerability and disturbance) that form a network of syndromes constituting an ethnopsychology.

In the next chapter, Alcántara and Lewis-Fernández examine the conditional risk of PTSD among Latino patients as compared to other groups. By conditional risk they mean the relative risk in one group as compared to other groups of developing any of the following after a trauma: a PTSD diagnosis, certain types of PTSD symptoms, more severe PTSD symptoms, or more persistent PTSD. In determining conditional risk, differences in trauma exposure are eliminated as a factor. The authors review the conditional risk literature in respect to the Latino population and find evidence for higher conditional risk for certain disorders after trauma, such as rates of PTSD. They examine possible reasons for possible increased conditional risk among the Latino population: peritraumatic responses, cultural syndromes (e.g., *ataque de nervios*), expressive style, and uneven distribution of social disadvantage. For example, as other chapters in the book suggest, if panic attacks are more prominent in a cultural group owing to ongoing stress combined with catastrophic cognitions about somatic symptoms, then the panic attacks may result in higher levels of arousal symptoms and more severe and persistent PTSD. Or it may be that certain groups react to a trauma with different coping styles—for example, derealization and dissociation—and this may influence course and symptomatology. It may be that a group has specific cultural syndromes that shape how the group reacts to trauma events and symptoms resulting from trauma: Latinos tend to use an "*ataque de nervios*" as a response to trauma, which will tend to guide distress in the direction of dissociation and panic attacks, and this in turn may predispose them to certain types of PTSD symptoms and to a certain recovery course. It may be that certain groups like Latinos have a different expressive style so that the relationship to symptoms is changed and so too the reporting of them. Or it may be that cultural values influence the experiencing of PTSD—among Latinos, fatalism may shape the sense of self upon being traumatized and influence the recovery course. And it may be that socioeconomic position, poverty, and discrimination, which are major issues in Latino communities, result in vulnerability, specific symptoms, and a certain recovery course.

Kohrt, Worthman, and Upadhaya present a biocultural approach to PTSD in terms of child experiences, pretrauma vulnerabilities, trauma event variables, and posttrauma variables. As an example of a pretrauma vulnerability, they review the literature that shows that there may be biological predisposition to a hyperreactivity to stressors among those with a short allele of the serotonin gene. They argue that certain cultural environments may lead to stressors and trauma that shape the local bio-ontology of trauma. They review the literature that experiencing stress prior to and following a trauma may impact greatly on its course. They also discuss other culture-determined vulnerabilities: certain cultures seem to be more protective toward women and children. Kohrt and his colleagues describe how the emotional impact of trauma may be shaped by local meanings. They review studies showing that arousal symptoms caused by trauma may be labeled as possession or panic, creating biolooping (or what might also be called bio-attentional looping), which amplifies certain symptoms and thereby shapes symptomatology (on biolooping, see Hinton and Good [Chapter 1]). And they discuss how certain locally specific variables may influence recovery, such as the degree of stress in the community and how a person's trauma is framed culturally by those in the community.

In their chapter, Ball and O'Nell examine "historical trauma" among Native American communities. The authors argue that the creation of PTSD in the DSM-III (the post-Vietnam syndrome) as a diagnosis for Vietnam veterans allowed members of that group to speak of their traumas and current stresses, and that before the diagnosis was recognized, that substance abuse, anger, and other symptoms experienced by veterans were blamed on the veterans themselves rather than being attributed to past trauma and current adversity. According to the authors, Vietnam veterans were doubly victimized: by the original trauma and then by having their trauma-induced behaviors attributed to moral weakness. But Ball and O'Nell argue that the concept of historical trauma better describes the life situation of Native Americans than does PTSD. They consider the Native American situation to be one of complex PTSD that comes about as "a chronic reaction to genocide and oppression," and that the resulting symptoms and problems are broader than anxiety, depression, or PTSD because of the length of time that these traumas have lasted and because of other particularities of history that the authors depict in genograms.

Many chapters in this volume describe various types of adversity in lifeworlds marked by trauma, and Ball and O'Nell's chapter reveals how these lifeworlds of adversity may be complicated by historical trauma. The concept of historical trauma is much broader than PTSD—for example, it emphasizes vulnerability factors and not just trauma—and captures better the life situation of those in many Indian communities. In these communities, assessing for PTSD can be problematic; it leads to a neglect of other trauma-related problems such as substance abuse, depression, anomie, low self-esteem, and other key dimensions of psychopathology. Then PTSD acts as a reification of trauma's effects and hence prevents the scrutiny of other effects of trauma, which are broad and entail complex processes in time.

As one example of these complex processes in time, as described by Ball and O'Nell, there is cultural loss. Cultural loss can be seen as a trauma and as a vulnerability factor. The loss of traditional culture and healing ceremonies acts as a trauma, what might be called cultural loss trauma, with culture configured as the source of self-esteem, resilience, and recovery; and cultural loss may lead to vulnerability to trauma by causing anomie and a sense of loss of agency, to a sense of being unable to "cope," to the loss of recuperation-promoting ethnopsychologies, ethnospiritualities, practices, and rituals. Another key aspect of historical trauma is intergenerational trauma. As in other chapters of this volume, such as that of Jenkins and Haas (Chapter 5), intergenerational issues are revealed as keenly important; but here in Ball and O'Nell's chapter, intergenerational trauma is located within the context of historical trauma—though this type of analysis was also suggested by Jenkins and Haas's chapter, in which the two authors describe a locality of high levels of endemic substance abuse, trauma, mental illness, and acting out behaviors that create self-perpetuating cycles of worsening through the generations.

According to the historical trauma perspective, one must examine how multiple traumas, losses, and stresses across time may create and shape life-worlds. Seen from this perspective, using exclusively the PTSD concept to examine the Native American situation is a medicalization that ignores not only the origin of the symptoms in socioeconomic forces such as poverty but also the origins in historical trauma. And seen from this perspective, the definition of trauma in the DSM-5 conceptualization (viz., criterion A) is too narrow, ignoring issues like cultural loss and historical trauma more generally. And from this perspective, in the PTSD criteria, criterion A should include not only traumas of an individual but of an individual's community through time. This historical trauma matrix includes traumas, vulnerability factors, stressors, social and cultural structures, intergenerational dynamics, cultural loss trauma, behaviors like self-cutting, and diagnostic disorders such as substance abuse—these all interact through time to form the historical trauma ontology.

In many Indian communities, historical trauma is now a prominent part of the local ethnopsychology, a concept well known by many. Ball and O'Nell report on studies of historical trauma based on operationalization of the concept into instruments. In a previous study, Ball and others found that many Native Americans thought about historical traumas on a daily basis and that it brought about rage and poor sleep among other effects: the study found that 72 percent of the members of a tribe had PTSD when assessed in reference to the termination of the tribe in the 1950s. The group also had extremely high levels of trauma and rates of PTSD. Out of this research, Ball and others decided to therapeutically use historical genograms that summarize the traumas endured by two tribes. A genogram shows trauma in the broader history of a tribe, and presents this information according to Native American values: traumas are depicted in a circle in relation to other important events in the tribe's cultural history, with the creation myth being placed at the beginning and time flowing in a counterclockwise direction.

Like several authors in this volume, Ball and O'Nell scrutinize the utility of the PTSD concept from the perspective of its ability to promote recovery. They argue that the historical trauma construct better captures the trauma ontology of Native Americans, and has greater therapeutic effects. This edited volume shows several instances of how new trauma subjectivities are formed through therapeutic ideas: in Oaxaca (Duncan [Chapter 6]), the promoting of the notion of trauma and of the need for therapeutic processes like talking about the trauma and developing self-esteem and empowerment; and here in the case of Native Americans, there is the idea that recovery results from learning to view history through the lens of historical trauma. Acquiring a historical consciousness is healing among the Native American groups, according to Ball and O'Nell. The genograms help to put the self-image of trauma in the broader context of creation, ceremonies, and both negative and positive aspects of history. Healing is a cosmology making and self making, which are seen as closely related processes; healing from trauma involves a recontextualization of a trauma event—and related behaviors and symptoms—in a new explanatory frame and an attribution of dysfunctional behaviors and symptoms of those in the community to historical traumas. And as a further therapeutic process, healing involves using traditional ceremonies to help to redress the trauma of cultural loss. Healing is a re-ontologization, a remaking of the person according to the original cosmology, spiritual system, ethnopsychology, and system of therapeutics. This reontologization is said to undo cultural loss trauma, to increase a sense of agency, and to increase self- and group esteem.

James examines the social life of trauma in Haiti and argues that interventions aimed to treat PTSD are doomed to fail unless they take into account the Haitian understandings of personhood, embodiment, and trauma, and their lived experiencing of insecurity. According to James, there is a political economy of trauma in Haiti in which the PTSD construct is the source of supposed therapeutic competency and serves as the language of nongovernmental organizations (NGOs) and other interventions, but that PTSD has limited efficacy—it is a medicalization that obscures. This is particularly so in the Haitian context in which intervention organizations emerge for a day and then fade away, replaced by yet another NGO or other group. As an overarching analytic frame, James presents the idea of ontological insecurity—from poverty, to physical assault, to political insecurity, to assault by spirits—and the historical origins of that insecurity. This is a complementary analytic frame to that of historical trauma (see Hinton and Good [Chapter 1]). James argues that "treatment programs focusing on acute *individual* traumatic suffering will not be effective long-term unless *collective* security—political, economic, and social—is established and sustained in Haiti." This notion of insecurity can be expanded to encompass all ontological levels: from the physical to the spiritual (see Hinton and Good [Chapter 1]; see also Hinton et al. 2009).

Multiple local explanatory frames in Haiti are used to explicate trauma's occurrence and the meaning of the trauma event, to explicate PTSD and other trauma symptoms, and to attempt recovery, and these frames must be taken into account in interventions, according to James. There is, in a modernist, Western-influenced explanation, an examination of the effects of gender inequalities and of a predatory national state. There is an evangelical interpretation in which Haiti's individual and collective traumas are seen to result from involvement with *Vodou*, in particular the purported "diabolical pact" that Haitians made with Satan in 1791 to attain the powers required to overthrow French colonial forces. As another interpretive frame, there is an epistemology of the Vodou tradition that may identify the ultimate cause of affliction to be the failure to uphold kinship and other spiritual obligations or to be the result of the jealousy or malediction of others that results in sorcery. There are ideas about the fate of the dead: following past political events of violence, the inability to observe customary mortuary rites for those lost and presumed dead are among the most devastating experiences for Haitians and contribute to psychosocial trauma—ghosts and not just memories constitute part of the Haitian trauma ontology. This results in spiritual insecurity, in fears of ghost attack. To illustrate the key role of interpretive frames in processing trauma, particularly the ethnopsychology, ethnophysiology, and ethnospirituality frames, James presents cases. In one case, trauma results in psychosis, and seemingly the local ethnopsychology predisposes to a psychosis-like reaction to trauma; the ethnopsychology includes ideas about multiple and dislocatable selves, possession, and a dangerous heating of the head. Local therapeutic ideas shape the course of trauma treatment: if a man becomes agitated, a nurse may consider the man's head (*tèt*) to be hot (*cho*), and their ministrations may aim to reverse the flow of excess blood to the head that caused his outburst. Or as the cases also illustrate, in the traditional understandings of embodiment in Haiti, the condition of hot or bad blood, *move san*, could cause *endispozisyon* (indisposition)—spells of "falling out" or fainting and weakness—as well as other disordered states, seemingly resulting in these states being part of the local trauma ontology.

James argues for the importance of a genealogy of current ontological insecurity, a genealogy of a subjectivity marked by insecurity—a complementary optic to that of historical trauma. In respect to genealogy, whereas Foucault (1978) traces the historical emergence of a certain current sexuality, the formation of a certain sexual subjectivity, James traces the historical formation of the ontologically insecure subject. It is another take on

Heidegger's *Dasein*, but the insecure Dasein (Heidegger 1962)—being-there in which "there" is a place of profound threat, not just existential angst: being-there-in-danger. In her usage, *ensekirite* describes the experience of living at the nexus of multiple uncertainties—political, economic, environmental, interpersonal, physical, and spiritual. In Haiti, insecurities such as the threat of violence are ongoing—there is no "post" in the sense of PTSD. In such circumstances, hypervigilance would seem to be adaptive and appropriate to the ecological context. How is it to attempt to recover with a self that was formed in a past that was marked by multiple traumas and types of stress, with a self living under current threat of trauma and confronting multiple types of ongoing stress, and with a self that is anticipated to have such threats and stresses in the future? These three time perspectives—past horizon, current moment, and future horizon—shape the self. Does the Vodou cosmology of multiple exterior and interior selves in the individual—for example, the *gros bon ange* and the *petit bon ange* and the *lwa*—best convey this sense of a lived fractured history? On multiple levels, the Haitian ontology is marked by insecurities, and a genealogy of those insecurities is necessary to do justice to the actual workings of the trauma survivor's plight.

Good, Good, and Grayman describe the effects of trauma in post–Civil War Aceh based on over five years of work designing interventions in that locality. On an early visit they were traveling with a mobile clinic to a village and heard accounts of routinized, horrific trauma: of a man being hung from a rope like a goat and his head beaten, left for dead; and of a woman, along with her children, forced to watch her husband having his heart cut out. During the Acehnese conflict, there was also economic terror in the form of the destruction of home and livelihood. The authors review the literature claiming that psychological interventions in such settings are a sort of psychological imperialism, the imposition of an alien concept on the local populace in the name of humanitarian intervention—that PTSD is a pseudocondition. The authors respond that in their work they have found that many PTSD symptoms not only are present in the Acehnese context but are prominent, a key part of what matters to persons in the locality, a cause of great impairment, and an important treatment target. This suggests that the portrayal of PTSD as a pseudocondition risks to be a kind of orientalization (Said 1978), the positing of the other as an exotic radical "other" with this interpretation of radical otherness serving the supposed interpreter but not the group itself: the interpretive error leads to the group in question not receiving needed care. The orientalizer self-aggrandizes at the expense of the other. But Good et al. do concur that the remainders of violence in Aceh are broader than PTSD and include acute psychosis, depression, and a wide range of anxiety disorders such as panic disorder, and that they include many somatic complaints like weakness, pain, stomach problems, and heart sensations. Panic attacks with multiple somatic symptoms are particularly prominent. (On somatic symptoms and panic among trauma survivors and the concept of the arousal complex, see also Hinton and Good [Chapter 1].) The authors conclude that a concept like complex trauma is needed to describe the broad range of symptoms that are a core part of the trauma survivor's experience, particularly in settings of ongoing ontological insecurity.

Conclusion

This edited book brings together a set of historical and ethnographic studies of trauma, trauma-related syndromes, PTSD, and trauma treatment in highly diverse settings. It examines how the phenomenology of responses to violence has varied historically, and it analyzes the emergence of PTSD and trauma treatment as contingent historical realities. In many cases, the authors describe PTSD and its uses in settings in which traumatic violence is or has been endemic, leading to complex forms of trauma-related suffering. The chapters examine the phenomenology of the remainders of violence in particular life-worlds, raising questions about the cross-cultural validity of the PTSD construct. They focus in particular on the inadequacy of narrowly defined PTSD for settings in which insecurity and violence are pervasive. And the chapters describe how PTSD is made real in various settings—how PTSD has produced new ways of conceiving violence toward women in Oaxaca, how the construct has been used to organize care for a wide range of postconflict mental health problems in Aceh, Indonesia, and how PTSD serves as a mechanism for adjudicating who can receive compensation in Haiti. The book thus portrays PTSD in action, as a concept that produces a variety of effects as it is translated into practice.

The authors in this book demonstrate how a historically and culturally contextualized understanding of trauma survivors can help avoid dehumanization and interpretive violence. The goal is to advance a study of trauma survivors that does not distort the radical positionality that is one individual's experiencing of a trauma event. The goal is to examine trauma ontology in cross-cultural perspective, to determine experience-near categories of understanding of trauma's effects in those localities. The goal is to explicate what is at stake for local actors and to be aware both of their being victims of vectors of force and of their being agents with a creative response to traumatic experience. Authors of the volume try to accomplish this by examining the category of PTSD and its application to local contexts, all the while investigating the broader effects of trauma and examining those effects from the perspective of multiple types of contextualization.

The book calls for a multifaceted view of evaluation and treatment that is developmental and ecological, one that takes into consideration the issue of treatment of current distress as well as public health approaches to prevention. There is much debate about which treatments may be effective for PTSD across cultures, and why.[10] The current volume describes the multiple ontological levels on which trauma makes a mark, the many paths that trauma effects take, and the ways that local responses to trauma shape the trajectory of trauma's effects as well. The book calls for an engaged anthropology in which contextualization informs treatment and the understanding of the effects of trauma. Contextualization leads to insights about culturally distinctive mechanisms that amplify or reduce symptoms, and contextualization also helps to address the following questions, which are a contextualization in respect to epistemology, episteme, and the biopolitics of power—the study of the consequences of a certain medical gaze. What is considered the object of treatment, who does the treatment apparatus empower and disempower, what are the consequences of the interventions for individuals and social groups, and what are the social and moral implications of those treatments—these are key issues that a socially engaged anthropology must address (Fassin and Pandolfi 2010; Fassin and Rechtman 2009).

Our goal is to show how a historical, multifaceted, development-informed contextualization may contribute to the debates about trauma, long-term suffering, and care. The chapters bear witness to suffering, suggest possible targets of humane care, and provide insights into how those treatments might be developed. The volume thus calls for an anthropologically informed contextualization of PTSD and posttraumatic stress syndromes and suggests ways in which this might be accomplished.

Notes

1. On the mechanisms of possible efficacy, see Hinton and Kirmayer (2013), which is the introduction to a special issue on this topic in *Transcultural Psychiatry*.

2. Speaking to this issue of stigma and its contestation, the Purple Heart can be given to those with traumatic brain injury and other physical injuries, but not to those who claim that combat led to PTSD. As we will see in what follows, traumatic brain injury is not uncommonly a PTSD-like syndrome that is taken on to avoid stigma associated with a PTSD diagnosis. The regulation barring those with PTSD from getting the Purple Heart is currently being contested by mental health advocacy groups.

3. Based partly on cross-cultural considerations (for a review, see Hinton and Lewis-Fernández 2011), some changes were made from DSM-IV to DSM-5 in the PTSD criteria. For one, the nightmare criterion has been changed so that it does not have to be an exact replaying of the trauma but rather just has to evoke a sense of terror and negative emotion reminiscent of the event. Second, in the section of the DSM-5 PTSD criteria labeled "negative alterations in cognitions and mood associated with the traumatic event," in the criterion "persistent and exaggerated negative beliefs or expectations about oneself, others, or the world," it is now stated that this includes ideas about bodily damage from the event, which is fairly common in cross-cultural contexts and in past historical periods (see Hinton and Good [Chapter 1] and Boehnlein and Hinton [Chapter 4]). And third, the numbing (restricted range of affect) item was altered so that it is now specified as an anhedonia, depressive-type item; as discussed in chapter 1, the numbing item is often difficult to apply cross-culturally because of translation difficulties.

4. Typically items C3-C7 in the DSM-IV are considered numbing items, though some of the items are clearly depressive symptoms, and so the items would be best considered as dysphoria and numbing items (Friedman et al. 2011).

5. This last item is strongly shaped by cultural ideas about how trauma can damage the mind or body, such as a Latino's fearing that fright may dislodge the soul or a Cambodian's belief that overwork will permanently deplete and damage the body.

6. Some consider the amnesia item to be a numbing or avoidance item, claiming that amnesia results from the attempt to not recall a negative event. But factor analyses show amnesia loading with depression items suggesting that it is a depressive-type item in many cases: It may result from a sort of mental lethargy, faulty concentration, a torpor (e.g., Armour et al. 2012; Elhai and Palmieri 2011).

7. For an overview, see Hinton and Good (Chapter 1) on wind attacks or *khyâl* attacks; see also www.khyalattacks.com (Devon E. Hinton, M.D., Ph.D.).

8. Generalized anxiety disorder and major depression are highly correlated and share symptoms such as poor concentration.

9. Analogously, Charcot's grand hysteria patients were the prototypical cases of disorder in the second half of the nineteenth century. Hence, what serves as a prototype may be a historical construction. In other cases, actual physical illnesses like brain injury may serve as the prototypical case of what might result and then are imitated and so also become forms of psychological distress (see the Boehnlein and Hinton chapter on TBI [Chapter 4]).

10. For example, recent studies suggest that treatments that target the biology of trauma (viz., pharmacology) or treatments focused on certain psychological aspects of the disorder (viz., cognitive behavioral therapy) are effective treatments for the DSM-defined symptoms of PTSD, and even culturally specific symptoms, such as somatic symptoms (Bass et al. 2013; Hinton et al. 2012).

References

American Psychiatric Association
  1980 Diagnostic and Statistical Manual of Mental Disorders. 3rd edition. Washington, D.C.: American Psychiatric Association.
  1987 Diagnostic and Statistical Manual of Mental Disorders. 3rd edition. Text revision. Washington, D.C.: American Psychiatric Association.
  1994 Diagnostic and Statistical Manual of Mental Disorders. 4th edition. Washington, D.C.: American Psychiatric Association.
  2000 Diagnostic and Statistical Manual of Mental Disorders. 4th edition. Text revision. Washington, D.C.: American Psychiatric Association.
  2013 Diagnostic and Statistical Manual of Mental Disorders. 5th edition. Washington, D.C.: American Psychiatric Association.
Armour, Cherie, Siti Raudzah Ghazali, and Ask Elklit
  2012 PTSD's Latent Structure in Malaysian Tsunami Victims: Assessing the Newly Proposed Dysphoric Arousal Model. Psychiatry Research 206:26–32.
Armstrong, Louise
  1994 Rocking the Cradle of Sexual Politics: What Happened When Women Said Incest. Reading, MA: Addison-Wesley.
Barad, Mark, and Christopher K. Cain
  2007 Mechanisms of Fear Extinction: Toward Improved Treatment for Anxiety. In Understanding Trauma: Integrating Biological, Clinical, and Cultural Perspectives. Laurence J. Kirmayer, Robert Lemelson, and Mark Barad, eds. Pp. 78–97. New York: Cambridge University Press.
Bass, Judith K., Jeannie Annan, Sarah McIvor Murray, Debra Kaysen, Shelly Griffiths, Talita Cetinoglu, Karin Wachter, Laura K. Murray, and Paul A. Bolton
  2013 Controlled Trial of Psychotherapy for Congolese Survivors of Sexual Violence. New England Journal of Medicine 368:2182–91.
Bohacek, Johannes, Katharina Gapp, Bechara, J. Saab, and Isabelle M. Mansuy
  2013 Transgenerational Epigenetic Effects on Brain Functions. Biological Psychiatry 73:313–20.
Breslau, Naomi, and Ronald C. Kessler
  2001 The Stressor Criterion in DSM-IV Posttraumatic Stress Disorder: An Empirical Investigation. Biological Psychiatry 50:699–704.

Brewin, Chris R., Bernice Andrews, and John D. Valentine

2000 Meta-Analysis of Risk Factors for Posttraumatic Stress Disorder in Trauma-Exposed Adults. Journal of Consulting and Clinical Psychology 68:748–66.

Brown, Daniel P., Alan W. Scheflin, and D. Corydon Hammond

1998 Memory, Trauma Treatment, and the Law. New York: Norton.

Bryant, Richard A.

2010 The Complexity of Complex PTSD. American Journal of Psychiatry 167:879–81.

2012 Simplifying Complex PTSD: Comment on Resick et al. Journal of Traumatic Stress 25:252–53.

Cahill, Shawn P., Barbara O. Rothbaum, Patricia A. Resick, and Victoria M. Follette

2009 Cognitive Behavioral Therapy for Adults. *In* Effective Treatments for PTSD: Practice Guidelines from the International Society for Traumatic Stress Studies. Edna B Foa, Matthew J Friedman, and Judith A Cohen, eds. Pp. 139–222. New York: Guilford Press.

Carr, John E., and Peter P. Vitaliano

1985 The Theoretical Implications of Converging Research on Depression and the Culture-Bound Syndromes. *In* Culture and Depression: Studies in Anthropology and Cross-Cultural Psychiatry of Affect and Disorder. Arthur Kleinman and Byron J. Good, eds. Pp. 244–67. Berkeley: University of California Press.

Conte, J. R.

1991 Child Sexual Abuse: Looking Backward and Forward. *In* Family Sexual Abuse: Frontline Research and Evaluation. Michael Q. Patton, ed. Pp. 3–22. Newbury Park, Calif.: Sage.

Courtois, Christine A., and Julian D. Ford

2009 Treating Complex Traumatic Stress Disorders: Scientific Foundations and Therapeutic Models. New York: Guilford Press.

Cukor, Judith, Megan Olden, Francis Lee, and JoAnn Difede

2010 Evidence-Based Treatments for PTSD, New Directions, and Special Challenges. Annals of the New York Academy of Sciences 1208:82–89.

de Jong, Joop T., Ivan H. Komproe, Joseph Spinazzola, Bessel A. van der Kolk, and Mark H. Van Ommeren

2005 DESNOS in Three Postconflict Settings: Assessing Cross-Cultural Construct Equivalence. Journal of Traumatic Stress 18:13–21.

Didi-Huberman, Georges, and Jean-Martin Charcot

2003 Invention of Hysteria: Charcot and the Photographic Iconography of the Salpêtrière. Cambridge, Mass.: MIT Press.

Duffield, Mark

2001 Governing the Borderlands: Decoding the Power of Aid. Disasters 25:308–20.

Eisenberg, Leon

1977 Disease and Illness: Distinctions Between Professional and Popular Ideas of Sickness. Culture, Medicine, and Psychiatry 1:9–23.

Elhai, Jon D., and Patrick A. Palmieri
    2011 The Factor Structure of Posttraumatic Stress Disorder: A Literature Update, Critique of Methodology, and Agenda for Future Research. Journal of Anxiety Disorders 25:849–54.
Fassin, Didier, and Mariella Pandolfi
    2010 Contemporary States of Emergency: The Politics of Military and Humanitarian Interventions. Cambridge, Mass.: Zone.
Fassin, Didier, and Richard Rechtman
    2009 The Empire of Trauma: An Inquiry into the Condition of Victimhood. Princeton, NJ: Princeton University Press.
Foa, Edna B., Anke Ehlers, David M. Clark, David F. Tolin, and Susan M. Orsillo
    1999 The Posttraumatic Cognitions Inventory (PTCI): Development and Validation. Psychological Assessment 11:303–14.
Foa, Edna B., Terence M. Keane, Matthew J. Friedman, and Judith A. Cohen, eds.
    2009 Effective Treatments for PTSD: Practice Guidelines from the International Society for Traumatic Stress Studies. New York: Guilford Press.
Foucault, Michel
    1978 The History of Sexuality. New York: Pantheon.
Friedman, Matthew J., Jonathan R. T. Davidson, and Dan J. Stein
    2009 Psychopharmacotherapy for Adults. In Effective Treatments for PTSD: Practice Guidelines from the International Society for Traumatic Stress Studies. Edna B. Foa, Matthew J. Friedman, and Judith A. Cohen, eds. Pp. 245–68. New York: Guilford Press.
Friedman, Matthew J., Terence M. Keane, and Patricia A. Resick
    2014 Handbook of PTSD: Science and Practice. New York: Guilford Press.
Friedman, Matthew J., Patricia A. Resick, Richard A. Bryant, and Chris R. Brewin
    2011 Considering PTSD for DSM-V. Depression and Anxiety 28:750–59.
Green, Linda
    1999 Fear as a Way of Life: Mayan Widows in Rural Guatemala. New York: Columbia University Press.
Haskell, Yasmin Annabel
    2011 Diseases of the Imagination and Imaginary Disease in the Early Modern Period. Turnhout: Brepols.
Heidegger, Martin
    1962 Being and Time. New York: Harper.
Heim, Christine, D., Jeffrey Newport, Stacey Heit, Yolanda P. Graham, Molly Wilcox, Robert Bonsall, Andrew H. Miller, and Charles B. Nemeroff
    2000 Pituitary-Adrenal and Autonomic Responses to Stress in Women After Sexual and Physical Abuse in Childhood. Journal of the American Medical Association 284:592–97.
Herman, Judith L.
    1981 Father-Daughter Incest. New York: Basic.

1992 Trauma and Recovery. New York: Basic.

1993 Complex PTSD: A Syndrome in Survivors of Prolonged and Repeated Trauma. Journal of Traumatic Stress 5:377–91.

Hinton, Devon E., and Byron J. Good, eds.

2009 Culture and Panic Disorder. Palo Alto, Calif.: Stanford University Press.

Hinton, Devon E., Alexander L. Hinton, Dara Chhean, Vuth Pich, Reattidara J. R. Loeum, and Mark H. Pollack

2009 Nightmares Among Cambodian Refugees: The Breaching of Concentric Ontological Security. Culture, Medicine, and Psychiatry 33:219–65.

Hinton, Devon E., and Baland Jalal

2014 Parameters for Creating Culturally Sensitive CBT: Implementing CBT in Global Settings. Cognitive and Behavioral Practice 21:139–44.

Hinton, Devon. E., and Laurence J. Kirmayer

2013 Local Responses to Trauma: Symptom, Affect, and Healing. Transcultural Psychiatry 50:607–21.

Hinton, Devon E., Maria A. Kredlow, Eric Bui, Mark H. Pollack, and Stefan G. Hofmann

2012 Treatment Change of Somatic Symptoms and Cultural Syndromes Among Cambodian Refugees with PTSD. Depression and Anxiety 29:148–55.

Hinton, Devon E., and Roberto Lewis-Fernández

2011 The Cross-Cultural Validity of Posttraumatic Stress Disorder: Implications for DSM-5. Depression and Anxiety 28:783–801.

Hinton, Devon E., Edwin Rivera, Stefan G. Hofmann, David H. Barlow, and Michael W. Otto

2012 Adapting CBT for Traumatized Refugees and Ethnic Minority Patients: Examples from Culturally Adapted CBT (CA-CBT). Transcultural Psychiatry 49:340–65.

Horowitz, Mardi Jon

1976 Stress Response Syndromes. New York: J. Aronson.

James, Erica Caple

2008 Haunting Ghosts: Madness, Gender, and Ensekirite in Haiti in the Democratic Era. In Postcolonial Disorders. Mary Jo Good, Sandra T. Hyde, and Byron J. Good, eds. Pp. 132–56. Berkeley: University of California Press.

Jones, Edgar, and Simon Wessely

2005 Shell Shock to PTSD: Military Psychiatry from 1900 to the Gulf War. Hove, East Sussex: Psychology Press.

Kempe, C. Henry, Frederic N. Silverman, Brandt F. Steele, William Droegemueller, Henry K. Silver

1962 The Battered Child Syndrome. JAMA 181:17–24.

Kilshaw, S.

2009 Impotent Warriors: Gulf War Syndrome, Vulnerability, and Masculinity. New York: Berghahn.

Kirmayer, Laurence J., Robert Lemelson, and Mark Barad, eds.

2007 Understanding Trauma: Integrating Biological, Clinical, and Cultural Perspectives. New York: Cambridge University Press.

Kleinman, Arthur, Leon Eisenberg, and Byron J. Good

1978 Culture, Illness, and Care: Clinical Lessons from Anthropologic and Cross-Cultural Research. Annals of Internal Medicine 88:251–58.

Kugelmann, Robert

2009 The Irritable Heart Syndrome in the American Civil War. *In* Culture and Panic Disorder. Devon E. Hinton and Byron J. Good, eds. Pp. 85–112. Palo Alto, Calif.: Stanford University Press.

Ledoux, Joseph

1996 The Emotional Brain. New York: Simon and Schuster.

Lewis, Oscar

1959 Five Families: Mexican Case Studies in the Culture of Poverty. New York: Basic.

1966 La Vida: A Puerto Rican Family in the Culture of Poverty—San Juan and New York. New York: Random House.

Luxenberg, Toni, Joseph Spinazzola, Jose Hidalgo, Cheryl Hunt, and Bessel A. van der Kolk

2001 Complex Trauma and Disorders of Extreme Stress (DESNOS) Diagnosis, Part Two: Treatment. Directions in Psychiatry 21:395–415.

Luxenberg, Toni, Joseph Spinazzola, and Bessel A. van der Kolk

2001 Complex Trauma and Disorders of Extreme Stress (DESNOS) Diagnosis, Part One: Assessment. Directions in Psychiatry 21:373–94.

Mayer, Emeran

2007 Somatic Manifestations of Traumatic stress. *In* Understanding Trauma: Biological, Clinical and Cultural Perspectives. Laurence Kirmayer, Robert Lemelson, and Mark Barad, eds. Pp. 142–70. New York: Cambridge University Press.

Micale, Mark S., and Paul Frederick Lerner

2001 Traumatic Pasts: History, Psychiatry, and Trauma in the Modern Age, 1870–1930. New York: Cambridge University Press.

Nakimuli-Mpungu, Etheldreda, Stephen Alderman, Eugene Kinyanda, Kathleen Allden, Theresa S. Betancourt, Jeffrey S. Alderman, Alison Pavia, James Okello, Juliet Nakku, Alex Adaku, and Seggane Musisi

2013 Implementation and Scale-Up of Psycho-Trauma Centers in a Post-Conflict Area: A Case Study of a Private-Public Partnership in Northern Uganda. PLOS Medicine 10:1–8.

Pandolfi, Mariella.

2008. Laboratories of Intervention: The Humanitarian Governance of the Postcommunist Balkan Territories. *In* Postcolonial Disorders. Mary-Jo DelVecchio Good, Sandra Teresa Hyde, Sarah Pinto, and Byron J. Good, eds. Pp. 157–186. Berkeley: University of California Press.

Pupavac, Vanessa
  2001 Therapeutic Governance: Psycho-Social Intervention and Trauma Risk Management. Disasters. 25:358–72.
Quirk, Gregory, Mohammed R. Milad, Edwin Santini, and Kelimer Lebron
  2007 Learning Not to Fear: A Neural Systems Approach. *In* Understanding Trauma: Biological, Clinical and Cultural Perspectives. Laurence Kirmayer, Robert Lemelson, and Mark Barad, eds. Pp. 60–77. New York: Cambridge University Press.
Resick, Patricia A., Michelle J. Bovin, Amber L. Calloway, Alexandra M. Dick, Matthew W. King, Karen. S. Mitchell, Michael K. Suvak, Stephanie Y. Wells, Shannon W. Stirman, and Erika J. Wolf
  2012 A Critical Evaluation of the Complex PTSD Literature: Implications for DSM-5. Journal of Traumatic Stress 25:241–51.
Said, Edward W.
  1978 Orientalism. New York: Vintage.
Shalev, Arieh Y.
  2007 PTSD: A Disorder of Recovery? *In* Understanding Trauma: Biological, Clinical and Cultural Perspectives. Laurence Kirmayer, Robert Lemelson, and Mark Barad, eds. Pp. 207–24. New York: Cambridge University Press.
Silove, D.
  2007 Adaptation, Ecological Safety Signals, and the Trajectory of PTSD. *In* Understanding Trauma: Biological, Clinical and Cultural Perspectives. Laurence Kirmayer, Robert Lemelson, and Mark Barad, eds. Pp. 242–58. New York: Cambridge University Press.
Summerfield, Derek
  1999 A Critique of Seven Assumptions Behind Psychological Trauma Programmes in War-Affected Areas. Social Science and Medicine 48:1449–62.
  2000 Childhood, War, Refugeedom and "Trauma": Three Core Questions for Mental Health Professionals. Transcultural Psychiatry 37:417–33.
Theidon, Kimberly
  2013 Intimate Enemies: Violence and Reconciliation in Peru. Philadelphia: University of Pennsylvania Press.
van der Kolk, Bessel A.
  2007 The Developmental Impact of Childhood Trauma. *In* Understanding Trauma: Biological, Clinical and Cultural Perspectives. Laurence Kirmayer, Robert Lemelson, and Mark Barad, eds. Pp. 224–41. New York: Cambridge University Press.
van der Kolk, Bessel A., James W. Hopper, and Janet E. Osterman
  2001 Exploring the Nature of Traumatic Memory: Combining Clinical Knowledge with Laboratory Methods. Journal of Aggression, Maltreatment, and Trauma 4:9–31.

van der Kolk, Bessel A., and Onno van der Hart

  1989 Pierre Janet and the Breakdown of Adaptation in Psychological Trauma. American Journal of Psychiatry 146:1530–40.

Yehuda, Rachel, and Alexander C. McFarlane

  1995 Conflict Between Current Knowledge About Posttraumatic Stress Disorder and its Original Conceptual Basis. American Journal of Psychiatry 152:1705–13.

Young, Allan

  1995 The Harmony of Illusions: Inventing Post-Traumatic Stress Disorder. Princeton, N.J.: Princeton University Press.

CHAPTER 1

The Culturally Sensitive Assessment of Trauma: Eleven Analytic Perspectives, a Typology of Errors, and the Multiplex Models of Distress Generation

Devon E. Hinton and Byron J. Good

In this chapter we present several forms of analysis that can be used to assess trauma and its effects in a culturally sensitive way. These analytic lenses demonstrate cross-cultural variation in DSM-5-defined posttraumatic stress disorder (PTSD) symptoms and trauma-related disorder more broadly. The chapter also serves to situate the theoretical contributions of the chapters in this volume. The first section presents the eleven-dimension analysis of the trauma survivor that can be used to examine in a multidimensional ecological way the ontology of the trauma survivor (on the call to contextualism, see Good 1977; Kirmayer et al. 2007). The second section presents a typology of errors (Kleinman 1988) that should be avoided in order to evaluate trauma in a culturally sensitive manner. Throughout the chapter and in a third and final section we present multiplex models to show how trauma symptoms are generated through biocultural mechanisms and how trauma results in particular episodes of distress.

Eleven Analytic Perspectives: The Multiaxial Analysis of the Trauma Survivor

As indicated in Figure 1.1, trauma survivors and their key complaints can be examined in terms of eleven ontological dimensions that create a certain trauma subjectivity.

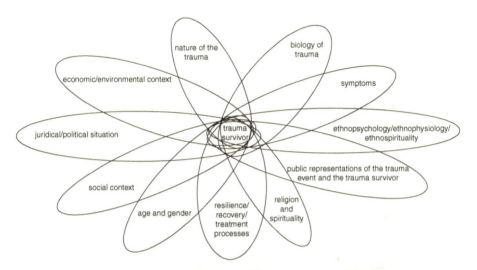

Figure 1.1. A multiaxial approach to the trauma survivor's ontology: Eleven analytic perspectives. The trauma survivor can be analyzed in terms of multiple ontological dimensions that range from biology to the justice situation.

The Type of Trauma and the Particularities of Effects

The term "trauma" is borrowed from the medical sciences, where it means a physical injury, and it is used to depict certain sorts of events that are deeply disturbing—to the point of causing permanent psychological harm, evidenced by perduring symptoms (McNally [Chapter 2]; Young and Breslau [Chapter 3]; see also Fassin and Rechtman 2009; Hollan 2013). The term "trauma" implies that some objectively verifiable damage has been sustained; the term "psychological trauma" suggests that whatever is upsetting to a certain degree is sufficient to traumatize and cause a long-lasting wound.[1]

There is great variability in the types of trauma, and the nature of the trauma event is a key part of every trauma survivor's subjectivity. Below we will discuss several classifications of trauma. Other types could also be identified. The trauma can be classified in the following ways, which are discussed in the rest of this section: the trauma can be classified by

- whether it is complex trauma;
- what are the trauma's general characteristics (e.g., physical assault, illness, observing a killing or a beating);

- whether it tends to induce strongly certain specific symptoms (e.g., anger or somatic symptoms) and how it does so;
- whether it has effects on the self-, interpersonal-, group-, and world-schema;
- whether it has intergenerational aspects;
- whether it occurs in the context of historical trauma;
- whether it is a social loss trauma (e.g., involves the death of a relative);
- whether it is a cultural loss trauma (e.g., involves the loss of cultural traditions);
- whether it is a ritual omission trauma (i.e., involves an inability to perform indicated rites);
- whether it is a social status loss trauma (i.e., involves a severe loss of social standing and status);
- whether it is an economic loss trauma (i.e., involves a severe loss of economic security); or
- whether it is episodic, endemic, or cohort in type.

In the trauma literature, one often finds the term "complex trauma," which may indicate either of the following or both (Bryant 2012; Friedman et al. 2011; Resick et al. 2012): a certain kind of trauma (viz., severe single trauma or repeated traumas) or trauma occurring during states of vulnerability (e.g., trauma at a particularly early age, trauma with genetic vulnerability, trauma with minimal social support, or trauma with ongoing stress). Of note, vulnerability factors said to result in complex PTSD are also recovery-inhibiting factors, like ongoing stress and broken social structures. Complex trauma is said to cause complex PTSD (Bryant 2012; Friedman et al. 2011; Resick et al. 2012), characterized by a recalibration of the nervous system to a state of hyperreactivity to a wide range of stimuli, such as to noises or visual reminders of the trauma, and by poor regulation of negative emotion, such as anger, and this hyperreactivity to stimuli and poor emotion regulation result in the frequent experiencing of symptoms such as anger, anxiety, and somatic symptoms (see Good and Hinton [Introduction]). Complex PTSD is described in many chapters in this volume (Jenkins and Haas [Chapter 5]; Duncan [Chapter 6]; Ball and O'Nell [Chapter 10]; Good, Good, and Grayman [Chapter 12]). As discussed throughout this volume, the exact nature of the traumas and vulnerability factors—and recovery inhibitors—needs to be carefully investigated.

On the most basic level, a trauma may be classified by the nature of the trauma event itself, such as torture, an illness, slave labor, starvation, or observing someone being beaten or killed. Each of these will have subtypes: torture will have subtypes depending on how it is perpetrated (Ursano and Rundell 1986). The type of trauma will result in specific effects and forms a key aspect of the local trauma ontology, and the ethnography of the trauma events and their classification is a key part of witnessing.

The type of trauma results in a specific trauma ontology in that it will tend to induce certain symptoms. Traumas can be classified and examined by the bodily and mental states they strongly induce, immediately in the event, and afterward. During the event certain emotions (e.g., anger) or specific symptoms (e.g., dizziness) may occur. Somatic symptoms are prominent in the trauma ontology of many cultural groups (for one review, see Hinton and Lewis-Fernández 2011): this is true of Cambodian survivors of the Pol Pot regime, and this was true of survivors of the Nazi concentration camps and other such internment settings, the term "concentration camp syndrome" being used after World War II to describe a cluster of symptoms found in those camp and internment survivors, one part of which was somatic symptoms (Bower 1994). This somatic symptom prominence in the trauma presentation seemingly results in part from the nature of the trauma that was experienced. Certain traumas strongly induce somatic symptoms, and so create a trauma ontology that includes prominent somatic symptoms along with frequent panic and arousal (Hinton et al. 2012, 2013b): this is because (1) experiencing the somatic symptoms for any reason leads to recall of past negative events encoded by those somatic symptoms, and then this recall of the somatic symptom-encoded negative events further evokes the somatic symptoms (both by somatic flashback and by the induction of arousal-inducing fear), creating vicious circles of worsening; or (2) the episode may begin by thinking of the trauma event, which then induces somatic symptoms by somatic flashback and by the induction of fear, also starting vicious circles of worsening.[2]

One can further classify and examine traumas from the perspective of the mechanism by which they cause somatic symptoms. For example, almost all Cambodian survivors of the Pol Pot period (1975–1979) experienced multiple events that brought about extreme somatic states. They had illness during the Pol Pot period that strongly induced symptoms: malaria, considered by them to be one of the worst traumas, in which the person had daily events of rigors (a feeling of extreme cold to the point of shaking along with panic-like

symptoms such as palpitations and dizziness) followed by a high tempera-
ture state, in which the person experienced strong palpitations, dizziness,
tinnitus, headache, and sweating. Cambodians usually had starvation-
induced edema alternating with extreme emaciation, accompanied by
stomach cramps, bodily coldness, numbness, and other dysphoric somatic
states. They had to do slave labor, often resulting in muscle soreness from
carrying weights at the shoulder, exhaustion, dizziness, and syncope. They
often saw corpses and mutilated bodies, inducing nausea and dizziness.
They were often beaten, causing headache and other pains. And they often
experienced fear, owing to all the traumas mentioned above, as well as
others—being threatened by death, observing others killed, being constantly
at risk of assault and death—with this fear resulting in muscle tension, palpitations, and other somatic symptoms.[3] All these traumas and somatic
states mark the space-time (chronotope) of the Pol Pot period, constitute a
somatic chronotope (Bahktin 1981) for the Cambodian refugee survivor,
contributing to somatic symptoms being a prominent aspect of their
trauma ontology. (Of note, somatic symptoms may be prominent in a group
simply from the severity of the cumulative trauma load—e.g., multiple
trauma events—rather from specific induction of somatic symptoms at the
time of the trauma.)

Traumas can also be classified by the effect on self-, interpersonal-, group-,
and world-schemas. Family-based violence—for example, parental abuse—
may destroy bonds of trust (Jenkins and Haas [Chapter 5]), shaping
interpersonal schemas, or the trauma, such as a genocide in which perpetrators are not punished, may result in a sense of a lack of justice and other effects that shape the world-schema (Foa et al. 1997, 1999). The trauma may
also be an assault on self- and group-schemas, on self- and group-esteem, and
the trauma may lead to stigmatization—both self-inflicted stigmatization and
other-inflicted stigmatization. That is, certain types of traumas like rape or
other acts of degradation may result in a sense of shame and in stigma, not
just in trauma symptoms like poor concentration. The nature of the trauma
that is recalled in memory will shape identity. When recalled to mind, the
trauma memory may bring about a strong sense of anger or shame, among
other emotions, may bring about a certain trauma-linked self-schema, or self-
image (Foa et al. 1997, 1999): some traumas may be especially shaming and
create what has been referred to as "humiliation memory" (Foa and Rothbaum 1998; Langer 1991) and these traumas may act as self-image violence.

Genocide and political terror may aim to create humiliation memory in the self- and/or group schema. In situations of genocide and political terror, perpetrators often purposefully use techniques to abuse and kill that will be the most upsetting in that cultural context; this increases terror and the sense of degradation and results in the recall of the trauma being extremely disturbing, a humiliation memory (Hagengimana and Hinton 2009; Hinton et al. 2013a, 2013c).[4] The perpetrators aim to create a negative self-image and a sense of shame for the targeted individual and that person's group more broadly, a kind of group-image violence, which may be perpetrated by symbolic violence. Such degrading imagery and experiences tend to create simultaneously a sense of rage and shame in the members of the targeted group. The tattoo of a number on the arm of the Jewish Holocaust survivor is an example of this kind of trauma, an attempt to impose an animal status on the other. Similarly, during the Rwandan genocide, the Hutu perpetrated violence against Tutsi guided by certain cultural schemas of what constitutes the abhorrent. The violence emphasized blocking imagery through the manner of killing, for example, impaling along the entire digestive tract, and through the manner of maiming, for example, truncating the breasts of women, castrating men, and cutting the person's Achilles tendon. This violence and the general rhetoric of the genocide seemingly attempted to represent the Tutsi in blocking imagery that resonated with other negative exemplars of blocking in the culture—for example, the witch was considered a blocking entity and was configured in such images[5]—and that contrasted with the positive exemplars of flow as health and prosperity in the Rwandan culture.

A trauma may be intergenerationally transmitted, and may have intergenerational effects. Trauma in one generation may be passed on to the next through multiple means: epigenetics; exposure to parental psychopathology, which may include anger and substance abuse; and parental downward economic and social mobility, which will create a certain life context for the child. Intergenerational trauma may play a key part in historical trauma. Historical trauma often refers to intergenerational trauma combined with other types of trauma as sustained by a group. Historical trauma refers to the fact that a traumatic event endured by an entire group—for example, a genocide that results in mass trauma in which local traditions are destroyed—may have effects through the generations by such means as impacting on social structures and the various sources of resilience and collective self-esteem, leading potentially to multiple negative outcomes that range from substance abuse, to violence, to PTSD-like symptoms (Ball and O'Nell [Chapter 10]).

Social loss is another type of trauma. "Social loss trauma" refers to the loss of significant others owing to death or separation by distance, for example, after migration, immigration, or forced relocation. The term "bereavement trauma" may be used to refer to the death of a loved one, which may be even more upsetting if circumstances prevented performing culturally indicated death rituals.

Some use the term "cultural bereavement" (Eisenbruch 1991), or what might be called cultural-loss trauma, to refer to the loss of cultural traditions owing to their purposeful destruction or to the traumatized having moved to a location where those cultural institutions are not present: cultural loss may range from diminished access to spiritual traditions to inability to maintain food traditions and traditional diet. In some cases there may be public displays of destruction of aspects of a culture's identity such as the burning of temples—at the extreme, there may be cultural violence to the point of cultural genocide. (See Duncan [Chapter 6] on how migration is locally considered a trauma that brings about loss of social and cultural structures, and see Ball and O'Nell [Chapter 10] on cultural loss processes in historical and intergenerational trauma.)

The forced omission of indicated rituals may constitute a trauma, and complicate other traumas: what is considered to be dangerous and damaging about the trauma event may be that it made it impossible to do certain rituals, what might be called ritual omission violence. In these cases, inability to perform time-sensitive rituals is considered a key part of what is upsetting about the trauma event, what might also be called ritual omission trauma. As one example, Cambodians were unable to conduct postpartum rituals such as "steaming" in the Pol Pot period. If a woman does not perform these rituals, she fears the vessels in her body may become permanently disordered and thereby predispose her to frequent *khyâl* attacks,[6] that is, an upward surge in the body of blood and khyâl, a wind-like substance, that may cause various bodily disasters. As another example of ritual omission trauma, it is often impossible to perform mortuary rites in situations of mass violence. In many cultural contexts, not conducting burial or other mortuary ceremonies is thought to result in the deceased's not being reborn but rather becoming a ghost-like entity, and it is often thought that the deceased's restless spirit may attack the living—often in a nightmare, with a nightmare often configured as the experiencing of the dreamer's wandering soul—and so may cause illness and even death (James [Chapter 11]; see also Hagengimana and Hinton 2009; Hinton et al. 2009a, 2013a, 2013c). These rebirth and attack concerns worsen bereavement and give rise to despair, guilt, and fear; and these concerns and cultural frames—along with the biology of trauma, which results in nightmares and sleep paralysis—seemingly lead to the encountering of the dead in nightmares and sometimes in sleep paralysis. Through these mechanisms, bereavement then becomes a key part of the trauma ontology of certain cultural groups such as Cambodians and Rwandans.

A trauma may involve a fall in social status and economic state. For example, in the Cambodian genocide and Chinese Cultural Revolution, there was a precipitous fall in social status and economic status of certain groups, who were often targeted for verbal abuse and various humiliations (Kleinman and Kleinman 1994). Or in Aceh, government forces often purposefully targeted economic resources of those considered to be rebellious (Good, Good, and Grayman [Chapter 12]).

A trauma may be further classified by degree of chronicity within a society. Several chapters document the repeated acts of violence that members of some societies and social classes confront, what might be called endemic trauma, that is, types of trauma frequently experienced by members of a society (Jenkins and Haas [Chapter 5]; Duncan [Chapter 6]), and cohort trauma, that is, a trauma like a genocide or 9/11 experienced by most in a society of a certain age (Pedersen and Kienzler [Chapter 7]; James [Chapter 11]; Good, Good, and Grayman [Chapter 12]). Episodic trauma is trauma that is not endemic or cohort in type, but much more sporadic, like a mugging in a wealthy suburb. As discussed in this and the following sections, there may be situations in which endemic trauma and cohort trauma co-occur in a situation of ongoing daily stressors such as poverty, resulting in what might be called a 1-2-3 punch of adversity. These might be called cultures of trauma and stress, of trauma and structural violence (Jenkins and Haas [Chapter 5]; Duncan [Chapter 6]; James [Chapter 11]).

Several chapters implicitly or explicitly invoke the concept of structural violence (Jenkins and Haas [Chapter 5]; Duncan [Chapter 6]; Ball and O'Nell [Chapter 10]). When using the term "structural violence," one should differentiate between the literal and metaphorical senses of the term. The term "structural violence" as usually defined suggests that endemic societal problems like poverty are a kind of trauma. It may be clearer to use the term "structural insecurity" to refer to economic insecurity and some other key aspects of what is usually meant by the term "structural violence," and for trauma experienced by a group that is meant in the literal sense to use the terms "endemic traumas" (for recurring traumas that afflict a group, e.g., gun violence, crime, and sexual violence) and "cohort traumas" (for traumas experienced by an age cohort, e.g., a war, genocide, or a major act of terrorism like 9/11 in the United States).

Biology of Trauma

Another key ontological dimension of the trauma survivor is trauma's effects on the nervous, endocrine, and other biological systems, and the actual wounds on the body such as permanently deformed limbs from torture or scars from shrapnel or other injury. The inner and outer body may be marked by trauma, and as is explained below, the biological legacies of trauma range from changes to genes owing to epigenetic mechanisms, to amygdala hyperreactivity, to amygdala-based memories, to vagal-tone-caused poor emotion regulation, to brain-based generation of orthostatic dizziness and sleep paralysis, to biology-based predisposition to migraine with aura, to long-term biological effects of starvation, to bodily deformations. And the biological effects of trauma may be much worsened by current stressors like poverty and the threat of violence while living in crime-marked urban areas (Hinton and Lewis-Fernández 2011).

The neurobiology of trauma will produce a certain potential set of symptoms, what might be called a trauma symptom pool, with each symptom being interpreted according to the local cultural context, as is depicted in Figure 1.2. (On the call for a neuroanthropology of PTSD, see Pedersen and Kienzler [Chapter 7]; Kohrt, Worthman, and Upadhaya [Chapter 9]; see also Collura and Lende 2012; Finley 2012; Hinton and Kirmayer 2013.) Trauma-caused biological changes include decreased vagal tone that brings about poor ability to regulate emotion (Blechert et al. 2007; Hinton et al. 2009b). The trauma memory itself is registered in the amygdala (Ledoux 1996). A key aspect of trauma is a biology-generated emotional and somatic hyperreactivity in response to negative emotions and ruminative states like worry and in response to various external cues such as a noise or to any reminder of the trauma. This hyperreactivity is characterized by the rapid induction of

Cultural interpretive processes

- The attribution of the symptom to a disturbance of mind, body, or spiritual state leading to:
  - catastrophic cognitions about the symptom's meaning, e.g., concerns that the symptom indicates a mental perturbation, physiological disturbance, or spiritual assault
  - scanning of the body and mind for symptoms thought to be caused by the feared disturbance
  - anticipatory fear about events, actions, and things thought to trigger bouts of the feared condition (e.g. standing up, engaging in worry, a loud noise, being in public)
  - attempts to treat the condition, e.g., through self-help methods, local healing traditions, and Western-type professional treatments
  - interpersonal, economic, identity, and stigma effects of self-labeling and other-labeling as having the condition

Negative memories

- The experiencing of a trauma memory, which may be triggered or worsened by the experiencing of a cue present during the trauma such as a negative emotion, a visual cue, or a somatic symptom: the experiencing of dizziness triggering recall of a trauma marked by dizziness

The trauma symptom pool

- DSM-5 PTSD symptoms: trauma recall, startle, poor concentration, hypervigilance, avoidance of reminders of trauma, insomnia, nightmare
- Various non-DSM symptoms:
  - somatic symptoms (e.g., dizziness, palpitations, headache), which may be triggered by emotional states (e.g., worry, anxiety, depression), external stimuli (e.g., sounds or odors), motion (e.g., riding in a car), actions (e.g., exertion or standing up), trauma recall, or prolonged stress resulting from adversity
  - arousal and panic attacks, which can be triggered by the same triggers mentioned for "somatic symptoms" (see Figure1.3)
  - "current problems–trauma" complex or "thinking a lot" complex (see Figure1.3)
  - sleep-related complaints: sleep paralysis, hypnopompic and hypnagogic hallucinations, nocturnal panic
  - cognitive-capacity complaints: forgetfulness (closely related to the DSM-5's PTSD symptom of poor concentration)
  - other symptoms not listed above: poor emotion regulation such as rapid induction of arousal during negative mood states; anxiety disorders such as panic attacks, panic disorder, and generalized anxiety disorder; impulsive, destructive behaviors such as suicidality, substance abuse, violence, and other risk behaviors; negative self-image (e.g., one of shame, of incompetence, of failure, of being damaged), spiritual-image, and world-image; bereavement; motion sickness; agoraphobia, and general sensitivity to external stimuli (e.g., to sounds, to complex visual environments, to smells); social withdrawal

Trauma-related biological processes

- Low vagal tone • Amygdalar hyperreactivity • Dysregulation of the cortisol axis

Figure 1.2. The multiplex trauma model: A biocultural model of cultural influences on trauma-related disorder. Feedback loops occur when cultural interpretive processes and negative memories increase arousal and distress and when cultural interpretive processes lead to bio-attentional looping such as surveying of the body for feared symptoms. The trauma symptom pool represents possible symptoms.

strong emotions and many somatic symptoms (Hinton et al. 2011). This hyperreactivity may begin in utero through intergenerational mechanisms: if a pregnant woman experiences trauma, it may cause certain shifts in the genes of the in utero child by epigenetic mechanisms, leading to hyperreactivity in many psychobiological respects, seemingly preparing the child for a hostile environment (Binder and Nemeroff 2010; Heim et al. 2000; Sherin and Nemeroff 2011; Yehuda and Bierer 2009).

The biology of trauma worsens the ability to handle current problems by several mechanisms, including by increasing reactivity (due to amygdalar reactivity) and diminishing psychological flexibility (due to amygdalar reactivity and diminished vagal tone). These coping difficulties predispose to the occurrence of distress episodes of the type depicted by the "current problems–trauma model" (Figure 1.3), this symptom complex forming one part of the trauma symptom pool. As shown in the model, when confronted by a problem, the trauma survivor may rapidly experience arousal that impairs the ability to consider other action options and compromises the ability to adjust to the situation. In addition, the mental and somatic symptoms induced by the distress experienced upon confronting the problem may give rise to catastrophic cognitions and may trigger trauma recall as well as negative memory more generally. Distress may rapidly escalate. The current problems–trauma model shows one aspect of the lifeworld of the traumatized person, a certain symptom complex: the frequent triggering by current life problems of severe episodes of distress through certain mechanisms, a multiplex model. Theorists increasingly advocate the need to show how specific PTSD symptoms and other symptoms interact in particular episodes (Borsboom and Cramer 2013; McNally 2012; van Os 2013), as this multiplex model does. Additionally, this multiplex model (Figure 1.3) demonstrates that trauma survivors don't simply have "symptoms," but experience certain symptom complexes, certain causal networks, which have a local trajectory.

The neurobiology of trauma may result in certain cross-cultural differences in symptomatology. Among Cambodian refugees, the biology of trauma conjoined with a seeming inborn predisposition plays a key role in producing orthostatic panic and sleep paralysis (Hinton et al. 2012). Orthostatic dizziness may result from trauma-caused impairment of the systolic blood pressure response to standing. Certain groups seem particularly prone to this effect, such as Cambodian refugees; and among Cambodian refugees, frequent orthostatic dizziness interacts with cultural syndromes to trigger panic on

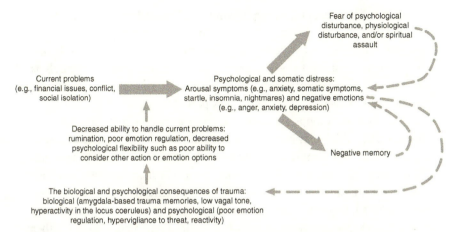

Figure 1.3. The "current problems–trauma" model. The model shows the key role of current problems in generating distress among traumatized populations, with problems meant in the broad sense ranging from current financial problems, concerns about personal safety, spiritual concerns (e.g., about the "rebirth" of a dead relative), to conflicts. Trauma will predispose to poor problem solving: rumination and the rapid induction of arousal. Once being confronted with a problem induces psychological and somatic distress, that distress may be interpreted as indicating the presence of a syndrome or some other disorder. Then bio-attentional looping may occur: fear of having a particular disorder (e.g., a cultural syndrome) will increase psychological and somatic distress, which in turn will worsen psychological and somatic distress, resulting in even more fear of having a disorder (e.g., a cultural syndrome), and so on. The figure also shows how psychological and somatic distress leads to the triggering of negative memory, which also leads to looping effects. As shown, in a feedback loop, psychological and somatic distress worsens the biological and psychological consequences of trauma; that in turn reduces the ability to handle current problems, which will lead to more psychological and somatic distress, and so on, in another vicious cycle.

standing, and too, the orthostatic dizziness brings about trauma recall, further worsening panic (e.g., fear of a khyâl attack; for a discussion of this syndrome, see the section below on ethnopsychology/ethnophysiology/ethnospirituality).

Sleep paralysis is a state of bodily paralysis conjoined with an inability to speak that occurs when falling asleep or awakening. Sleep paralysis is worsened by anxiety, and some groups have particularly high rates, such as Cambodian refugees, with the high rates seemingly resulting from a conjunction of anxiety and biological predisposition (Hinton et al. 2005a,b). Moreover, some groups, like Cambodian refugees, also have extremely high rates of hypnagogic and hypnopompic hallucinations during sleep paralysis, which consists of seeing a shadow or other form approach and then descend upon one's body during sleep paralysis, often accompanied by extreme shortness of breath. And among Cambodian refugees, sleep paralysis and the accompanying hallucinations are given elaborate cultural meanings, and so result in sleep paralysis being a key part of their trauma ontology.

Certain Asian groups appear to have an elevated predisposition to motion sickness, which may indicate a biologically based enhanced tendency to experience dizziness more generally and to be conditioned to dizziness cues (Hinton and Good 2009). This tendency to motion sickness combined with conditionability to dizziness cues—along with a tendency to have impaired orthostatic adjustment—may explain in part why dizziness is so prominent in the distress presentations of many traumatized Asian groups. As another example of biologically driven somatic symptoms, we have found that Cambodian refugees frequently have headaches induced by distress, for example, by worry, and that the headaches are frequently accompanied by migraine-like visual auras such as scintillating scotomas or phosphenes (Sacks 1985) as well as multiple panic-like symptoms. This is part of the Cambodian reactivity complex. This again points to the existence of local biologies of trauma.

Symptom Dimension

There has been much debate as to whether DSM-5 PTSD and its symptoms are present in other cultures or whether it and its symptoms are a culturally specific experiencing applicable only to the West, a sort of Western cultural syndrome or idiom of distress (Summerfield 1999; Watters 2010; Young 1995). Recent research clearly shows that many aspects of the PTSD construct do indeed represent a cross-cultural psychobiological fact (Good, Good, and Grayman [Chapter 12]; for a recent review, see Hinton and Lewis-Fernández 2011) and that many of the symptoms listed in the PTSD criteria capture certain key aspects of the effect of trauma across cultures: unwanted recall of past trauma events, flashbacks, recurring nightmares, hypervigilance, startle, and anger. However, there are some symptoms in the PTSD criteria in DSM-IV-TR (APA 2000) that seem less prominent or even absent in other cultures following trauma, namely, "amnesia," "numbing," and "a feeling of detachment or estrangement from others," and several of these are difficult to translate and evaluate in another cultural context, specifically, the numbing and detachment items (Hinton and Lewis-Fernández 2011).[7] In DSM-5, the numbing item has been replaced by a much more easily translated item, namely, an inability to experience pleasure, but the other problematic items have been retained.

The prominence of PTSD symptoms (and other symptoms) in a group's trauma ontology will vary. This variation results from the types of trauma commonly experienced, the local biology of trauma, and the various dimensions of the cultural meaning of symptoms. Let us take the case of the cultural meaning of the symptom. The symptom may be attributed to a local cultural syndrome (Hinton et al. 2012), and more generally, in each culture, certain PTSD symptoms may be considered especially indicative of a disturbance of psychology or physiology or of a comprised spiritual status such as a spiritual attack. For example, Cambodian refugees often attribute startle to a physiological problem such as heart weakness, and they usually attribute nightmares to be the actual negative experiencing of the dreamer's wandering soul such as encountering the dead and being attacked by hostile spirits (Hinton et al. 2009a).

As a major limitation of the PTSD approach, certain symptoms and psychopathological dimensions commonly found in other cultures that result from trauma are not listed in the PTSD criteria; the spectrum of trauma symptoms is much broader than PTSD as defined in the DSM (see McNally [Chapter 2]; Young and Breslau [Chapter 3]). Trauma survivors have a wide range of possible symptoms, what we have called the trauma symptom pool. If any of those symptoms are common in a certain group's trauma presentation, failing to assess those symptoms results in an underinclusion error, that is, in category truncation, and results in a lack of "content validity" (Keane et al. 1996).

As one example, somatic symptoms are not in the DSM-5 criteria for PTSD but are a common reaction to trauma in many cultural contexts: among traumatized Cambodians, dizziness and neck soreness are highly endorsed complaints (Hinton and Lewis-Fernández 2011; Jenkins 1996; Kirmayer 1996a; Mayer 2007). The reasons for certain somatic symptoms being so prominent in the trauma presentation of a certain group are multifactorial. They range from the nature of the trauma event; to the encoding of certain trauma memories in terms of somatic sensations; to great chronic arousal and frequent panic owing to a biological recalibration of the nervous system; to catastrophic cognitions about somatic symptoms such as attribution to certain cultural syndromes; to the symptoms being prominent in local metaphors used to express dysphoria, resulting in metaphor-guided somatization; to the role of certain somatic symptoms as an idiom of distress in the culture in question (e.g., Good, Good, and Grayman [Chapter 12]; see also Hinton et al. 2012, 2013b). For example, among Cambodian refugees, a particular cultural syndrome is one reason dizziness and several other somatic symptoms are prominent: the syndrome referred to as "khyâl attacks" gives rise to multiple catastrophic cognitions about somatic symptoms, creating a hypervigilant surveying of the body for them, particularly for dizziness, in multiple situations said to trigger the khyâl attacks, such as engaging in worry or standing up.

Other than somatic symptoms, the following are some examples of symptoms and symptom complexes common in many traumatized populations but that are not in the DSM-5 criteria:

- Sleep paralysis is often a key symptom around which are centered an elaborate set of practices and beliefs (Hinton et al. 2005b).
- Substance abuse and acting out (externalizing) behaviors are also very common conditions among trauma victims but are not in the DSM PTSD criteria.
- Complicated bereavement is not in the PTSD criteria but is often a key issue, especially in situations of mass violence where brutal and widespread deaths occurred and where indicated rituals could not be performed.
- Cultural syndromes may constitute a key part of the local response to trauma (see the next section below on ethnopsychology/ethnophysiology/ethnospirituality) and result in trauma causing certain unique symptom clusters that relate to the cultural syndrome; these cultural syndromes, which are produced by the interaction of the biology of trauma and a set of expectations, among other variables, form a key part of the local presentation and experiencing of trauma.
- Multiple anxiety disorders, in particular panic disorder, panic attacks, and generalized anxiety disorder (GAD)-type worry, often co-occur with PTSD, and worsen one another (see also Good, Good, and Grayman [Chapter 12]).
- A general reactivity to worry and other negative emotional states is common in many traumatized groups, that is, the rapid induction of distress, arousal, and somatic symptoms.
- Frequent experiencing of the current problems–trauma complex (Figure 1.3), resulting in difficulties resolving problems, arousal,

and in much worsening of trauma-related disorder (Hinton et al. 2008, 2011).

- Frequent experiencing of the "thinking a lot" complex, that is, the hypercognizing complex, is common among traumatized groups (see the following section on ethnopsychology/ethnophysiology/ethnospirituality).

As indicated in this section and throughout this chapter and volume, the effects of trauma are broad, particularly when seen in cross-cultural perspective, and are much broader than the DSM-5 PTSD criteria. Hence our use of the terms "posttraumatic stress syndrome," or "trauma-related disorder" to indicate trauma symptoms in the broad sense. The particular symptom saliences and complaints typically found in trauma-related disorder in a certain group can be specified. In the Cambodian posttraumatic stress syndrome, prominent complaints include various somatic symptoms such as dizziness and migraine-type headache with aura; sleep paralysis; trauma recall; multiple somatic symptoms and panic triggered by many cues (e.g., standing up, encountering certain smells, engaging in worry, experiencing any strong emotion); bereavement and related practices; nightmares that are interpreted as the visitation by dead relatives; and syndromes such as khyâl attacks, heart weakness, and "thinking a lot," with the complaint of "thinking a lot" usually indicating the presence of—that is, episodes of—the "current problem-trauma" symptom complex, as shown in Figure 1.3 (Hinton et al. 2012, 2013b). The Cambodian posttraumatic stress syndrome, or trauma assemblage, also includes the local consequences of having the disorder (economic and interpersonal course) and ways of seeking treatment, for example, "coining" or meditation. In the Cambodian case, these complaints and symptoms, consequences, and ways of seeking recovery all also form key aspects of the lifeworld of trauma, of the biocultural ontology of trauma.[8]

The Meaning of the Trauma Event and Resulting Symptoms According to the Local Ethnopsychology/Ethnophysiology/Ethnospirituality

The local conceptualization of the nature of mental processes, bodily functioning, and the spiritual domain: all these will result in ideas about which symptoms will be caused by trauma, the meaning of those symptoms, and how they should be treated. These understandings will amplify and even induce—through self-surveillance—certain symptoms following trauma. A key part of the trauma event memory is what the person thinks the trauma did to him or her, a key determinant of which is the syndrome that the person thinks to be caused by that trauma. There may result a certain trauma-based identity or self-schema, and there may result a certain spiritual-schema, such as the conceptualization of the spiritual status of those who died during a genocide. The syndromes that a group considers to be caused by a trauma event form a key part of the trauma meaning space, shape how trauma is en-minded and embodied, and lead to particular ideas about the trauma's dangerousness, to a certain self-imagery of damage. Even if trauma-caused symptoms like startle and somatic distress are not linked in that cultural group to trauma, that is, the symptoms are not thought to be caused by trauma, those trauma-caused symptoms will be interpreted according to the local meaning systems. Consequently, the local ethnopsychology, ethnophysiology, and ethnospirituality will have a profound effect on the trajectory of trauma in a given context and on how the symptoms of trauma are experienced and treated and these understandings and actions will form a key component of the trauma ontology (Pedersen and Kienzler [Chapter 7]).

Experiencing trauma-related symptoms as "weak heart" in Cambodia will result in a very different trauma ontology than experiencing them as "PTSD" in the United States—different emphasized symptoms, different interpersonal effects, different identity effects, different ideas about the psychology and physiology generating symptoms, and different ways of attempting treatment (Hinton et al. 2002). The entirety of syndromes that are said to be caused by trauma in a culture along with all the syndromes to which trauma-caused symptoms are attributed might be called the network of trauma syndromes. This is illustrated in Figure 1.4 for Cambodian refugees (for the case of Quechua speakers in the Peruvian Andes, see Pedersen and Kienzler [Chapter 7, Figure 7.4]). More broadly, since Figure 1.4 also depicts ideas about the spiritual status of the dead and ideas about spiritual assault, it might be called the depiction of the spiritual and syndromic effects of trauma. As shown in Figure 1.4 and in Figure 7.4 in Pedersen and Kienzler (Chapter 7), often the syndromes and various idioms are thought to be interconnected in a causal network, and the network constitutes a local ethnotheory of trauma effects. These various syndromes—and the associated ethnopsychology, ethnophysiology, and ethnospirituality—are the matrix in which the trauma symptoms are interpreted.

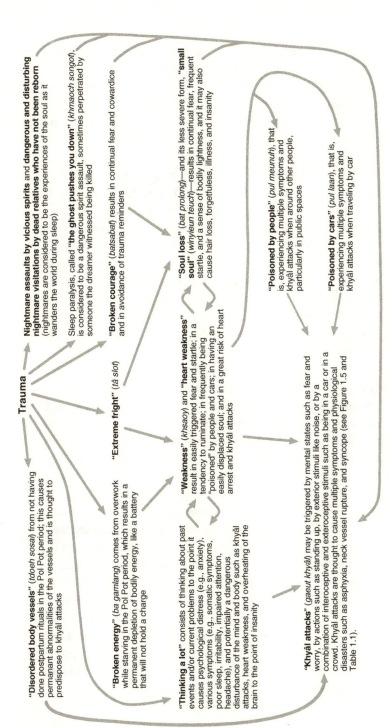

Trauma

"Disordered body vessels" (*tdoeh sosai*) from not having done postpartum rituals in the Pol Pot period; this causes permanent abnormalities of the vessels and is thought to predispose to khyâl attacks

"Broken energy" (*ba gamlang*) comes from overwork while starving in the Pol Pot period, which results in a permanent depletion of bodily energy, like a battery that will not hold a charge

"Thinking a lot" consists of thinking about past events and/or current problems to the point it causes psychological distress (e.g., anxiety), various symptoms (e.g., somatic symptoms, poor sleep, irritability, impaired attention, headache), and potentially a dangerous disturbance of the mind and body such as khyâl attacks, heart weakness, and overheating of the brain to the point of insanity

"Khyâl attacks" (*gaeut khyâl*) may be triggered by mental states such as fear and worry, by actions such as standing up, by a combination of interoceptive and exteroceptive stimuli such as being in a car or in a crowd. Khyâl attacks are thought to cause multiple symptoms and physiological disasters such as asphyxia, neck vessel rupture, and syncope (see Figure 1.5 and Table 1.1).

"Extreme fright" (*tâ slot*)

"Weakness" (*khsaoy*) and "heart weakness" result in easily triggered fear and startle; in a tendency to ruminate; in frequently being "poisoned" by people and cars; in having an easily displaced soul; and in a great risk of heart arrest and khyâl attacks

Nightmare assaults by vicious spirits and dangerous and disturbing nightmare visitations by dead relatives who have not been reborn (nightmares are considered to be the experiences of the soul as it wanders the world during sleep)

Sleep paralysis, called "the ghost pushes you down" (*khmaoch songob*), is considered to be a dangerous spirit assault, sometimes perpetrated by someone the dreamer witnessed being killed

"Broken courage" (*batsabat*) results in continual fear and cowardice and in avoidance of trauma reminders

"Soul loss" (*bat prolong*)—and its less severe form, "small soul" (*winyiewn teuch*)—results in continual fear, frequent startle, and a sense of bodily lightness, and it may also cause hair loss, forgetfulness, illness, and insanity

"Poisoned by people" (*pul meunuh*), that is, experiencing multiple symptoms and khyâl attacks when around other people, particularly in public spaces

"Poisoned by cars" (*pul laan*), that is, experiencing multiple symptoms and khyâl attacks when traveling by car

Figure 1.4. The trauma syndrome network among Cambodian refugees. This figure shows a syndrome network, a form of semantic network; moreover, it is a causal semantic network. The figure shows the causal network of closely related syndromes that shapes the Cambodian conceptualization of the effects of trauma. The figure depicts the processes of "circular causation" as conceptualized by Cambodians: "thinking a lot" causes weakness (e.g., it directly exhausts and impairs sleep and appetite), which then produces a predisposition to "thinking a lot," and so on. As another example, "soul loss" causes weakness, which then predisposes to soul loss, and so on.

In a particular cultural group, specific syndromes will be thought to be caused by trauma, such as PTSD in the United States or *susto* in certain Latin American countries. In other cultural contexts, what we in the United States would call a psychological trauma—seeing someone killed, being in a nearly fatal accident, being beaten—may not be considered permanently damaging with specific long-term symptoms. In the United States, bracket creep has resulted in increasingly minor events being considered traumatic and capable of causing the PTSD syndrome. The layperson's understanding results in PTSD serving for some as a sort of idiom of distress rather than a neurobiologically driven process (McNally [Chapter 2]; Young and Breslau [Chapter 3]): the person may label an event as traumatic and wonder about having PTSD, and then through self-surveillance come to take on the category's symptoms, even though most of the symptoms are due to anxiety and depression rather than to trauma. Whereas in the United States there is the idea that even minor trauma may produce PTSD, in some cultures, as in the Oaxacan (Duncan [Chapter 6]), the opposite seems to be the case: domestic abuse is not thought to cause PTSD. On the other hand, in Oaxaca events like humiliations or migration are increasingly considered to be traumatic and to induce PTSD and other disorders, with this new trauma ontology or episteme formed in large part by recent public awareness campaigns.

In many other cultural and historical contexts, events that in the modern West would be considered psychologically traumatizing are thought to cause psychological damage not because of their emotional impact but rather because of their directly damaging effects on the body; the bodily damage syndromes have psychological symptoms as secondary symptoms. These might be called physiopsychological syndromes, or somatopsychic trauma syndromes, in which DSM-type PTSD symptoms and other symptoms caused by the biology of psychological trauma are given a pathomechanic explanation involving initial damage to the body. Bodily damage explanations of the effects of trauma were very prominent in industrialized Western societies in the past (McNally [Chapter 2]; Young and Breslau [Chapter 3]; Boehnlein and Hinton [Chapter 4]), for instance, railroad spine in the nineteenth century in the United States. Or in some past wars, what was considered to cause PTSD-type symptoms like startle or constant fear were bodily damaging events (Kugelmann 2009): in the Civil War, exertions like carrying knapsacks were thought to damage the heart, or in World War I, exposures to blasts from bombs to damage the nervous system—and these bodily defects were thought to cause what would now be considered anxiety and other psycho-logical distress symptoms like startle or hypervigilance. In the ongoing wars in Iraq and Afghanistan, many are said to have traumatic brain injury (TBI), a disorder that has among its diagnostic criteria PTSD-like symptoms such as poor concentration and anger; but in a considerable number of cases the TBI-like symptoms seem to actually result from psychological traumas and daily stresses, from PTSD or general distress like anxiety and depression (Boehnlein and Hinton [Chapter 4]).

By way of contrast to these physiopsychological syndromes of trauma, current scientific theories of PTSD in the United States posit a psycho-somatic-psychic causality (psychic event → brain changes → psychological symptoms), and this forms a common model in the lay psychology. Accord-ing to this theory, a psychologically upsetting event is seared into the amyg-dala, and the amygdala and other brain structures will tend to cause all the psychological symptoms associated with trauma and the various reactivities such as startle (Ledoux 1996). This physiological model of trauma's effects is increasingly prominent in the Western imaginary of trauma, as found in representational spaces from talk shows to self-help books—plastic models of the amygdala held in the hand during explanations, the supposed loca-tion of trauma's central wound.

Cultural ideas shape the perceived dangerousness and specific effects of trauma, so that some types of trauma events may be locally interpreted as being more damaging than they would be in another cultural context. Cam-bodians consider that working while starving during the Pol Pot period had an especially debilitating effect on the body—that it made the body to be like a battery that cannot hold a charge—and so resulted in a permanent state of bodily weakness and heart weakness (*khsaoy beh doung*), with that heart weakness thought to result in PTSD-like symptoms such as startle, fear, and hypervigilance and in a predisposition to heart arrest and khyâl attacks. In terms of spiritual schemas, as discussed above, Cambodians and Rwandans consider that certain types of death as well as not performing indicated mor-tuary rituals may cause the deceased's spirit to enter a miserable state and to possibly become dangerous to the living. More generally, the inability to per-form a ritual may lead to a sense of disorder in the mental, bodily, or spiri-tual realms, what we have referred to as ritual omission trauma. As another example of this, a Cambodian woman may believe that failure to do postpar-tum rituals during the Pol Pot period has damaged her vessels and predisposed her to khyâl attacks, which may lead her to interpret trauma-related arousal from any trigger—like dizziness or palpitations that result from startle—as indicating the onset of a khyâl attack.

In the U.S. military, certain syndromes have shaped views about the dangerousness of war theater events. The Gulf War syndrome caused veterans of that conflict to fear that exposure to fumes might cause bodily harm and various symptoms, when in fact those symptoms resulted from anxiety and depression; as a result, veterans often came to reframe psychological distress as the Gulf War syndrome (Cohn et al. 2008; Jones and Wessely 2005; Kilshaw 2009). A veteran of the Iraqi war will expect that a trauma event involving explosions may bring about traumatic brain injury and those fears will cause him or her to be hypervigilant for amnesia, poor concentration, forgetfulness, headache, and certain other symptoms associated with TBI (Boehnlein and Hinton [Chapter 4]); consequently, among those having no actual brain trauma but who attribute psychological distress symptoms (e.g., those generated by PTSD and general anxiety and depression) to TBI, those psychological and somatic symptoms that have an equivalent in TBI will be emphasized (e.g., forgetfulness, poor concentration, headache), and there will be self-imagery of permanent damage. As these examples show, there is not just the trauma event itself but what the survivor thinks that the trauma did to him or her.[9]

The symptoms caused by trauma may be attributed to a syndrome that is not specifically caused by trauma according to the local understanding. That is, often the trauma-caused symptoms will be attributed to a cultural syndrome without trauma itself being perceived as the syndrome's cause. Much of the Cambodian experiencing of trauma-related experiencing plays out through the attribution of trauma-related symptoms to various syndromes, as indicated in Figure 1.4, and events of these syndromes in many cases will not be attributed to trauma:[10] startle and arousal-caused symptoms may be attributed to heart weakness, without trauma being thought to be the cause of the reactivity or symptoms. Or trauma symptoms may be attributed to spiritual assault rather than trauma. In several cultural contexts in Africa, the symptoms caused by trauma—from tinnitus to nightmare to sleep paralysis—are often thought to be brought about by spiritual assault and possession (see the next section on the religious/spiritual dimension).

Somatic symptoms are a key part of the presentation of trauma in many groups, and the interpretation of those somatic symptoms in terms of the local ethnophysiology, ethnopsychology, and ethnospirituality—and related syndromes—will result in a specific trauma ontology (for one review, see Hinton and Lewis-Fernández 2011).[11] These attributions often lead to great concerns about imminent danger: if a Cambodian attributes arousal-caused somatic symptoms to "soul loss," heart weakness, or "thinking a lot" (see Figure 1.4), this will increase the perceived degree of dangerousness of those symptoms—and determine the indicated treatments. Let us examine in more detail a syndrome that greatly shapes the Cambodian experiencing of trauma-related somatic symptoms and that leads to severe catastrophic cognitions about those symptoms.

In the Cambodian context, trauma-caused arousal symptoms are often thought to be caused by a khyâl attack. Traumatized Cambodian refugees often have somatic symptoms brought about by various types of triggers: by triggers that are in the PTSD criteria such as trauma recall, anger, fear, nightmare, and sounds that startle, and by other types of triggers such as standing up, encountering certain smells, traveling in a car, entering complex visual and multisensorial environments (e.g., the mall or the temple), worry, and emotions such as sadness. The resulting arousal and somatic symptoms are often labeled as a khyâl attack, which leads to fears that the symptoms are produced by a dangerous dysregulation of khyâl, a wind-like substance said to flow alongside blood in the body (Figure 1.5, Table 1.1). Those catastrophic cognitions often lead to anxious self-surveying of the body for khyâl attack symptoms and the catastrophic cognitions lead to great fear upon seemingly discovering such a symptom. According to the Cambodian ethnophysiology, khyâl attack should be treated in certain ways, most often "coining," which entails pushing down the edge of a medication-dipped coin on the skin and dragging it outward such as down along the arms to help the flow of khyâl and its egress from the body (for a detailed description of khyâl attacks, including film footage of their traditional treatment, viz., coining, see www .khyalattack.com). The construct of khyâl attacks, in interaction with the biology of trauma, leads to the Cambodian trauma ontology prominently featuring bouts of arousal labeled as a khyâl attack: these bouts are triggered by what are considered typical triggers of khyâl attacks such as fright, worry, standing up, entering crowded spaces, and exertion, with the resulting arousal-caused somatic symptoms being labeled as khyâl attack symptoms, and with the sufferer of the bout attempting treatment in indicated ways, for example, by coining—and prevention by indicated means. (And

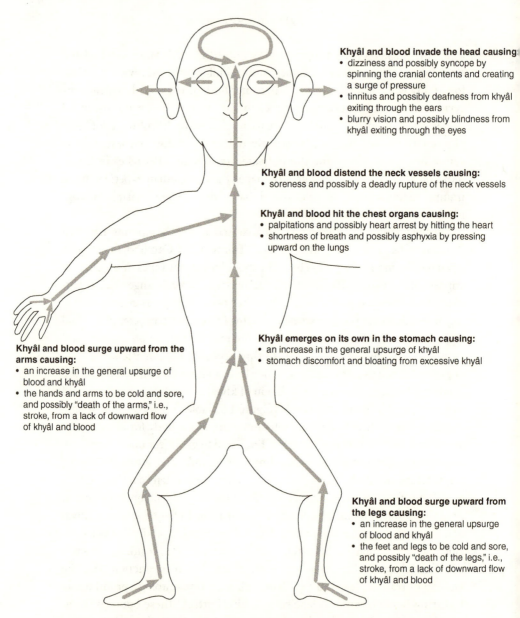

Khyâl and blood invade the head causing:
- dizziness and possibly syncope by spinning the cranial contents and creating a surge of pressure
- tinnitus and possibly deafness from khyâl exiting through the ears
- blurry vision and possibly blindness from khyâl exiting through the eyes

Khyâl and blood distend the neck vessels causing:
- soreness and possibly a deadly rupture of the neck vessels

Khyâl and blood hit the chest organs causing:
- palpitations and possibly heart arrest by hitting the heart
- shortness of breath and possibly asphyxia by pressing upward on the lungs

Khyâl and blood surge upward from the arms causing:
- an increase in the general upsurge of blood and khyâl
- the hands and arms to be cold and sore, and possibly "death of the arms," i.e., stroke, from a lack of downward flow of khyâl and blood

Khyâl emerges on its own in the stomach causing:
- an increase in the general upsurge of khyâl
- stomach discomfort and bloating from excessive khyâl

Khyâl and blood surge upward from the legs causing:
- an increase in the general upsurge of blood and khyâl
- the feet and legs to be cold and sore, and possibly "death of the legs," i.e., stroke, from a lack of downward flow of khyâl and blood

Figure 1.5. A khyâl attack: Ethnophysiology, symptoms, and associated disasters. The arrows represent the flow of khyâl and blood upward in the body during a khyâl attack. During the healthy state, khyâl and blood flow downward in the direction opposite to the arrows, with khyâl exiting the body through the hands and feet, through bodily pores, and down through the gastrointestinal tract, but during a khyâl attack, khyâl and blood surge upward in the body to cause the disasters outlined above.

Table 1.1. The Interpretation of Somatic Symptoms in Terms of a Khyâl Attack:
Correlated Physiological State and Feared Consequence

Symptom	Physiological state generating the symptom	Symptom-related fears (see Figure 1.5)
Dizziness	A surge of khyâl and blood into the head	Syncope owing to khyâl and blood shooting into the cranium, and concerns that dizziness indicates the occurrence of a "khyâl attack" and associated bodily disasters, the most severe type of khyâl attack being called "khyâl overload"
Tinnitus	A pressure-like escape of khyâl from the ears; reflecting this, tinnitus is called "khyâl exits from the ears" (khyâl ceuny taam treujieu)	Deafness owing to khyâl shooting out of the ears, and concerns that tinnitus indicates the occurrence of a khyâl attack and associated bodily disasters
Blurry vision	A pressure-like escape of khyâl from the eyes	Blindness owing to khyâl shooting out the eyes, and concerns that blurry vision indicates the occurrence of a khyâl attack and associated bodily disasters
Headache	An upsurge of khyâl and blood into the head and its vessels	Syncope, and concerns that a headache (especially migraine-type headache with aura) indicates the occurrence of a khyâl attack and associated bodily disasters
Neck soreness	An upsurge of surge of khyâl and blood into the neck vessels	Bursting of the neck vessels, and concerns that neck soreness indicates the occurrence of a khyâl attack and associated bodily disasters
Nausea	An excessive accumulation of khyâl in the stomach and abdomen	Emesis that may "burst the gall bladder," and concerns that the khyâl may move up from the stomach to cause a khyâl attack and associated bodily disasters

(continued)

Table 1.1. (continued)

Symptom	Physiological state generating the symptom	Symptom-related fears (see Figure 1.5)
Palpitations	An upsurge of khyâl and blood that presses on the heart and interferes with its pumping; also, as part of a khyâl attack, there are blockages in the vessels in the limbs, so the heart must work furiously to pump blood and khyâl through the vessels, another cause of palpitations	Cardiac arrest, and concerns that palpitations indicate the occurrence of a khyâl attack and associated disasters
Shortness of breath	An upsurge of khyâl and blood that presses on the lungs and interferes with breathing	Asphyxia, and concerns that shortness of breath indicates the occurrence of a khyâl attack and khyâl overload and associated disasters
Soreness in the legs or arms	A blockage of the flow of khyâl and blood through the vessels in the limbs, particularly at the joints; reflecting this, "sore joints" are called "plugged vessels" (cok sosai) or "blocked khyâl" (sla khyâl)	"Death of the limbs" from a lack of outward flow along the limbs, and a surge of khyâl and blood upward in the body to cause various disasters
Cold hands or feet	A blockage of the flow of khyâl and blood through the vessels in the limbs	"Death of the limbs" from a lack of outward flow along the limbs, and a surge of khyâl and blood upward in the body to cause various disasters
Poor appetite	A direct effect of excessive bodily khyâl	Bodily weakness, including heart weakness, owing to poor appetite resulting in bodily depletion. Heart weakness results in disasters like heart arrest and produces khyâl attacks by causing poor circulation that results in plugs in the limbs

Table 1.1. (continued)

Symptom	Physiological state generating the symptom	Symptom-related fears (see Figure 1.5)
Energy depletion	Excessive bodily khyâl depletes energy directly; it also depletes energy indirectly as well by causing poor sleep and poor appetite	Bodily weakness, especially heart weakness, owing to bodily depletion. Heart weakness results in disasters like heart arrest and produces khyâl attacks by causing poor circulation that results in plugs in the limbs

too, dizziness and arousal present in panic attacks, such as those labeled as khyâl attacks, will often trigger trauma recall and negative memory more generally; see the multiplex models.)

A cultural syndrome that is prominent among the traumatized in many countries across the globe is "thinking a lot" (see Pedersen and Kienzler [Chapter 7]; see also Hinton et al. 2011, 2012, in press; Kaiser et al. 2014; Patel et al. 1995). "Thinking a lot" might also be called a hypercognizing syndrome, or a hypercognizing symptom complex. In many cultures, "thinking a lot" forms a local sociosomatic theory that links social distress to the experiencing of psychological and bodily distress (Kirmayer 2001; Kleinman and Becker 1998).[12] A bout often starts by "thinking a lot" about current problems, that is, by worrying about something (e.g., having money for rent, a child's truancy, health of relatives, or one's own health), but also may begin with other types of thoughts: depressive thoughts (e.g., thinking about past failures or those who have died), anger issues (e.g., thinking with anger about what a child has done), or trauma recall (e.g., recall of being beaten or doing slave labor while starving). Thus, what is "thought a lot" about is not only worry but also depressive and other types of cognitions, with all these types of thinking often coming one after the other in an escalating episode of distress. Among traumatized populations, "thinking a lot," whether it be worry, depressive thoughts, anger thoughts, or trauma recall, often induces mental and somatic symptoms, which then give rise to trauma associations, catastrophic cognitions, and certain ideas about treatment. For example, Cambodians consider that "thinking a lot" (kut caraeun) may bring about insanity and permanent forgetfulness through overheating the brain and may cause death through the triggering of a serious khyâl attack; and Cambodians consider "coining" as a way of treating acute episodes and meditation as a way to prevent them.

There are several reasons why the "thinking a lot" syndrome is prominent among traumatized populations in countries having that idiom of distress. Trauma victims have a general tendency to engage in negative cognizing, with such episodes being labeled as "thinking a lot." Also, trauma victims often have many reasons to "think a lot," such as the trauma itself, having lost loved ones in a genocide, or being upset that the perpetrator has not been punished. As another reason for the prominence of "thinking a lot" syndromes in traumatized groups, "thinking a lot" syndromes often are centered on "thinking a lot" about a current problem, that is, worrying. Worry episodes, which will usually be labeled by the experiencer as "thinking a lot," are common and produce much distress among traumatized populations for the following reasons:

- Traumatized persons often live in difficult circumstances and so have multiple concerns that give rise to worry, and this worry will be labeled as "thinking a lot."
- Trauma results in a tendency to worry owing to trauma-caused hypervigilance to threat and difficulty in disengaging from negative states like worry.
- Trauma results in emotional and physiological reactivity to worry so that engaging in worry will lead to arousal and to multiple somatic symptoms such as palpitations, muscle tension, headache, and dizziness.
- Trauma increases catastrophic cognitions about the effects of worry and the induced mental and somatic symptoms owing to a general hypervigilance to threat.
- Many traumatized groups have catastrophic cognitions about the effects of worry: Cambodian refugees fear that worry-caused mental symptoms like poor concentration and forgetfulness will be permanent and lead to insanity and that worry-caused somatic symptoms like neck tension or dizziness indicate the onset of a khyâl attack.
- As we described above in the current problems–trauma complex (Figure 1.3), worry will result in bio-attentional looping processes and vicious cycles of worsening (on cultural syndromes, PTSD, and

looping, see Hinton and Lewis-Fernández 2011; Hinton et al. 2010; Kirmayer and Sartorius 2007). Thus, often a key part of trauma is not just the current problems–trauma complex but the hypercognizing-trauma complex, or "thinking a lot"–trauma complex, another key part of the trauma symptom pool.

Many chapters in this volume describe how cultural syndromes amplify and even induce the symptoms that are thought to be caused by the syndrome in question. Bio-attentional looping may occur as a result of a syndrome that shapes the experiencing of distress—for example, through the cultural syndrome amplifying and even inducing symptoms. See Figure 1.6 for a general model of how the cultural syndromes—including local lay understanding of a scientific syndrome—come to be enminded and embodied, become "forms of life" (Kishik 2008), lived ontologies. This model can be used for any of the syndromes discussed in this chapter, such as khyâl attacks.

To illustrate the processes in Figure 1.6, let us take the case of DSM-5-defined PTSD in those contexts where it is a diagnosis known by the local lay population. Increasingly as the DSM-defined PTSD construct has become known by laypersons in Western and non-Western cultural contexts, the understanding of the PTSD construct among professionals and laypersons in the society in question shapes the local trauma ontology. The Western concept of PTSD as understood in the particular cultural context in question shapes how trauma is experienced, how it is enminded and embodied, how it results in a certain social and economic course. PTSD as locally understood may come to be an idiom of distress as well—consequently, it may even be enacted during states of distress that are not produced by trauma. How does this induction and amplification of symptoms occur in the case of a cultural category or syndrome?

At the time of trauma, or at a later point, the person may experience upset and dysphoria and may wonder whether he or she has, or soon will have, any of the PTSD symptoms. If that person self-surveys for certain mental and physical symptoms such as jumpiness and hypervigilance or anger, then these symptoms may soon be discovered through a sort of attentional amplification; the symptoms may be induced by the expectation of their occurrence—the expectation of being in a state of hypervigilance, of reacting with startle to a noise, of responding to minor annoyance with anger, and of various triggers such as watching scenes of war evoking trauma memory. If that person keeps conjuring to mind a certain traumatic event, ruminates on it,

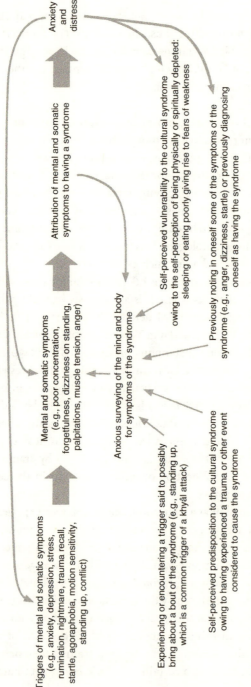

Figure 1.6. A multiplex model of the generation of a cultural syndrome. A trigger (e.g., anxiety, standing up, a conflict) brings about an initial symptom. Next, the attribution of a symptom to a syndrome will bring about more scrutinizing of the mind and body for syndrome-associated symptoms. This attribution often gives rise to catastrophic cognitions that result in anxiety and distress, and that anxiety and distress may lead to more mental and somatic symptoms, which in turn creates more fear of having a syndrome. As indicated, hypervigilant surveying of the mind and body for symptoms results from several processes, such as experiencing a trigger that is known to cause a bout of the syndrome. This multiplex model is nested: it shows the importance of the reaction of the social network to the person having the syndrome and its symptoms as well as the economic effects and the effects of treatments that are self-administered, sought out, and received owing to labeling symptoms as a certain kind of disorder. Of note, in some cases a syndrome may not lead to anxiety and distress, but rather it may just serve as an explanatory frame for behaviors such as anger, even a justificatory frame, that is, a frame that excuses behaviors. But the rest of the model still applies.

continually views it with pained fear as being a pathogenic event that now explains all his or her woes and the tragic trajectory of life events, and if that person gives it a central piece in his or her life narrative, then the image may seem vivid and loom large in his or her mind. If the person hears others recounting such a narrative, and if the disorder and its symptoms are depicted in publically advertised medical literature, movies, TV, talk shows, and media, if having PTSD is seen as positively valenced, if having the disorder has positive economic effects (e.g., receiving monthly benefits), then the tendency to enmind and embody PTSD will be increased (McNally and Frueh 2013).

These same processes of culturally shaped bio-attentional looping will take place with all cultural syndromes attributed to trauma (for a description of how these issues play out among veterans of the Iraq war, see Finley 2011). To give the example of another contemporary war syndrome involving these types of processes, consider the case of "mimicked TBI" as a cultural distress syndrome, that is, the case of army personnel who have psychological distress without actual brain trauma but consider themselves to have traumatic brain injury (TBI). In such cases, a psychological syndrome masquerades as brain injury, and symptoms like poor concentration, poor memory, and poor anger control are sought out in self-surveillance, resulting in their amplification and induction, and those symptoms come to be framed in terms of a trauma ontology focused on that diagnosis. This model also applies to other war syndromes such as the Gulf War syndrome, in which olfactory sensitivity and other specific symptoms are emphasized (Cohn et al. 2008; Jones and Wessely 2005; Kilshaw 2009).

Religious/Spiritual Dimension

Religion and spirituality may be the main domain in which trauma events, trauma symptoms, and recovery play out (James [Chapter 11]). A religious frame may be used to comprehend violence and suffering as survivors seek explanations of why the trauma occurred, what the meanings of the symptoms are, and how the resulting suffering might be remedied. As indicated above, trauma-related symptoms like nightmares, somatic symptoms, and sleep paralysis may be shaped by and interpreted according to local religious ideas such as spiritual assault (Hinton et al. 2005a, 2009a): when a distressed Vietnamese survivor of trauma attributes somatic symptoms to the embodying of the wounds of the deceased through possession, or when a traumatized individual from Guinea Bissau attributes tinnitus, palpitations, cold extremities, or racing thoughts to possession (de Jong and Reis 2010, 2013; Gustafsson 2009). Seen globally, trauma often plays out in a possession idiom (de Jong and Reis 2010; Igreja et al. 2010; Neuner et al. 2012; Reis 2013; van Duijl et al. 2010). Treatment of trauma-related symptoms may involve local religious traditions such as meditation and making merit in a Buddhist context or purification and possession rituals in certain animistic or shamanistic traditions (Gustafsson 2009; Hinton and Kirmayer, 2013; Nickerson and Hinton 2011; Reis 2013). Buddhism explains trauma and suffering in terms of karma; monks may also help people cope with their suffering by reciting scripture and by providing ritual objects and ceremonies thought to alleviate suffering.

Religious beliefs influence how a person deals with the death of others, memorializes and commemorates the dead, and imagines what happens to a person after death (Hinton et al. 2013c; Reis 2013). What is thought to occur after a person dies a certain kind of death, and what are the indicated rituals to ensure auspicious rebirth: these often have a profound effect on the meaning of a particular death. In many cultural contexts, the manner of death and the lack of death rituals may prevent the deceased from reaching the next spiritual level, may cause the deceased to become vengeful and dangerous rather than protective. Such beliefs may lead to bereavement causing more anxiety and fear than depression and to a sense of imminent assault and a lack of spiritual protection. For these reasons, mourning and issues of complicated bereavement, and trauma-related disorder more generally, may play out in an idiom of spirits—of attack by spirits, of placation of spirits, of making offerings and conducting ceremonies for spirits. Trauma-related disorder may be driven by bereavement issues such as when there is great concern that the deceased has not been reborn and when dreams of the deceased are deeply upsetting because they are considered to indicate the deceased is in a difficult spiritual place; in these ways, bereavement concerns and dreams may form a key part of local trauma ontology and a key cog in the generation of PTSD-like distress.

Public Representation of the Trauma Event and the Trauma Survivor

Every society will represent the trauma event and the trauma survivor in certain ways. These narratives of the event and the descriptions of the trauma survivor will be found in a variety of domains that include public memorials, commemorative holidays and events, the visual arts, newspapers, books, television, state rhetorics, and public rituals. These representations shape how survivors view themselves and how they are viewed by others (Gustafsson 2009; Hagengimana and Hinton 2009; Hinton et al. 2013c; Kwon 2006, 2008; Perera 2001).

The survivor of certain kinds of trauma may be stigmatized in various ways, for example, as being somehow responsible for the event or being considered "polluted" afterward. The survivor's trauma symptoms may be said to result from weakness or malingering, or some other defect. In some cases, the trauma symptoms that seemingly relate to trauma—for example, substance abuse or self-cutting as a result of extreme distress following trauma—may not be recognized as resulting from a trauma, so that there is a blaming of the victim and a lack of awareness of the cause of disorder (Good and Hinton [Introduction]).[13] Trauma-type symptoms may be attributed to a combination of the trauma and "weakness," so that the condition is still stigmatizing (see Ball and O'Nell [Chapter 10] for a discussion of these issues as pertain to the veteran and Native American experience: the genogram and historical trauma as a compelling alternative public representation of the Native American trauma survivor).

The public representation of the trauma survivor will include the cultural syndromes associated with the trauma and its symptoms, both syndromes attributed to trauma and those not attributed to trauma but that are the common interpretations of trauma symptoms. These syndromes will create expectations about the individual that then take on a self-fulfilling role. Namely, these syndromes will create expectations about the individual in the form of symptoms, behaviors, and indicated interventions, and they will result in the person having a certain syndrome-based identity (Hollan 2004). To give some historical examples, three disorders were common PTSD-like presentations in World War I, and each was a radically different representation of the effects of war, and each created a radically different syndrome-based identity: shell shock was a war syndrome in which exposure to bombs seemingly "shattered" the nervous system, leading to certain stereotypical movements among other symptoms, and the disorder suggested cowardice; other guises of trauma-related disorder in that war were soldier's heart and neurasthenia, but these conditions were less stigmatizing (Jones and Wessely 2005; Kugelmann 2009). To take the example of a more recent war, the diagnosis of Gulf War syndrome was less stigmatizing than that of anxiety or depression, and having the syndrome had different interpersonal, economic, and identity effects. In the public media representation of the Iraqi war, PTSD and TBI seem to be two highlighted disorders, with a conflation of constituting symptoms often occurring. In the case of public representation of both TBI and PTSD resulting from the Iraqi war, through newspaper media and such movies as the *The Hurt Locker* (Bigelow 2008), there are salientized a certain sensitivity of the nervous system, poor concentration, forgetfulness, and predisposition to anger.

Public representations are not static but continuously enacted and created in various settings including institutional ones. Take the case of an event the first author (Hinton) witnessed at the Vietnam War Memorial in Washington, D.C. When the first author visited that memorial, the guide, a Vietnam veteran, said that the tactile sense he experienced upon rubbing his finger across the names of the victims chiseled in marble had the power to evoke the sensory-scape of Vietnam: the sounds of planes, the smell of sulfurous bombs, and the image of bloody bodies. In this narrative there is an interaction of the space of remembering, the specificity of the memorial, the biology of trauma, and expectations about what passing through a trauma event will do to the individual. This veteran is producing at the space of the memorial a common public representation of the effects of the Vietnam War, according to which continued sensorial reliving in memory is a prominent aspect of that war's effects. The inner-seared image that is continually relived is like another memorial to the events, an inner badge. In certain war syndromes, anger or startle may play a similar role: icons of having endured an unutterable horror, of having carried the burden of a nation, of having made a supreme sacrifice.

Age and Gender Space

Age and gender influence trauma exposure, structural violence, stigmatization upon being traumatized, and ability to recover from trauma. There may be age- and gender-based vulnerabilities to encountering traumas and to its negative effects, and age and gender will influence the experiencing and trajectory of trauma-related disorder (Jenkins and Haas [Chapter 5]; Duncan [Chapter 6]). Early trauma predisposes to the development of a general reactivity and severe posttraumatic stress syndrome (Farmer 1997; Honwana

2006; Straker 1992; Suleiman 2006; Trawick 2007). Youth may be exposed to intergenerational trauma, such as having traumatized parents who exhibit mood extremes and have an impaired ability to nurture. Also, traumas such as spousal abuse and sexual violence may vary by gender, and gender may influence the stigmatization resulting from trauma: a rape victim being blamed for what occurred and being labeled as "polluted" (Coulter 2009). Also, age and gender may impact exposure to structural violence and the ability to recover after mass violence: in certain cultural contexts, a woman may have especially poor economic prospects after the death of a spouse during a genocide, and she may face cultural prohibitions against remarriage for women.

Social Dimension

Violence and its aftermath are situated in given social contexts, ones that may undergo significant transformation through trauma (Hobfoll 2012; Lischer 2005; Lubkemann 2008). Trauma survivors reside in a certain family and social structure, and it is there that trauma's main effects may be felt, and the trauma events themselves may emerge in the family itself in the form of spousal or child abuse (see Jenkins and Haas [Chapter 5]; Duncan [Chapter 6]). Trauma may shatter a family through the trauma-caused anger of the parent, spouse, or child or through trauma-caused silences and nonverbal behaviors (Argenti and Schramm 2010; Hinton et al. 2009c). On a group level, trauma may have its effects through the social interactions and social structures brought about by drug use, violence, and defeatism (Jenkins and Haas [Chapter 5]; see also Evans-Campbell 2008; Gone 2009). Trauma symptoms and syndromes are treated and reacted to at the level of family, creating a certain interpersonal course of trauma symptoms: Cambodian refugees often consider anxiety symptoms and panic attacks to be a khyâl attack—that is, a surge of khyâl and blood upward in the body that compresses the lungs, causing asphyxia, and hits the heart, causing palpitations (see Figure 1.5 and Table 1.1), among other disorders—and they often ask family members to treat the symptoms by coining and by other methods, including massage.

The intactness of the family and its manner of functioning will impact on resilience and current levels of stress. There may be a loss of relatives and friends, for example, owing to a genocide or to living in a community marked by drug overdoses, violence, and poor medical care. There may be social abandonment as a result of parental separation, which is all too common in settings of poverty (Jenkins and Haas [Chapter 5]; James [Chapter 11]). A person displaced from a country or community owing to civil war or other reasons will lose the support of friends and others (Hinton et al. 2010). There may be loss of connection with deceased ancestors, a key issue in cultural groups that emphasize that the dead interact with the living; in those cultural contexts the social network includes not only the living but the dead.

Idioms of distress and the local sociosomatics are also an important aspect of the social dimension. Within a particular group, certain syndromes or somatic symptoms will be considered key idioms of distress, that is, typical complaints of those under great stress, and thus indicators of ongoing interpersonal and other social problems (Kirmayer 2001). The cultural syndrome of "thinking a lot" functions as an idiom of distress in many cultural contexts, with "thinking a lot" often centering on worry and problems with the social context: a conflict with a child or spouse. The complaint evokes a certain theory of sociosomatics, according to which social problems may cause mental distress and somatic symptoms, possibly even death or insanity (see Figure 1.3). Or many somatic symptoms will be understood by members of a social group on a metaphoric level. In the United States, a trauma victim's complaint of back pain may be understood by others as indicating the person to be "overburdened" in the metaphoric sense (Hinton and Lewis-Fernández 2010). Dizziness has multiple metaphoric resonances in the Cambodian context and is a key presentation of social distress (Hinton et al. 2012), as is the case in China (Kleinman and Kleinman 1994; Park 2009).

Economic-Environmental Context

Each person inhabits a certain economic and environmental space. The person's economic-environmental situation includes the safety of self and family members (e.g., the probability of assault), level of income, housing, and access to water and food. These issues impact on ontological security (Pedersen and Kienzler [Chapter 7]; James [Chapter 11]; see also Green 1999; Hinton et al. 2009a; Hobfoll 2012).[14] If concerns about these life domains are acute, then this may intensify the effects of trauma by bringing about repeated activation of the autonomic nervous system and an emergency mode. This will worsen PTSD symptoms, for example, trauma recall, irritability, hypervigilance, and nightmare, and other symptoms as well, like sleep paralysis, somatic symptoms, and panic attacks (on such symptoms, see Cougle et al. 2010; Friedman and McEwen 2004; Hinton et al. 2005b); and then these symptoms—and others of the arousal complex[15]—may have reverberating effects on the other ontological levels such as that of the family. Additionally, those with fewer economic resources often have varying knowledge of, access to, and options for health care, resulting in health insecurity, with higher loads of health care burden—another stress and topic of worry. Above we provided a model of how worry, stress, and ontological insecurity worsen symptomatology, creating vicious circles of worsening (see Figure 1.3), a model of how current life stresses produce somatic symptoms and disorder. The economic dimension also drives which treatments are locally offered, be they pharmacologic interventions by firms, new paradigms of treatment produced by researchers who are funded by national agencies, or humanitarian interventions.

Juridical and Political Space

How the effects of trauma play out will be influenced by juridical and political issues. In the case of mass violence or acts of violence that are endemic in a society, whether perpetrators are punished may influence symptoms, in particular the degree of anger of survivors (see McNally [Chapter 2]; Ball and O'Nell [Chapter 10]). There is also the key issue of what compensation is given to the trauma survivor such as disability payments and whether asylum status will be granted (Fassin and Rechtman 2009). How these justice issues are handled will vary across societies. So too will the specific juridical processes by which this occurs, processes that produce a certain public representation of trauma survivors; for example, those persons having certain traumas and symptoms may obtain disability benefits and refugee status. These determination processes will involve institutional-based rules and dramas of adjudication, which shape public representations of the traumatized and lead to certain sets of traumas and symptoms as scripts that the trauma survivor may tend to enmind, embody, and enact—or at least emphasize among other possible presentations. These scripts will shape the experiencing and presentation of the trauma survivor.

Resilience/Recovery/Treatment Dimension

The course of trauma-related disorder and its symptoms will be highly influenced by sources of resilience, recovery processes, and treatment sought and obtained for the condition (Collura and Lende 2012; Hinton and Kirmayer 2013). How the person attempts to deal with the trauma and to recover from its symptoms will vary greatly and will be profoundly influenced by cultural context (Ball and O'Nell [Chapter 10]; Good, Good, and Grayman [Chapter 12]). The trauma events and the resulting symptoms will lead the person to consider him- or herself to have some sort of disorder, which will result in certain treatments and attempts at recovery. The group may provide a source of resilience in various domains such as in ethnopsychology: in Cambodian Buddhism, many Buddhist-inspired idioms help to distance from negative affect ("you should stay far from your mood" [*niw chagnay pii arom*] or "you should change your attentional focus" [*gat ceut*]), and so too many proverbs such as "keeping yourself from getting excessively angry once will gain you a hundred days of happiness" (Nickerson and Hinton 2011). Public health announcements on television about the effects of trauma and about trauma-related symptoms may influence whether treatment is sought; self-help books or CDs may be used. Specialized mental health facilities may provide treatment, which may consist of receiving a selective serotonin reuptake inhibitor (SSRI), for example, Prozac, or receiving cognitive-behavioral therapy that involves the repeated discussion of the trauma event. Local healing traditions may be sought out for treatment of symptoms: Cambodian refugees may label somatic symptoms like dizziness and palpitations experienced upon trauma recall as a khyâl attack and ask a family member to do coining (Hinton et al. 2010), or a Cambodian may interpret a nightmare as a spiritual assault and consult with monks and perform religious rituals (Hinton et al. 2009a).

Each person is in a certain trauma-recovery space. How recovery plays out will depend in large part on the professional and lay syndromes that become frames of understanding and experiencing; those syndromes result in certain types of help seeking on the part of the individual and certain institutional-based interventions. In the cultural context, the trauma recovery episteme, that is, the conceptualization of how treatment should occur for trauma-caused symptoms, will have both professional and lay versions, each of which will be heterogeneous as well, such as multiple professional subdivisions. The trauma-recovery apparatus (*dispositive*) is formed by the actual recovery processes that are available from the level of local ethnopsychology, to traditional healers, to medical treatment centers.

Ethnography should be done to determine how persons with psychological trauma tend to recover on their own (e.g., sources of resilience), where they tend to receive treatment, and how they typically present to get treatment (the gateway distress presentation), such as with a somatic complaint to the primary care physician or with spirit possession to a local healer. The trajectory of trauma symptomatology depends on the part of the trauma recovery apparatus the person is engaged in, which will have variable effects on that individual and that individual's familial and general existential situation. If the psychological trauma is labeled as PTSD and treated with a selective serotonin reuptake inhibitor (SSRI), for example, Paxil, and given by a particular person in the health care system, what are the effects (Jenkins 2011)? How is the treatment described to the person and what is the person's understanding of the given diagnosis and medication, and does this create a new explanatory frame that is a key part of the hybrid trauma ontology? Does the pharmacological treatment result in medicalization, that is, using pills to treat symptoms that ultimately result from current issues of stress such as lack of housing, without addressing that problem? And even if the economic-environmental origins, such as poor housing, are not addressed, does the medication help the person improve to the point of coping better and hence aid recovery (Good, Good, and Grayman [Chapter 12])? Or does the medication do no good? How much does ontological security—such as economic insecurity and ongoing threat of spousal abuse and other forms of violence—persist and make recovery impossible?

The global trauma industry alters local recovery processes through advertisement, clinical trials, efficacy claims, and the actual effects of medications and other treatments it offers (Pedersen and Kienzler [Chapter 7]; Good, Good, and Grayman [Chapter 12]). Governmental agencies fund certain types of research, resulting in the production of certain types of knowledge about trauma, and pharmacological companies will conduct studies and try to create markets for their products (Jenkins 2011). Therapy trial results may make their way into journals and physician trainings and ultimately daily practice. News outlets like the *New York Times* publish stories about the struggles of particular war veterans and other trauma survivors, and about novel treatments and treatment trials. In international contexts, humanitarian agencies and others often follow the flow of money to conduct studies desired by national and international agencies, which will lead to certain types of interventions being implemented and certain ways of determining effectiveness. These various agencies—the pharmaceutical industry, foundations, national agencies—constitute another set of institutions, explanatory frames, and zones of trauma ontology production (Fassin and Pandolfi 2010; Fassin and Rechtman 2009).

A Typology of Errors

In this section we outline certain mistakes the researcher may make when studying trauma-related disorder in another cultural context.

Decontextualization Error

To fail to examine the situation of trauma victims and their key symptoms in terms of the eleven analytic dimensions is to commit an error of decontextualization.[16] Learning to contextualize trauma survivors and their complaints in respect to these eleven analytic dimensions is to acquire "contextual competency." Let us take an example of a symptom decontextualization. If the investigator ignores the ethnopsychology, ethnophysiology, and ethnospirituality according to which a presenting symptom—whether it be dizziness, startle, poor concentration, nightmare, or some other symptom—is understood by the experiencer, the investigator commits a decontextualization error, a semantic-type decontextualization.[17] Of note, the origins of symptoms in each of the ontological zones, as well as the effects in each of the zones, should also be assessed.

Medicalization Error

Medicalization is one type of decontextualization in which the clinician focuses on the patient's presenting complaint solely in terms of nosological categories and the related putative biological origin.[18] The clinician considers symptoms only from the perspective of DSM categories, tracing the disorder from abnormalities of brain chemistry to psychological and somatic symptoms, and ignores other possible causes such as social conflict, poverty, and community violence—and the clinician neglects to consider the effects of symptoms in other ontological domains, such as how trauma-caused anger results in family level effects. To determine the dimensions omitted through such medicalization, the researcher can use the eleven-dimension analysis. It may not be possible to intervene in other dimensions, or at least not immediately, but all these levels should be examined, what might be called cultivating "places for listening" (Fassin 2012).

Neglect of the Interaction Across Ontological Levels

An intervention at any one of the ontological levels affects the others. Even a narrow medical intervention may have effects throughout the different levels. The biology of trauma produces certain symptoms that if addressed by medication may lead to improvement in other ontological dimensions (see Good, Good, and Grayman [Chapter 12]). If a pill such as a selective serotonin reuptake inhibitor (SSRI), for example, Paxil, helps a person to sleep better and be less irritable, then that individual may cope better with current life issues and have less interpersonal conflict.

Neglect of Ontological Security and Its Genealogy

This chapter and others in the book illustrate ontological security to be a key analytic dimension (see too Green 1999; Hinton et al. 2009a; Hobfoll 2012; James 2008). Ontological security ranges from bodily health to spiritual, financial, and personal safety. Trauma victims are very sensitive to issues of ontological security. After a trauma, the survivor will continue to have a sense of being under threat, to have the feeling that a trauma or some other dangerous event is about to occur; consequently, the survivor will have a hyperreactive response to a threat, for example, the rapid induction of strong physiological arousal as well as recall of past traumas. Owing to being in this state, if the trauma survivor experiences actual current threats to security, those threats will greatly worsen trauma-related disorder through these multiplicative processes.

One way to assess ontological security is to profile current worry.[19] To do so, as a first step, the researcher should analyze the types and content of worry (Hinton et al. 2011). Next the researcher should try to construct causal models of the relationship of worry to PTSD and other aspects of trauma-related disorder, which can be based on the current problems–trauma model (see Figure 1.3): investigating such variables as symptoms induced by worry and catastrophic cognitions about those symptoms as well as determining how the symptoms are locally treated. Such multiplex models of worry (Figure 1.3) reveal a more complex and dynamic view of trauma-related disorder, situating it within the frame of ontological security.[20]

The genealogy of the current ontological security situation, its historical origins, should also be elucidated, as several chapters in this volume illustrate (Jenkins and Haas [Chapter 5]; Ball and O'Nell [Chapter 10]).[21] This includes the study of the intergenerational transmission of psychopathology, disadvantage, and suffering—what might be called micro-history as compared to macro-history. The dangers and difficulties in the local context—from stresses to traumas—may result from historical conditions of trauma and insecurity. The delineation of this genealogy may have a direct therapeutic effect for the population in question. By highlighting the dynamic origins of the current situation of ontological insecurity, genealogy gives insight into needed changes and how they may be brought about. When persons in these contexts become aware of this history and see themselves as partially the products of those forces, that historical consciousness may lead to a new sense of agency and self-esteem (Ball and O'Nell [Chapter 10]). Also, ways can be designed to attempt to address aspects of historical trauma, such as re-enculturing (e.g., revival of key cultural traditions) to address the loss of cultural traditions, thereby bringing a new group- and self-image and making available a new mode of being-in-the-world that may promote healing (see also Gone 2013; Hinton and Kirmayer 2013). (Though some have argued, such as Fassin and Rechtman 2009, that the belief in historical origins may give rise to a sense of profound victimhood and a justificatory frame for current dysfunction

that seemingly impedes recovery, particularly if economically or otherwise reinforced.)

Overinclusion Error

The investigator commits this sort of error upon assuming that a symptom
that is part of psychological distress in one cultural context exists in another
when in fact it is not present or minimally so. For example, in the DSM-IV
PTSD category, one finds certain symptoms—amnesia for a trauma, estrangement and detachment from others, or numbing (and all these symptoms
except "numbing" are found in the DSM-5 criteria)—that may not be present prominently in many other cultural contexts.[22] It is very difficult to
translate to other languages the PTSD criterion of feeling of detachment or
estrangement; the item suggests a sort of derealization or depersonalization
that is part of a certain history of theorizing in the West about trauma's effects. Likewise, it is very difficult to translate the term "emotional numbing"
to other languages; again, the idea of emotional numbing seems to arise from
the particular history of trauma in the Western context guided by theories
of the cause of trauma-related disorder (as noted above, numbing is a PTSD
criterion in DSM-IV but not in DSM-5).[23] (The overinclusion error, and the
following errors, for example, category truncation error and salience error,
parse different types of "category errors" [Kleinman 1988].)

Category Truncation Error

When a researcher does not assess a symptom or syndrome that is a key part
of a construct in a certain location, for example, a salient somatic symptom
or an important cultural syndrome, we refer to this as a category truncation
error. This type of error results in a lack of "content validity" in assessing
trauma-related disorder in the locality (Hinton and Lewis-Fernández 2011),
a truncation error. A prominent part of the trauma response in a locality may
extend beyond PTSD symptoms, as indicated in Figure 1.2 in the box labeled
"the trauma symptom pool"; for example, the trauma response may include
somatic symptoms, cultural syndromes, panic attacks, panic disorder, uncontrollable worry, substance abuse, low self-esteem, complicated bereavement,

and disrupted family bonds (see McNally [Chapter 2]; Young and Breslau [Chapter 3]; Jenkins and Haas [Chapter 6]). The centrality of these other trauma-related symptoms can be examined by various means: factor analyses of the PTSD items along with these other trauma-related symptoms (e.g., somatic symptoms) may reveal that these other symptoms are the highest loading items in one-factor solutions (e.g., as we found for "thinking a lot" among Cambodian refugees; see Hinton et al. [in press]).

Salience Error

When assessing PTSD symptoms and trauma symptoms more generally, researchers often disregard differences in salience, namely, of frequency and intensity. We refer to this as a salience error. A difference in symptom salience may result from profound cultural differences, such as from any of the eleven dimensions discussed above (see Figure 1.1).[24] Ongoing threat and danger may lead to arousal symptoms like startle being prominent. Anger may be prominent owing to a perceived lack of justice, both in the sense of the perpetrator not being punished and the victim not receiving what he or she considers just—social security disability or citizenship (McNally [Chapter 2]). Many trauma symptoms will be more salient in a particular cultural context owing to their attribution to certain cultural syndromes and to their centrality in the local ethnopsychology, ethnophysiology, or ethnospirituality (for these issues, see also Pedersen and Kienzler [Chapter 7]; Alcántara and Lewis-Fernández [Chapter 8]): if a culture gives elaborate meaning to nightmares—such as considering them to indicate the spiritual status of the deceased—then nightmares may take on particular salience and become a key part of the trauma ontology in that context (Hinton et al. 2009a).

To avoid a salience error, the investigator should first examine the spectrum of responses to trauma in a locality because there is a wide range of possible symptoms other than DSM-5 symptoms as indicated in Figure 1.2 in the box labeled "trauma symptom pool"[25] (doing so also prevents a category truncation error). Next the investigator should determine whether any of these are especially salient aspects of trauma-related disorder in a particular context. For example, drug abuse or self-cutting may be highly salient symptoms in one context (Jenkins and Haas [Chapter 5]), and suicidality or depression in another. Once such saliences are discovered, the mechanisms causing those differences need to be examined (see below, the sections "biocultural causal model" and "local causal model"): in the Cambodian case, examining why somatic symptoms, panic attacks, such as those triggered by standing up and by worry, and panic disorder are such prominent aspects of their trauma-related disorder.

Let us examine how a salience error can be committed in assessing somatic symptoms. From a cross-cultural perspective, somatic symptoms are prominent in trauma presentations, and certain somatic symptoms will be salient in a particular cultural context. Four types of salience errors can be made in respect to somatic symptoms. One error is not to assess somatic symptoms and note their salience in a group. Another error is not to assess subtypes, such as pain symptoms versus panic-type symptoms. Yet another error is to not assess the saliency of particular symptoms; as part of the assessment of the trauma response, not just somatic symptoms in general but specific somatic symptoms should be profiled, that is, not only rates and severity of aggregate symptoms but also rates and severity of individual symptoms. And finally, the frequency of types of particular subtypes of a symptom, such as dizziness that is triggered in particular ways, for example, by standing up, should be assessed (see the section "abstraction error"): in the Cambodian context, dizziness is a frequent and severe symptom, and so too dizziness on standing (Hinton et al. 2012, 2013b). To not assess individual salient symptoms is to commit an abstraction error (see the section "abstraction error"), that is, to commit the error of examining a broader category, when differences will only be found when examining particular items: this occurs if the investigator determines somatic symptoms as a whole, such as on a scale, and does not scrutinize individual symptoms such as dizziness.

Abstraction Error

Researchers commit this type of error when they examine a general class rather than its subunits, the concrete exemplars, for example, "somatic symptoms" rather than specific somatic symptoms. Individuals do not experience somatic symptoms but rather specific symptoms such as dizziness, and not just dizziness, but dizziness of a certain type—such as that having a certain quality (e.g., true vertigo or a sense of imbalance) and that having a certain trigger (e.g., standing up or fear)—and these are the true forms of actual experiencing, the units of actual phenomenological experiencing, the experience-near categories (Kleinman 1988). And an abstraction error is also committed when a symptom like anger or dizziness is not contextualized in respect to the local semantic and causal networks. For example, there will be local terms for anger, often several types, each of which may have a slightly different meaning, different metaphors. There will be a certain ethnopsychology and ethnophysiology of anger. There will be certain common causes of anger in the cultural group. There will be certain ways of treating it. Likewise, a somatic symptom can be so examined, contextualizing it in its semantic networks—and causal networks (see the following two sections on "causal models"). In this way an abstraction error is avoided.

Not Assessing Biocultural Causal Models

Often researchers describe an idiom of distress or syndrome without exploring its semantic network (Good 1977), and often without showing how the idiom of distress or syndrome involves multiple interacting processes that may unfold in specific episodes as depicted in what we have called multiplex models (e.g., Figures 1.3 and 1.6). This might be called a semantic-type and a dynamism-type abstraction, and it is an abstraction from psycho- and bio-pathological processes that occur in time. Biocultural causal models show the interaction of various types of processes in time, such as triggers, cultural models, trauma associations, catastrophic cognitions, and somatic symptoms that are induced by arousal. The models reveal how idioms of distress and syndromes form dynamic networks and particular episodes that unfold in time. These multiplex models, for example, the current problems–trauma model (Figure 1.3), depict symptom complexes, causal networks, that are key aspects of trauma-related disorder in a locality. One needs to examine not just symptoms, but these causal networks.

Not Assessing Local Causal Models

The researcher needs to determine the local causal network models that articulate how a complaint is locally understood. To give an example, the symptom of worry can only be understood in the context of "thinking a lot," because this is the way that local populations often label events of worry. The model of the Cambodian conceptualization of "thinking a lot" is shown in Figure 1.7. This might be called a local causal network model of a syndrome

Treating "thinking a lot" and its induced symptoms by various methods such as attentional control, mindfulness, obeisance to the Buddha, coining, "cracking" the joints, and taking tonics and sleep and appetite promoters

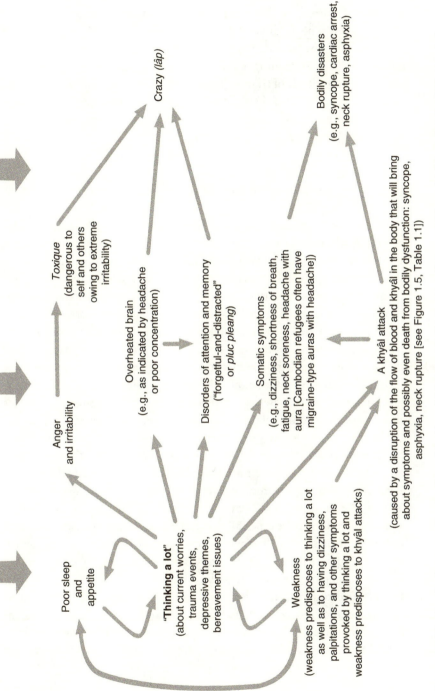

Figure 1.7. The Cambodian causal network model of how "thinking a lot" generates distress and how thinking a lot should be treated.

or idiom of distress, in that it shows the Cambodian conceptualization of what the syndrome or idiom of distress causes and what it is caused by, and how it is should be treated.[26] In turn, "thinking a lot" can be situated in the more general understanding of how syndromes occur (Figure 1.6), and local ideas about the effects of trauma (Figure 1.4; cf. Pedersen and Kienzler, Figure 7.4 [Chapter 7]). These kinds of models combine semantic network analysis and episode analysis in order to avoid both a semantic-type error and a dynamism error, both abstraction errors.

Multiplex Models of the Effects of Trauma

In this chapter, we presented dynamic biocultural models of how distress and cultural syndromes are generated in traumatized populations (see Figures 1.2, 1.3, and 1.6), as well as dynamic models showing how local populations consider different types of distress to be generated (see Figures 1.4 and 1.7). Elsewhere we have referred to these as multiplex models, which are characterized by bio-attentional looping that leads to vicious circles of worsening: attentional focus on feared symptoms amplifies them, what might be called attentional amplification, and the increased symptom leads to more fear, and fear itself activates the biology of anxiety that increases symptoms by mechanisms such as the activation of the autonomic nervous system—and increased symptoms and fear lead to more catastrophic cognitions about somatic symptoms and attentional scanning of the body for symptoms, and so on.[27]

The first multiplex model we presented (see Figure 1.2), the multiplex trauma model, is a cultural cognitive neuroscience model of trauma-related disorder. The model demonstrates how several trauma-related biological and psychological processes produce a certain potential trauma symptom pool (see too, Good, Good, and Grayman [Chapter 12]; see also Shorter 1992). Some symptoms may be especially amplified, and so set up vicious circles of worsening. This amplification occurs through bio-attentional looping, which results in large part from cultural processes, for example, the interpretation of anxiety symptoms in terms of the local ethnophysiology, ethnopsychology, and ethnospirituality. The biocultural multiplex models are nested (this nesting is shown most clearly in Figure 1.6) and so take into account the interpersonal and economic effects of the complaint, the role of the complaint as idiom of distress, and the resulting treatment course, all of which might be called socio-cultural pragmatics.

Thus, a biocultural multiplex model (e.g., Figures 1.2, 1.3, and 1.6) emphasizes multiple processes—bio-attentional looping, cultural interpretation of symptoms, trauma associations, socio-cultural pragmatics—and the importance of episode analysis, that is, the ethnography of particular distress episodes (Hinton et al. 2012). A biocultural multiplex model is a dynamic comorbidity model in that it assumes that among trauma victims often multiple psychopathological dimensions and types of symptoms—like worry, somatization, panic attacks, PTSD, depression, and panic disorder—will co-occur and worsen one another. Increasingly, the elucidation of these sorts of causal networks models is considered to be an important way to understand how psychopathology occurs (Borsboom and Cramer 2013; McNally 2012; van Os 2013). More generally, there needs to be a complex view of "symptoming," that is, the occurrence of a symptom as a dynamic event that involves multiple processes in interaction, and of "syndroming," likewise considered as a dynamic event. Our models try to capture symptom and syndrome as event.

In this chapter, we presented multiplex models that incorporated current psychobiological theories of psychopathology (see Figures 1.2, 1.3, and 1.6), and we presented local causal network models that articulate how the local population views distress to be generated (see Figures 1.4 and 1.7). That is, one type of multiplex model (a biocultural causal-network model) showed how general psychobiological processes could be hypothesized to interact with local idioms and syndromes to create a certain illness reality, whereas the other type of multiplex model (a local causal-network model) showed the local conceptualization of disorder. These two types of multiplex models, the general biocultural model and the local model, give key insights into how local biologies and local psychopathologies are formed. These two types of causal network models capture in a contextualized and dynamic way the key role of idioms of distress and syndromes (cultural concepts of distress) in local biocultural ontologies.

Conclusion

This chapter has provided three analytic optics—the eleven analytic perspectives, the typology of errors, and the multiplex models—to use in examining trauma-related disorder. These three types of analytic optics help to situate the chapters of this volume in theoretical context and suggest theoretical frameworks for the cross-cultural study of trauma-related disorders.

Through these three analytic optics, local trauma ontologies can be delin-
eated, and the cross-cultural study of those ontologies advanced. Otherwise
the performed analysis risks being decontextualized and abstracted, a sort
of interpretive violence (Bibeau and Corin 1995; Nations 2008)—only the
semblance of understanding the experiential space of the trauma survivor.
Through these three analytic optics, the researcher becomes aware of key
processes to target in interventions that seek to alleviate distress and build
resilience of individuals and communities.

Notes

1. In addition to these metaphor issues, the term "psychological trauma" is problematic in that it suggests that trauma impacts only on the psychological domain, when
clearly it has reverberating effects on multiple existential levels—the family, the society itself, spirituality (Jenkins and Haas [Chapter 5]; Ball and O'Nell [Chapter 10]; James
[Chapter 11]).

2. Traumas that strongly induce certain somatic symptoms may create a trauma ontology that includes prominent somatic symptoms along with frequent panic and arousal
(Hinton et al. 2012, 2013b). This is because whenever the somatic symptom is experienced it may trigger trauma recall, and whenever trauma recall occurs it may trigger the
somatic symptom. In groups with traumas strongly paired to somatic symptoms, those
somatic symptoms may evoke memories of past traumas and fear that involve particular
events featuring that somatic sensation and possibly entire time periods encoded by that
somatic sensation. In the latter case, the somatic symptom acts as a somatic chronotope
evoker, a somatic marker of an entire time period. The term "chronotope" is taken from
Bakhtin (1981), indicating a certain space-time. Jane Yager (2009) in her review of Karl
Schlögel's *Moscow Dreams* (2008), a book on Moscow during the time of the Stalinist terror, describes Schlögel's use of the term "chronotope" in the following way, which is very
close to the usage we intend here: "the Moscow of 1937 as a chronotope, a specific and
inextricable bundle of time and space whose defining features are despotic arbitrariness,
suddenness, shock, attack out of nowhere, disappearance and the blurring of the line between reality and phantasm." We argue that certain images and somatic symptoms have
the power to evoke such a space-time, a specific chronotope.

3. Below we provide a more detailed typology of traumas based on how they induce
somatic symptoms, providing Cambodian examples. Many Cambodian refugees, survivors of the Pol Pot genocide which occurred 1975–79, have had all these types of traumas,
which explains in part why Cambodian refugees have such prominent somatic symptoms.

- *Fear-inducing events.* Somatic symptoms such as palpitations and sweating
  may result from the fear response during traumas—for example, when be-

ing beaten or threatened or when observing others being hit or killed—such as through autonomic arousal from activation of the sympathetic nervous system. Repeated severe fear was commonly experienced in the Pol Pot genocide. (The following traumas are almost all fear-inducing events as well as trauma events having other specific effects, so that they induce somatic symptoms both by a fear response and by specific effects, thus acting as a somatic symptom–inducer in two ways.)

- *Blow to the body and bodily injury.* Symptoms like headache and backache may result directly from being beaten. Such blows were common during the Pol Pot genocide, for example, punishments for perceived slowness in work. Scars and bodily shrapnel may even remain.
- *Illness.* Symptoms like nausea may result from illnesses such as cancer or malaria. In the Pol Pot period, Cambodian refugees often endured untreated illnesses that induced somatic symptoms: malarial illness was extremely common, usually lasting for months, and it produced almost daily rigors that featured palpitations, dizziness, and other symptoms—that is, malarial illness was a biology-induced event causing symptoms also found in a panic attack, a kind of malaria-caused panic attack.
- *Poisoning.* Various symptoms like nausea may result from poisoning. Cambodians often inadvertently consumed toxins when surreptitiously eating raw plants or uncooked meats in the Pol Pot period (e.g., certain kinds of roots must be cleaned a long time to rid them of toxins before eating, but often there was not time to do this for fear of being caught), and the toxins commonly would induce dizziness, nausea, palpitations, and other symptoms.
- *Starvation.* Weakness, dizziness, palpitations, and other symptoms may result from a lack of vitamins, protein, and calories. In the Pol Pot period, most Cambodian refugees experienced protein and calorie starvation, which caused weakness, severe edema, and palpitations on the slightest effort. These starvation effects were much worsened by beriberi from thiamine deficiency.
- *Slave labor.* A variety of symptoms, including palpitations, dizziness, weakness, and syncope may be experienced during slave labor, and particularly if doing this labor while starving. In the Pol Pot period, Cambodians were forced to do slave labor while starving: in the most typical form of labor, dam building, the laborer carried a basket heavy with dirt at each end of a pole that was balanced at the shoulder, which caused bodily soreness, particularly neck soreness, dizziness, and extreme exhaustion.
- *Viewing dismembered bodies, blood, and corpses, or consuming corpse-contaminated water.* Nausea, disgust, and other symptoms may result from encountering corpses, seeing severed limbs and blood, or consuming contaminated foodstuffs. In the Pol Pot period, Cambodians often came upon corpses in a state of decay, infested by maggots, and they often

inadvertently consumed water from sources containing corpses; and often they saw bombing victims who were eviscerated and whose limbs had been severed.

- *Near drowning.* Asphyxia may result from near drowning while traversing water or from torture methods. Cambodians are often unable to swim, and they have frequently experienced near drowning, particularly in the Pol Pot period when forced to work in deep water and to cross rivers; some were tortured by having their heads forced into water containers.

4. On "humiliated" memory, see Langer (1991), and also Kirmayer (1996b). As an example of humiliated memory, the person may recall being beaten or having to live without bathing, in filthy and tattered clothes, and with the body infested by vermin.

5. In addition to the manner of trauma acting as an assault on group self-esteem, the cultural encoding of the trauma events as "blocked flow" also contributed to the prominence of shortness of breath and gastrointestinal complaints among those Rwandans who survived the genocide, with these two somatic complaints each being a somaticized image of blockage, seemingly demonstrating the process of metaphor-guided somatization (Hagengimana and Hinton 2009).

6. On khyâl attacks, see below (viz., the section on ethnopsychology/ethnophysiology/ethnospirituality), and see also the DSM-5 (American Psychiatric Association 2013), in which khyâl attacks are one of the nine cultural concepts of distress.

7. These items may appear to be artificially elevated in surveys for several reasons. For one, an item that is poorly understood may be endorsed at the same level as the previously answered item, what might be called response perseveration. Second, misconstrual of meaning may lead to incorrect responses to an item. As an example, though amnesia does not seem to result commonly in other cultures following trauma, it may still be endorsed at a high rate owing to a lack of specification: the question about amnesia may be misconstrued as asking about poor memory in general, which is a common symptom of depression, that is, misconstrued as asking about poor memory in general rather than the memory of a particular trauma event. And third, there may be problems in translating a term that has no equivalency in another language. "Numbing" is a difficult term to translate and often must be rendered as an absence of pleasurable feelings as well as sad feelings. It would seem the use of the term "numbing" to describe an emotional state is a Western idiom of distress that poorly translates to many cultures; that is, the physical state of numbing cannot be used as a metaphor to describe an emotional state in many cultural contexts. Likewise detachment, a dissociation-type symptom, is difficult to translate and seemingly emerges from particularities of the U.S. context rather than a universal fact of biology.

8. Here we consider a syndrome as a "symptom" in the sense of an indicator of the presence of trauma-related disorder.

9. There are processes of *Nachträglichkeit* or *après-coup*, that is, afterwardness (Eickhoff 2006). If the person thinks that a trauma like torture has caused a symptom such

as back pain, then this produces a certain identity and relationship to the trauma event and shapes the survivor (Kirmayer 2008). The symptom may serve as self-identity and self-presentation and may impact on obtaining asylum and benefits. In terms of self-fashioning, metaphoric and other meanings come into play as well: back pain and imagery of burden. In such cases, how much the actual trauma event caused the symptom and how much the symptom resulted from processes of amplification—metaphoric resonance amplification and attentional amplification, for example—is hard to disentangle.

10. Some examples of these syndromes in the Cambodian context are the following (see also Figure 1.4):

- "Soul loss," a type of syndrome common in many cultures in various forms (Rubel et al. 1984), is considered by Cambodians to occur when a trauma or any fright displaces the soul; this leads to symptoms like startle and a general state of hypervigilant fear. Cambodians often attribute symptoms like startle, hypervigilance, poor concentration, forgetfulness, and avoidance of trauma reminders to the soul's not being secured in the body or being displaced from it. This soul "dislocation" is thought to be caused by a great fright such as upon being threatened with death by a Khmer Rouge soldier, seeing a ghost, hearing a sudden loud noise, or having a nightmare (Chhim 2012; Hinton et al. 2013b).
- "Heart weakness" is considered by Cambodians to cause startle, palpitations, irritability, excessive worry, and poor concentration, among other symptoms. It may be caused by a great fright, weakness itself (e.g., owing to poor sleep and appetite), or an inborn trait.
- "Thinking a lot" is considered by Cambodians to cause many symptoms that Western psychology would classify as trauma symptoms such as inability to distance from current problems and issues, irritability, insomnia, a reactivity to worry and other negative emotions, and "thinking a lot" is considered to bring about dangerous mental states and physical perturbations, such as permanent forgetfulness, insanity, and a dangerous weakness, as well as khyâl attacks. Cambodians believe that "thinking a lot" may be caused by many processes such as being weak, thinking about current life distress issues like poverty, or ruminating about losses or past traumas.
- Khyâl attacks are considered by Cambodians to be triggered by multiple causes such as standing up or fright, and those attacks are thought to result in physiological perturbations that bring about symptoms like dizziness, palpitations, and neck soreness as well as possibly death owing to syncope, heart arrest, neck vessel rupture, or other causes.

11. As emphasized in this chapter, a somatic symptom may have metaphoric resonances and a role as an idiom of distress as well, both of which contribute to the symptom's meaning.

12. "Thinking a lot" also involves other types of cognizing as well, such as cognizing about depressive themes such as being left by a wife for another man or being separated from relatives. These other types of negative cognizing may trigger many of the same processes as outlined for worry-type cognitions, such as the induction of multiple somatic symptoms. Additionally, "thinking a lot" may consist of other kinds of thoughts, such as thoughts of the past, another reason for the syndrome's commonality among trauma victims.

13. That is, it may be that individuals in a society have trauma symptoms that are not attributed to trauma, and the investigator must determine how those symptoms and persons are represented in a particular society.

14. Insecurity may also arise from a feeling of being in a vulnerable physical, psychological, or spiritual state, for example, of being at risk of assault by spirits. For a discussion of this type of insecurity, see the section on ethnopsychology/ethnophysiology/ethnospirituality and that on religion/spirituality.

15. This might also be called the reactivity–dysregulation complex, in that there is both reactivity to multiple triggers and poor ability to regulate the states of distress. The biological causation will be multiple, such as autonomic arousal and low vagal tone.

16. In medicine, these are referred to as "contextual errors" (Weiner et al. 2010).

17. As outlined in this chapter, there are many types of desemantization errors. Though not emphasized in this chapter, failing to consider metaphoric dimensions is another sort of semantic-type decontextualization of a symptom (Hinton et al. 2012).

18. Focusing on just one dimension is a myopia: attending only to the biological dimension is a simplistic "biologization" (cf. to the term "medicalization").

19. We presented a model that illustrated how worry generates trauma-related disorder (Figure 1.3). As Figure 1.3 illustrates, having experienced trauma in the past may result in worry having a far greater tendency to induce somatic symptoms and negative affective states (e.g., anxiety, depression, and panic), and this vulnerability may set up various looping processes. According to this biocultural model, past trauma results in the laying down of memory in the amygdala and biological shifts that may result in a state of rapidly induced arousal, increased reactivity to stress, and impaired ability to adapt. Engaging in worry may then set up various vicious circles that are depicted in Figure 1.3.

20. As we have discussed, "thinking a lot" is a common presentation of distress in many cultural contexts, and often the content of "thinking a lot" involves current concerns. The close relationship of ontological security to trauma-related symptoms is articulated in many ethnopsychologies, as shown in this chapter and in others in this volume (Pedersen and Kienzler [Chapter 7]). We have discussed the centrality of "thinking a lot" to trauma-related disorder among Cambodian refugees in this chapter, and noted that "thinking a lot" often begins upon thinking about current life problems (Figure 1.3). In order for Figure 1.3 to fully apply to "thinking a lot," it needs some modification. Besides beginning by thinking about current problems, the episodes

may commence upon thinking about depressive themes (e.g., separation and past failures), traumas, or anger issues. So in Figure 1.3, "Current Problems" would be replaced by "Negative Cognizing (e.g., thinking about current problems; separation from a loved one owing to death, distance, or break up; failures; conflicts; and/or past negative events)." Many of these kinds of thoughts are often present together bringing about escalating distress. "Thinking a lot" syndromes often articulate a local theory of the key relationship of current life distress to symptomatology, including trauma-related symptoms; the syndromes constitute a local theory of trauma somatics, of trauma sociosomatics, in which ontological security plays a key role.

21. On genealogy, see also Foucault (1978) and Fassin and Rechtman (2009).

22. Such overinclusion may not be detected for reasons of misassessment: if a person does not understand a questionnaire item, he or she may endorse having the same level of severity of that item as he or she had for the previous item, what we referred to above as a confusion-caused perseveration error, a form of response perseveration (see McNally [Chapter 2]). Then the item will seem to be prominent in a context when in fact it is not. See note 7 in this chapter for further discussion.

23. In the United States, the complaint of numbness by a trauma victim seemingly has metaphoric dimensions, a statement about an existential location. The idea that numbing is a key symptom of trauma also relates to a certain history of theorizing about pathophysiology: the opiate theory of numbing and PTSD (Glover 1993; van der Kolk et al. 1985). Here the scientific theory of pathophysiology seemingly shapes the theory of symptom profile.

24. The salience issue can be examined by techniques like latent variable analysis.

25. Some examples, grouped by type, are the following: DSM-type PTSD symptoms (e.g., anger and startle); somatic symptoms; behaviors (e.g., self-cutting, substance abuse, suicide gestures); psychopathology dimensions (e.g., worry, panic attacks); symptom complexes (e.g., the current problems–trauma complex); and diagnostic categories (e.g., panic disorder and major depression).

26. Figure 1.3 could be considered a biocultural multiplex model of one key aspect of the "thinking a lot" syndrome: that aspect of it focused on current concerns. Local network models consider only the local cultural model of disorder, whereas the biocultural multiplex models take into account the local conceptualization of disorder as well as current theories of biological and psychological processes.

27. The biolooping processes are more clearly shown in the biocultural models, but these same processes will also play a key role in local causal networks.

References

American Psychiatric Association
    2000 Diagnostic and Statistical Manual of Mental Disorder. 4th edition. Text revision. Washington, D.C.: American Psychiatric Association.

2013 Diagnostic and Statistical Manual of Mental Disorders. 5th edition. Washington, D.C.: American Psychiatric Association.

Argenti, Nicolas, and Katharina Schramm
2010 Remembering Violence: Anthropological Perspectives on Intergenerational Transmission. New York: Berghahn.

Bakhtin, M. M.
1981 The Dialogic Imagination: Four Essays. Austin: University of Texas Press.

Bibeau, Gilles, and Ellen E. Corin
1995 Beyond Textuality: Asceticism and Violence in Anthropological Interpretation. Berlin: Mouton de Gruyter.

Bigelow, Kathryn, dir.
2008 The Hurt Locker. Summit Entertainment. Calif.

Binder, Elisabeth B., and Charles B. Nemeroff
2010 The CRF System, Stress, Depression and Anxiety-Insights from Human Genetic Studies. Molecular Psychiatry 15:574–88.

Blechert, Jens, Tanja Michael, Paul Grossman, Marta Lajtman, and Frank H. Wilhelm
2007 Autonomic and Respiratory Characteristics of Posttraumatic Stress Disorder and Panic Disorder. Psychosomatic Medicine 69:935–43.

Borsboom, Denny, and A. O. Cramer
2013 Network Analysis: An Integrative Approach to the Structure of Psychopathology. Annual Review of Clinical Psychology 9:91–121.

Bower, Herbert
1994 The Concentration Camp Syndrome. Australian and New Zealand Journal of Psychiatry 28:391–97.

Bryant, Richard A.
2012 Simplifying Complex PTSD: Comment on Resick et al. (2012). Journal of Traumatic Stress 25:252–53.

Chhim, Sotheara
2012 Baksbat (Broken Courage): The Development and Validation of the Inventory to Measure Baksbat, a Cambodian Trauma-Based Cultural Syndrome of Distress. Culture, Medicine, and Psychiatry 36:640–59.

Cohn, Simon, Clare Dyson, and Simon Wessely
2008 Early Accounts of Gulf War Illness and the Construction of Narratives in UK Service Personnel. Social Science and Medicine 67:1641–49.

Collura, Gino L., and Daniel H. Lende
2012 Post-Traumatic Stress Disorder and Neuroanthropology: Stopping PTSD Before It Begins. Annals of Anthropological Practice 36:131–48.

Cougle, Jesse R., Matthew T. Feldner, Meghan E. Keough, Kirsten A. Hawkins, and Kristin E. Fitch
2010 Comorbid Panic Attacks Among Individuals with Posttraumatic Stress Disorder: Associations with Traumatic Event Exposure History, Symptoms, and Impairment. Journal of Anxiety Disorders 24:183–88.

Coulter, Chris
2009 Bush Wives and Girl Soldiers: Women's Lives Through War and Peace in Sierra Leone. Ithaca, N.Y.: Cornell University Press.

de Jong, Joop, and Ria Reis
2010 Kiyang-Yang, A West-African Postwar Idiom of Distress. Culture, Medicine, and Psychiatry 34:301–21.
2013 Collective Trauma Resolution: Dissociation as a Way of Processing Post-War Traumatic Stress in Guinea Bissau. Transcultural Psychiatry 50:644–61.

Eickhoff, Friedrich-Wilhelm
2006 On Nachträglichkeit: The Modernity of an Old Concept. International Journal of Psychoanalysis 87:1453–69.

Eisenbruch, Maurice
1991 From Post-Traumatic Stress Disorder to Cultural Bereavement: Diagnosis of Southeast Asian Refugees. Social Science and Medicine 33:673–80.

Evans-Campbell, T.
2008 Historical Trauma in American Indian/Native Alaska Communities: A Multi-level Framework for Exploring Impacts on Individuals, Families, and Communities. Journal of Interpersonal Violence 23:316–38.

Farmer, Paul
1997 On Suffering and Structural Violence: A View from Below. *In* Social Suffering. Arthur Kleinman, Veena Das, and Margaret Lock, eds. Pp. 261–84. Berkeley: University of California Press.

Fassin, Didier
2012 Humanitarian Reason: A Moral History of the Present. Berkeley: University of California Press.

Fassin, Didier, and Mariella Pandolfi
2010 Contemporary States of Emergency: The Politics of Military and Humanitarian Interventions. Cambridge, Mass.: Zone.

Fassin, Didier, and Richard Rechtman
2009 The Empire of Trauma: An Inquiry into the Condition of Victimhood. Princeton, N.J.: Princeton University Press.

Finley, Erin P.
2011 Fields of Combat: Understanding PTSD Among Veterans of Iraq and Afghanistan. Ithaca, N.Y.: Cornell University Press.
2012 War and Dislocation: A Neuroanthropological Model of Trauma Among American Veterans with Combat PTSD. *In* The Encultured Brain: An Introduction to Neuroanthropology. Daniel H. Lende and Greg Downey, eds. Pp. 263–90. Cambridge, Mass.: MIT Press.

Foa, Edna B., Laurie Cashman, Lisa Jaycox, and Kevin Perry
1997 The Validation of a Self-Report Measure of Posttraumatic Stress Disorder: The Posttraumatic Diagnostic Scale. Psychological Assessment 9:445–51.

Foa, Edna B., Anke Ehlers, David M. Clark, David F. Tolin, and Susan M. Orsillo
    1999 The Posttraumatic Cognitions Inventory (PTCI): Development and Valida-
    tion. Psychological Assessment 11:303–14.
Foa, Edna B., and Barbara Olasov Rothbaum
    1998 Treating the Trauma of Rape: Cognitive-Behavioral Therapy for PTSD. New
    York: Guilford.
Foucault, Michel
    1978 The History of Sexuality. 3 vols. New York: Pantheon.
Friedman, Matthew J., and Bruce S. McEwen
    2004 Posttraumatic Stress Disorder, Allostatic Load, and Medical Illness. In Trauma
    and Health: Physical Health Consequences of Exposure to Extreme Stress. Paula
    P. Schnurr and Bonnie L. Green, eds. Washington, D.C.: American Psychological
    Association.
Friedman, Matthew J., Patricia A. Resick, Richard A. Bryant, and Chris R. Brewin
    2011 Considering PTSD for DSM-V. Depression and Anxiety 28:750–59.
Glover, H.
    1993 A Preliminary Trial of Nalmefene for the Treatment of Emotional Numbing
    in Combat Veterans with Post-Traumatic Stress Disorder. Israel Journal of Psy-
    chiatry and Related Sciences 30(4):255–63.
Gone, Joseph P.
    2009 A Community-Based Treatment for Native American Historical Trauma:
    Prospectes for Evidence-Based Practice. Journal of Consulting and Clinical Psy-
    chology 77:751–61.
    2013 Redressing First Nations Historical Trauma: Theorizing Mechanisms for Indig-
    enous Culture as Mental Health Treatment. Transcultural Psychiatry 50:683–706.
Good, Byron J.
    1977 The Heart of What's the Matter: The Semantics of Illness in Iran. Culture,
    Medicine, and Psychiatry 1:25–58.
Green, Linda
    1999 Fear as a Way of Life: Mayan Widows in Rural Guatemala. New York: Colum-
    bia University Press.
Gustafsson, Mai Lan
    2009 War and Shadows: The Haunting of Vietnam. Ithaca, N.Y.: Cornell University
    Press.
Hagengimana, Athanase, and Devon E. Hinton
    2009 Ihahamuka, a Rwandan Syndrome of Response to the Genocide: Blocked
    Flow, Spirit Assault, and Shortness of Breath. In Culture and Panic Disorder.
    Devon E. Hinton and Byron J. Good, eds. Pp. 205–29. Stanford, Calif.: Stanford
    University Press.
Heim, Christine, D. Jeffrey Newport, Stacey Heit, Yolanda P. Graham, Molly Wilcox,
    Robert Bonsall, Andrew H. Miller, and Charles B. Nemeroff

2000 Pituitary-Adrenal and Autonomic Responses to Stress in Women After Sexual and Physical Abuse in Childhood. Journal of the American Medical Association 284:592–97.

Hinton, Devon E., Nigel P. Field, Angela Nickerson, Richard Bryant, and Naomi Simon
2013a Dreams of the Dead Among Cambodian Refugees: Frequency, Phenomenology, and Relationship to Complicated Grief and PTSD. Death Studies 37:750–67.

Hinton, Devon E., and Byron J. Good
2009 A Medical Anthropology of Panic Sensations: Ten Analytic Perspectives. *In* Culture and Panic Disorder. Devon E. Hinton and Byron J. Good, eds. Pp. 57–81. Stanford, Calif.: Stanford University Press.

Hinton, Devon E., Alexander Hinton, Dara Chhean, Vuth Pich, Reattidara J. R. Loeum, and Mark H. Pollack
2009a Nightmares Among Cambodian Refugees: The Breaching of Concentric Ontological Security. Culture, Medicine, and Psychiatry 33:219–65.

Hinton, Devon E., Alexander L. Hinton, Kok-Thay Eng, and Sophearith Choung
2012 PTSD and Key Somatic Complaints and Cultural Syndromes Among Rural Cambodians: The Results of a Needs Assessment Survey. Medical Anthropology Quarterly 29:147–54.

Hinton, Devon E., Susan Hinton, Khin Um, Audria Chea, and Sophia Sak
2002 The Khmer "Weak Heart" Syndrome: Fear of Death from Palpitations. Transcultural Psychiatry 39:323–44.

Hinton, Devon E., Stefan G. Hofmann, Roger K. Pitman, Mark H. Pollack, and David H. Barlow
2008 The Panic Attack–PTSD Model: Applicability to Orthostatic Panic Among Cambodian Refugee. Cognitive Behaviour Therapy 27:101–16.

Hinton, Devon E., Stefan G. Hofmann, Mark H. Pollack, and Michael W. Otto
2009b Mechanisms of Efficacy of CBT for Cambodian Refugees with PTSD: Improvement in Emotion Regulation and Orthostatic Blood Pressure Response. CNS Neuroscience and Therapeutics 15:255–63.

Hinton, Devon E., and Laurence J. Kirmayer
2013 Local Responses to Trauma: Symptom, Affect, and Healing. Transcultural Psychiatry 50:607–21.

Hinton, Devon E., M. Alexandra Kredlow, Vuth Pich, Eric Bui, and Stefan G. Hofmann
2013b The Relationship of PTSD to Key Somatic Complaints and Cultural Syndromes Among Cambodian Refugees Attending a Psychiatric Clinic: The Cambodian Somatic Symptom and Syndrome Inventory (SSI). Transcultural Psychiatry 50:347–70.

Hinton, Devon E., and Roberto Lewis-Fernández
2010 Idioms of Distress Among Trauma Survivors: Subtypes and Clinical Utility. Culture, Medicine, and Psychiatry 34:209–18.

2011 The Cross-Cultural Validity of Posttraumatic Stress Disorder: Implications for DSM-5. Depression and Anxiety 28:783–801.

Hinton, Devon E., Angela Nickerson, and Richard A. Bryant
2011 Worry, Worry Attacks, and PTSD Among Cambodian Refugees: A Path Analysis Investigation. Social Science and Medicine 72:1817–25.

Hinton, Devon E., Sonith Peou, Siddharth Joshi, Angela Nickerson, and Naomi Simon
2013c Normal Grief and Complicated Bereavement Among Traumatized Cambodian Refugees: Cultural Context and the Central Role of Dreams of the Deceased. Culture, Medicine, and Psychiatry 37:427–64.

Hinton, Devon E., Vuth Pich, Dara Chhean, and Mark H. Pollack
2005a "The Ghost Pushes You Down": Sleep Paralysis–Type Panic Attacks in a Khmer Refugee Population. Transcultural Psychiatry 42:46–78.

Hinton, Devon E., Vuth Pich, Dara Chhean, Mark H. Pollack, and Richard J. McNally
2005b Sleep Paralysis Among Cambodian Refugees: Association with PTSD Diagnosis and Severity. Depression and Anxiety 22:47–51.

Hinton, Devon E., Vuth Pich, Luana Marques, Angela Nickerson, and Mark H. Pollack
2010 Khyâl Attacks: A Key Idiom of Distress Among Traumatized Cambodia Refugees. Culture, Medicine, and Psychiatry 34:244–78.

Hinton, Devon E., Andrew Rasmussen, Leakhena Nou, Mark H. Pollack, and Mary-Jo DelVecchio Good
2009c Anger, PTSD, and the Nuclear Family: A Study of Cambodian Refugees. Social Science and Medicine 69:1387–94.

Hinton, Devon E., Ria Reis, and Joop de Jong
in press The "Thinking a Lot" Idiom of Distress and PTSD: An Examination of Their Relationship Among Traumatized Cambodian Refugees Using the "Thinking a Lot" Questionnaire. Medical Anthropology Quarterly.

Hobfoll, Stevan E.
2012 Conservation of Resources and Disaster in Cultural Context: The Caravans and Passageways for Resources. Psychiatry 75:227–32.

Hollan, Douglas
2004 Self Systems, Cultural Idioms of Distress, and the Psycho-Biology Consequences of Childhood Suffering. Transcultural Psychiatry 41:62–79.
2013 Coping in Plain Sight: Work as a Local Repsonse to Event-Related Emotional Distress in Contemporary U.S. Society. Transcultural Psychiatry 50:726–43.

Honwana, Alcinda Manuel
2006 Child Soldiers in Africa. Philadelphia: University of Pennsylvania Press.

Igreja, Victor, Beataarice Dias-Lambranca, Douglas A. Hershey, Limore Racin, Annemiek Richters, and Ria Reis
2010 The Epidemiology of Spirit Possession in the Aftermath of Mass Political Violence in Mozambique. Social Science and Medicine 71:592–99.

James, Erica Caple
  2008 Haunting Ghosts: Madness, Gender, and Ensekirite in Haiti in the Democratic Era. *In* Postcolonial Disorders. Mary-Jo DelVecchio Good, Sandra T. Hyde, and Byron J. Good, eds. Pp. 132–56. Berkeley: University of California Press.
Jenkins, Janis H.
  1996 Culture, Emotion, and PTSD. *In* Ethnocultural Aspects of Posttraumatic Stress Disorder: Issues, Research, and Clinical Applications. Anthony J. Marsella, Matthew J. Friedman, Ellen T. Gerrity, and Raymond M. Scurfield, eds. Pp. 165–82. Washington, D.C.: American Psychological Association.
  2011 Pharmaceutical Self: The Global Shaping of Experience in an Age of Psychopharmacology. Santa Fe, N.M.: School for Advanced Research Press.
Jones, Edgar, and Simon Wessely
  2005 Shell Shock to PTSD: Military Psychiatry from 1900 to the Gulf War. Hove, East Sussex: Psychology Press.
Kaiser, Bonnie, Kristen E. McLean, Brandon. A. Kohrt, Ashley K. Hagaman, Bradley H. Wagenaar, Nayla M. Khoury, and Hunter M. Keys
  2014 *Reflechi Twòp*—Thinking too Much: Description of a Cultural Syndrome in Haiti's Central Plateau. Culture, Medicine, and Psychiatry 38:448–72.
Keane, Terence M., Danny G. Kaloupec, and Frank W. Weathers
  1996 Ethnocultural Considerations on the Assessment of PTSD. *In* Ethnocultural Aspects of Posttraumatic Stress Disorder: Issues, Research, and Clinical Applications. Anthony J. Marsella, Matthew J. Friedman, Ellen T. Gerrity, and Raymond M. Scurfield, eds. Pp. 183–208. Washington, D.C.: American Psychological Association.
Kilshaw, Susie
  2009 Impotent Warriors: Gulf War Syndrome, Vulnerability, and Masculinity. New York: Berghahn.
Kirmayer, Laurence J.
  1996a Confusion of the Senses: Implications of Ethnocultural Variations in Somatoform and Dissociative Disorders for PTSD. *In* Ethnocultural Aspects of Posttraumatic Stress Disorder: Issues, Research, and Clinical Applications. Anthony J. Marsella, Matthew J. Friedman, Ellen T. Gerrity, and Raymond M. Scurfield, eds. Pp. 131–64. Washington, D.C.: American Psychological Association.
  1996b Landscapes of Memory: Trauma, Narrative and Dissociation. *In* Tense Past: Cultural Essays in Trauma and Memory. Paul Antze and Michael Lambek, eds. Pp. 173–98. London: Routledge.
  2001 Cultural Variations in the Clinical Presentation of Depression and Anxiety: Implications for Diagnosis and Treatment. Journal of Clinical Psychiatry 13:22–28.
  2008 Culture and the Metaphoric Mediation of Pain. Transcultural Psychiatry 45:318–38.

Kirmayer, Laurence J., Robert Lemelson, and Mark Barad, eds.
    2007 Understanding Trauma: Integrating Biological, Clinical, and Cultural Per-
    spectives. New York: Cambridge University Press.
Kirmayer, Laurence J., and N. Sartorius
    2007 Cultural Models and Somatic Syndromes. Psychosomatic Medicine 69:832–40.
Kishik, David
    2008 Wittgenstein's Form of Life (To Imagine a Form of Life, I). London: Con-
    tinuum.
Kleinman, Arthur
    1988 Rethinking Psychiatry: From Cultural Category to Personal Experience. New
    York: Free Press.
Kleinman, Arthur, and Anne E. Becker
    1998 "Sociosomatics": The Contributions of Anthropology to Psychosomatic Medi-
    cine. Psychosomatic Medicine 60:389–93.
Kleinman, Arthur, and Joan Kleinman
    1994 How Bodies Remember: Social Memory and Bodily Experience of Criticism,
    Resistance, and Delegitimation Following China's Cultural Revolution. New Lit-
    erary History 25:707–23.
Kugelmann, Robert
    2009 The Irritable Heart Syndrome in the American Civil War. In Culture and
    Panic Disorder Devon E. Hinton and Byron J Good, eds. Pp. 85–112. Palo Alto,
    Calif.: Stanford University Press.
Kwon, Heonik
    2006 After the Massacre: Commemoration and Consolation in Ha My and My Lai.
    Berkeley: University of California Press.
    2008 Ghosts of War in Vietnam. Cambridge: Cambridge University Press.
Langer, Lawrence L.
    1991 Holocaust Testimonies: The Ruins of Memory. New Haven, Conn.: Yale Uni-
    versity Press.
Ledoux, Joseph
    1996 The Emotional Brain. New York: Simon and Schuster.
Lischer, Sarah Kenyon
    2005 Dangerous Sanctuaries: Refugee Camps, Civil War, and the Dilemmas of Hu-
    manitarian Aid. Ithaca, N.Y.: Cornell University Press.
Lubkemann, Stephen C.
    2008 Culture in Chaos: An Anthropology of the Social Condition in War. Chicago:
    University of Chicago Press.
Mayer, Emeran
    2007 Somatic Manifestations of Traumatic Stress. In Understanding Trauma: Bio-
    logical, Clinical and Cultural Perspectives. Laurence Kirmayer, Robert Lemel-
    son, and Mark Barad, eds. Pp. 142–70. New York: Cambridge University Press.

McNally, Richard

2012 The Ontology of Posttraumatic Stress Disorder: Natural Kind, Social Construction, or Causal System? Clinical Psychology Science and Practice 19(3):220–28.

McNally, Richard. J., and Bartley C. Frueh

2013 Why Are Iraq and Afghanistan War Veterans Seeking PTSD Disability Compensation at Unprecedented Rates? Journal of Anxiety Disorders 27(5):520–26.

Nations, Marilyn K.

2008 Infant Death and Interpretive Violence in Northeast Brazil: Taking Bereaved Cearense Mothers' Narratives to Heart. Cadernos de Saude Publica 24:2239–48.

Neuner, Frank, Anett Pfeiffer, Elisabeth Schauer-Kaiser, Michael Odenwald, Thomas Elbert, and Verena Ertl

2012 Haunted by Ghosts: Prevalence, Predictors and Outcomes of Spirit Possession Experiences Among Former Child Soldiers and War-Affected Civilians in Northern Uganda. Social Science and Medicine 75(3):548–54.

Nickerson, Angela, and Devon E. Hinton

2011 Anger Regulation in Traumatized Cambodian Refugees: The Perspectives of Buddhist Monks. Culture, Medicine, and Psychiatry 35:396–416.

Norris, Fran H., Julia L. Perilla, Gladys E. Ibanez, and Arthur D. Murphy

2001 Sex Differences in Symptoms of Posttraumatic Stress: Does Culture Play a Role? Journal of Traumatic Stress 14:7–28.

Park, Lawrence

2009 Dizziness and Panic in China: Organ and Ontological Disequilibrium. In Culture and Panic Disorder. Devon E. Hinton and Byron J. Good, eds. Pp. 157–82. Palo Alto, Calif.: Stanford University Press.

Patel, Vikram, E. Simunyu, and F. Gwanzura

1995 Kufungisisa (Thinking Too Much): A Shona Idiom for Non-Psychotic Mental Illness. Central African Journal of Medicine 41(7):209–15.

Perera, Sasanka

2001 Spirit Possessions and Avenging Ghosts: Stories of Supernatural Activity as Narratives of Terror and Mechanisms of Coping and Remembering. In Remaking a World: Violence, Social Suffering, and Recovery. Veena Das, Arthur Kleinman, Margaret Lock, Mamphela Ramphele, and Pamela Reynolds, eds. Pp. 157–200. Berkeley: University of California Press.

Reis, Ria

2013 Children Enacting Idioms of Witchcraft and Spirit Possession in Response to Trauma: Therapeutically Beneficial, and for Whom? Culture, Medicine, and Psychiatry 50:622–43.

Resick, Patricia A., Michelle J. Bovin, Amber L. Calloway, Alexandra M. Dick, Matthew W. King, Karen S. Mitchell, Michael K. Suvak, Stephanie Y. Wells, Shannon W. Stirman, and Erika J. Wolf

2012 A Critical Evaluation of the Complex PTSD Literature: Implications for DSM-5. Journal of Traumatic Stress 25(3):241–51.

Rubel, Arthur J., Carl W. O'Nell, and Rolando Collado-Ardón
1984 Susto: A Folk Illness. Berkeley: University of California Press.

Sacks, Oliver W.
1985 Migraine: Understanding a Common Disorder. Berkeley: University of California Press.

Sherin, Jonathan E., and Charles B. Nemeroff
2011 Post-Traumatic Stress Disorder: The Neurobiological Impact of Psychological Trauma. Dialogues in Clinical Neuroscience 13(3):263–78.

Shorter, Edward
1992 From Paralysis to Fatigue: A History of Psychosomatic Illness in the Modern Era. Toronto: Maxwell Macmillan.

Shrestha, Nirakar M., Bhogendra Sharma, Mark Van Ommeren, Shyam Regmi, Ramesh Makaju, Ivan H. Komproe, Ganesh B. Shrestha, and Joop de Jong
1998 Impact of Torture on Refugees Displaced Within the Developed World: Symptomatology Among Bhutanese Refugees in Nepal. Journal of the American Medical Association 280:443–48.

Straker, Gill
1992 Faces in the Revolution: The Psychological Effects of Violence on Township Youth in South Africa, Cape Town. Athens: Ohio University Press.

Suleiman, Susan Rubin
2006 Crises of Memory and the Second World War. Cambridge, Mass.: Harvard University Press.

Summerfield, Derek
1999 A Critique of Seven Assumptions Behind Psychological Trauma Programs in War-Affected Areas. Social Science and Medicine 48:1449–62.

Trawick, Margaret
2007 Enemy Lines: Childhood, Warfare, and Play in Batticaloa. Berkeley: University of California Press.

Ursano, Robert J., and James R. Rundell
1986 The Prisoner of War. In Coping with Life Crises: An Integrated Approach. Rudolph H. Moos and Jeanne A. Schaefer, eds. Pp. 431–54. New York: Plenum Press.

van der Kolk, Bessel, Mark S. Greenberg, Helene Boyd, and John H. Krystal
1985 Inescapable Shock, Neurotransmitters, and Addiction to Trauma: Toward a Psychobiology of Post Traumatic Stress. Biological Psychiatry 20(3):314–25.

van Duijl, Marjolein, Ellert Nijenhuis, Ivan H. Komproe, Hajo B. Gernaat, and Joop T. de Jong
2010 Dissociative Symptoms and Reported Trauma Among Patients with Spirit Possession and Matched Healthy Controls in Uganda. Culture, Medicine, and Psychiatry 34(2):380–400.

van Os, Jim
    2013 The Dynamics of Subthreshold Psychopathology: Implications for Diagnosis and Treatment. American Journal of Psychiatry 170(7):695–98.
Watters, Ethan
    2010 Crazy Like Us: The Globalization of the American Psyche. New York: Free Press.
Weiner, Saul J., Alan Schwartz, Frances Weaver, Julie Goldberg, Rachel Yudkowsky, Gunjan Sharma, Amy Binns-Calvey, Ben Preyss, Marilyn M. Schapira, Stephen D. Persell, Elizabeth Jacobs, and Richard I. Abrams
    2010 Contextual Errors and Failures in Individualizing Patient Care: A Multicenter Study. Annals of Internal Medicine 153(2):69–75.
Yager, Jane
    2009 Review of "Moscow Dreams." Times Literary Supplement. May 29.
Yehuda, Rachel, and Linda M. Bierer
    2009 The Relevance of Epigenetics to PTSD: Implications for the DSM-V. Journal of Traumatic Stress 22(5):427–34.
Young, Allan
    1995 The Harmony of Illusions: Inventing Post-Traumatic Stress Disorder. Princeton, N.J.: Princeton University Press.

PART II

Historical Perspectives

CHAPTER 2

Is PTSD a Transhistorical Phenomenon?

Richard J. McNally

Controversy has haunted the diagnosis of posttraumatic stress disorder (PTSD) ever since its appearance in the *Diagnostic and Statistical Manual of Mental Disorders* (DSM) more than thirty years ago (American Psychiatric Association [APA] 1980; Brewin 2003; McNally 2003b). One persistent concern is whether PTSD is a timeless, psychobiological entity, a natural kind discovered by astute clinicians, or whether it is a socially constructed phenomenon arising in the wake of the Vietnam War (Summerfield 2001). Most traumatologists—clinicians and scientists who study or treat the effects of psychological trauma—favor the first view. As Osterman and de Jong (2007) put it, we should "end the debate about the validity of the diagnosis of PTSD" (439), asserting that the disorder "appears to be a universal reaction to severe stressors that has transcultural diagnostic validity" (435). Hence, although the disorder has social *causes*, such as rape and combat, its resultant symptomatic profile is not a social *construction*, according to this view.

Other scholars, often historians or anthropologists, have favored the second view. As Young (1995) expressed it: "The disorder is not timeless, nor does it possess an intrinsic unity. Rather, it is glued together by the practices, technologies, and narratives with which it is diagnosed, studied, treated, and represented and by the various interests, institutions, and moral arguments that mobilized these efforts and resources" (5). He added, "traumatic memory is a man-made object. It originates in the scientific and clinical discourses of the nineteenth century; before that time, there is unhappiness, despair, and disturbing recollections, but no traumatic memory, in the sense that we know it today" (141).

As sometimes occurs in the social constructionist literature (McNally 2011:129), Young appears to conflate concept with referent, diagnosis with disorder. It is trivially true that all diagnostic concepts, including that of traumatic memory and PTSD itself, are man-made, but this does not necessarily mean that the phenomena to which they refer are also products of culture. Scientists constructed the periodic table, but the chemical elements themselves are not social constructs. They discovered the elements; they did not construct them. In fact, culture penetrates the symptomatic core of different DSM syndromes to varying degrees (McNally 2011:128–58).

These ambiguities notwithstanding, views such as Young's often incite anger among traumatologists because he seems to unmask PTSD as an artifact, a product of culture, not nature. This might not be such a problem if he were considering other anxiety disorders that do not imply the moral categories of innocent victim and perpetrator. If someone develops panic disorder or spider phobia, there is no one to blame. Yet when someone develops PTSD, there is almost always someone or something to blame for the suffering of victims. As Hayek (1978:31) observed, only when adverse outcomes arise from human conduct can we deem them morally unjust and not merely undesirable. Hence, traumatologists seemingly presuppose that to question the status of PTSD as a natural kind and to assert its artifactual character delegitimizes the suffering of victims, aligning the skeptic with the perpetrators.

Accordingly, traumatologists have sought to rebut social constructionist interpretations of PTSD in three ways. First, they have adduced biological data in support of the claim that PTSD is a natural kind, sometimes drawing moral conclusions from this research. As Yehuda and McFarlane (1997) said, "biological findings have provided objective validation that PTSD is more than a politically or socially motivated conceptualization of human suffering" (xv). They added that biological research provides "concrete validation of human suffering and a legitimacy that does not depend on arbitrary social and political forces. Establishing that there is a biological basis for psychological trauma is an essential first step in allowing the permanent validation of human suffering" (xv).

It is unclear how one can draw moral conclusions from biological research. Certainly, empathy for victims did not have to await the discoveries of biological psychiatry, and the reality of suffering does not depend on these discoveries. In fact, claims that biological research validates human suffering conflate the ontological and epistemic senses of subjectivity and objectivity.

Pain is ontologically subjective, but epistemically objective (Searle 1992:14). Accessible only to sufferers, pain is irreducibly a first-person phenomenon, but it is no less real for that fact. First-person phenomena, such as pain, fear, emotional numbing, and so forth, are emergent properties of the brain and hence epistemically objective facts about the world. Yet for something to be real, it does not have to be accessible to all observers. Biological studies concern third-person phenomena publically accessible to other observers, and hence ontologically objective. If the research is methodologically sound and free of bias, then it is empirically objective as well. But the reality of ontologically subjective suffering does not require ontologically objective biological data to validate it as a real feature of the world.

Second, traumatologists have conducted cross-cultural studies seeking to test whether PTSD occurs in non-Western societies (Osterman and de Jong 2007). Many of these studies involve the translation of standardized questionnaires and structured interviews from English to local languages around the globe. This systematic approach has great strengths, but it runs the risk of investigators missing posttraumatic symptoms that fall outside the DSM criteria. Having respondents provide answers to open-ended questions prior to having them respond to standardized inquiries would permit detection of local idioms of distress missed by our structured approaches. Another problem that can arise is that respondents may misunderstand the purpose of standardized assessments. For example, survivors of the tsunami in Sri Lanka thought that they had to provide the "correct" answer to assessment questions to receive much-needed clothing, food, and other forms of material aid (Watters 2010:65–125).

Third, traumatologists have sought to identify instances of PTSD throughout history. Many have argued that syndromes, such as shell shock in World War I and battle fatigue in World War II, were really PTSD under different names. Some have recognized the symptoms of PTSD in fictional characters such as Hotspur in Shakespeare's *Henry IV, Part I* (Kulka et al. 1990:284–85), and Achilles in Homer's *Iliad* (Shay 1994). If PTSD emerges in historical settings drastically different from our own, then the claim that it is solely a social product of the post–Vietnam War culture would be incorrect.

Yet a failure to detect PTSD throughout history is not necessarily fatal to claims about its validity. There are genuine disease entities that do not appear transhistorical despite their worldwide prevalence today. One example is AIDS, and another is schizophrenia. A comprehensive search of historical, medical, and fictional literature in Greek and Roman antiquity uncovered

clear descriptions of epilepsy, alcoholism, mania, delirium, and social phobia, but no descriptions of schizophrenia (Evans et al. 2003). In fact, few, if
any, convincing descriptions of schizophrenia appear prior to the nineteenth century (Hare 1988). Schizophrenia is seemingly a disease of recent
origin whose prevalence increased throughout the nineteenth-century Western world, remaining rare elsewhere until the twentieth century. Hence,
there is an asymmetry in how we interpret the historical data. Recognizing
a syndrome throughout time supports its validity, whereas noting its recent
appearance does not necessarily undermine such claims. Some genuine diseases are of recent vintage.

The chapters in this volume chiefly concern the transcultural character
of PTSD, whereas my chapter concerns its transhistorical character. I consider the limited data bearing directly on this issue, and I discuss the conceptual challenges that confront anyone asking whether PTSD is a timeless
syndrome.

Historical Findings

At least since the American Civil War, doctors have documented anxiety,
nightmares, guilt, depressed mood, and difficulty concentrating among psychiatrically troubled combat veterans (Dean 1997:91–114). Most military
physicians who treated psychologically disturbed soldiers during World Wars
I and II were convinced that traumatic stress reactions waned shortly after
the soldier left the battlefield. The stress of combat alone, they believed, was
insufficient to cause lasting psychological damage in normal men. They interpreted persistent, chronic psychiatric disability as indicative of psychological
vulnerability, preexisting psychopathology, or malingering. Furthermore, if
a soldier emerged from war psychologically intact, he was very unlikely to
suffer war-related symptoms later in life (Wessely 2005).

America's experience in Vietnam dramatically transformed these views
even though psychiatric casualties were strikingly rare during the war itself.
The rate was only 12 per 1,000 men, whereas it got as high as 101 per 1,000
during World War II (Dean 1997:40). Moreover, the vast majority of these
problems were unrelated to combat. Only 3.5 percent of all psychiatric casualties in Vietnam received a diagnosis of combat exhaustion (Marlowe 2001:86).

However, many veterans began experiencing serious and persistent
problems months and years after their return home. As Marlowe (2001:73)

observed, "Vietnam produced an extremely low proportion of proximate combat stress casualties and produced or is claimed to have produced massive numbers of postcombat casualties. Therefore, Vietnam breaks with the past normative pattern of combat and war zone stress casualty production."

To account for this historically unprecedented pattern, antiwar psychiatrists, such as Shatan (1973) and Lifton (1973) argued that the Vietnam War produced a new kind of traumatic stress disorder that had a delayed onset and a chronic course. They viewed the Vietnam War as an immoral conflict that fostered atrocities that later haunted the American soldiers who committed them. Moreover, because the conflict did not afford soldiers the opportunity to grieve for their dead comrades, they developed psychic numbing during the war and began to suffer other symptoms of traumatic stress only after their return to civilian life. Instead of viewing troubled veterans as suffering from preexisting problems merely exacerbated by the war, Shatan and Lifton argued that the war itself could produce lasting psychological harm.

Throughout the 1970s, Shatan, Lifton, and other clinicians joined forces with leaders of Vietnam veterans' organizations to urge the APA to include a new diagnosis of post-Vietnam syndrome in the then-forthcoming DSM-III. Troubled veterans needed such a delayed-onset stress diagnosis in the manual; without it, they would be ineligible to receive treatment and service-connected disability payments from the Veterans Administration (VA; Sparr and Pitman 2007). As Shatan emphasized, Vietnam veterans "can expect little help from the VA without proof that their affliction is 'service-connected' and can be diagnosed according to the revised APA classification" (i.e., DSM-II; quoted in Nicosia 2001:178).

Members of the DSM-III task force were initially resistant to recognizing post-Vietnam syndrome in the new manual. Some thought that combinations of established diagnoses covered the problems of veterans, thus making the new diagnosis unnecessary. Furthermore, one goal of the new manual was to develop a descriptive diagnostic system unburdened by etiological assumptions. Yet etiology was essential to the post-Vietnam syndrome. Finally, the notion of including a medical diagnosis arising from a specific historical event was odd.

Advocates for the new diagnosis accomplished their aim, but only after altering their strategy. They abandoned the idea of a disorder confined to Vietnam veterans, and they joined forces with mental health professionals who had been working with survivors of natural disasters, rape, and the Nazi Holocaust. They now argued that any terrifying, life-threatening event

occurring outside the range of everyday life could produce a chronic syndrome like the one exhibited by traumatized Vietnam veterans. One influential member of the DSM-III task force concurred, noting how she had
observed strikingly similar traumatic stress symptoms in her patients who
had suffered extreme burns. The DSM-III committee rejected post-Vietnam
syndrome but included PTSD in the new manual. Unlike the historically
situated post-Vietnam syndrome, PTSD was a universal syndrome arising
from exposure to any kind of traumatic stressor. Fulfilling the aims of Shatan,
Lifton, and the veterans' organizations, Congress listed PTSD as a disorder
compensable by the VA after its formal recognition in DSM-III. Importantly,
DSM-III specified that the syndrome could have a delayed onset, thereby enabling veterans to have access to VA treatment and compensation, even when
symptoms surfaced years after their return to civilian life.

The political story behind the recognition of PTSD invites a social constructionist interpretation of the disorder, but it does not confirm it. The political dimension does not mean that the disorder is nothing but a cultural
artifact. Political factors figured in the recognition of AIDS, and no one
doubts the validity of this disease entity. In fact, in the case of PTSD, the political forces aligned to support its recognition in DSM-III encountered a federal government reluctant to acknowledge the expensive psychiatric damage
associated with the war. Therefore, one could argue that a powerful political
movement was vital to overcoming opposing political forces aiming to downplay the psychiatric consequences of the conflict.

There is a growing consensus that PTSD possesses cross-cultural validity (Osterman and de Jong 2007). Ironically, the historical record provides
less support for the hypothesis that PTSD is a timeless universal response to
trauma. Indeed, differences in psychiatric symptoms among trauma victims
across time are striking (Jones and Wessely 2005). For example, shell shock
victims in World War I exhibited symptoms suggestive of neurological disease, such as paralysis, tremor, inability to walk, and inability to speak. These
abnormalities have rarely appeared in traumatized veterans of subsequent
wars. The Persian Gulf War of 1991 resulted in British and American veterans complaining of a baffling array of medically unexplained symptoms perhaps suggestive of exposure to toxins.

British researchers, led by the historian Edgar Jones and the psychiatrist
and epidemiologist Simon Wessely, have done rigorous empirical work on the
historicity of PTSD. They examined the British military medical files of 1,856
men evaluated for service-connected disability pensions (Jones et al. 2003).

These men had received annual evaluations of their postcombat symptoms until their symptoms remitted or stabilized. For some veterans, the archival data included a decade of annual assessment reports. The troubled veterans described the full range of their psychological and somatic symptoms. Jones and his colleagues developed a checklist of PTSD symptoms, noting which ones appeared in each veteran's file. They were especially interested in seeing whether flashbacks—vivid, involuntary, seemingly unchanging sensory memories of combat—appeared in the archives.

Although flashbacks are a hallmark symptom of PTSD today (Brewin 2011), they almost never receive mention in the medical records of British military psychiatric cases until the Persian Gulf War. For example, only 3 of the 640 cases from World War I reported phenomena suggestive of flashbacks (0.5 percent), and only 5 of 367 cases from World War II did so (1.4 percent). None of the 428 psychiatric casualties of the Victorian campaigns and the Boer War complained of flashbacks. However, 36 of the 400 Persian Gulf War veterans experienced them (9 percent).

Moreover, if anything, Jones and his colleagues were too liberal when interpreting problems as flashbacks. They may have overestimated their frequency prior to the Persian Gulf War. For example, one World War I shell shock victim complained of vertigo, tremors, headaches, weakness, irritability, depressed mood, poor sleep, claustrophobia, loss of interest in people, dreams about the war, and "flashbacks." Jones's research team classified the following phenomenon as a flashback. The veteran complained about awakening from sleep, seeing people standing in his bedroom, and experiencing fear.

It is doubtful that these experiences qualify as flashbacks. There is no mention of vivid, sensory memories erupting when he awakened from sleep. Indeed, there is no reference to the war at all.

Most likely, the veteran was suffering from episodes of isolated sleep paralysis, not flashbacks (Hufford 1982; McNally and Clancy 2005a). These events are akin to a hiccup in the architecture of rapid eye movement (REM) sleep, the stage of sleep when we do most of our dreaming. During REM sleep, people experience full body paralysis (except for their eyes), but they do not realize this because they are asleep. However, during one of these episodes, the cognitive and muscular aspects of REM become desynchronized. That is, the sleeper awakens while muscle paralysis remains in effect, thereby terrifying the person. In many cases, the person experiences the intrusion of REM mentation into emerging wakefulness, experiencing hypnopompic ("upon awakening") hallucinations, as intruders in the person's bedroom. Usually these episodes last for a few minutes, at most, before the paralysis wanes, the hallucinations vanish, and the terror-stricken person is left wondering what just happened.

Although the British veteran did not mention an inability to move, his experience is far more suggestive of an isolated sleep paralysis episode than a sensory flashback of a battle scene. Sleep paralysis episodes are especially common in adults who report having been sexually abused as children (McNally and Clancy 2005b), and in people with anxiety disorders (Otto et al. 2006), especially those with chronic PTSD (Hinton et al. 2005). Erratic sleeping patterns increase the likelihood of isolated sleep paralysis, and this may explain why people with trauma histories, anxiety disorders, or both have them more than other people do.

Of the 1,007 psychiatric casualties from World Wars I and II, only 8 had flashbacks (liberally defined), and only 5 of these men appear to have qualified for DSM-IV-TR (APA 2000) PTSD. Indeed, in the entire data set, core PTSD symptoms, such as intrusive memories and avoidance of reminders, were uncommon. These findings prompted Jones et al. (2003) to conclude that PTSD may be a "contemporary culture-bound syndrome" (162).

What are the implications of these findings for the historicity of PTSD? If a veteran does not *express* certain symptoms, does that mean that he did not *experience* them? Does the historical niche constrain experience as well as expression of symptoms by influencing the probability of a trauma survivor experiencing certain symptoms that people throughout history have always been capable of experiencing?

One cannot prove the null hypothesis that traumatized soldiers in the past did not experience certain symptoms. The absence of evidence is not evidence of absence. Yet as Jones et al. emphasized, veterans interviewed for disability pensions were highly motivated to describe the full range of their symptoms, especially dramatic ones such as flashbacks. Nevertheless, the most stringent test would have involved doctors explicitly asking about certain symptoms that patients might not have expressed.

For example, Hinton et al. (2005) found that Cambodian refugees living in America who had developed chronic PTSD following the trauma of the Pol Pot regime did not mention their frequent, terrifying episodes of isolated sleep paralysis until asked about the phenomenon directly. These patients had described other symptoms of PTSD, including nightmares, but they never mentioned having awakened at night, experiencing paralysis, and seeing threatening demons, Khmer Rouge cadres, or ghosts of those who died during the Pol Pot terror. In fact, 76 percent of the PTSD patients, relative to 25.9 percent of psychiatric patients with non-PTSD diagnoses, reported at least one episode of isolated sleep paralysis during the previous twelve months. Despite their failure to mention these episodes spontaneously to the doctor, perhaps because they viewed the phenomenon as supernatural rather than medical, 65 percent of the PTSD patients had sleep paralysis at least once per month, the highest rate in the psychiatric literature.

In another study of the British military medical records, Jones et al. (2002) identified three partly overlapping clusters that have occurred among psychiatric casualties from the Boer War through the Persian Gulf War. The "debility" cluster included complaints about weakness, chronic fatigue, anxiety, and breathlessness. The "somatic" cluster comprised symptoms such as anxiety, rapid heart rate, dizziness, and breathlessness. The "neuropsychiatric" cluster included anxiety, depression, fatigue, sleep difficulties, irritability, startle responses, personality changes, and chronic pain. The upshot is that chronic psychobiological problems arising in response to the trauma of war have varied widely throughout history. None of these statistically identified syndromes map onto PTSD as we understand it today.

In fact, our concept of PTSD has evolved since Shatan (1972) described the hallmark symptoms of post-Vietnam syndrome. Shatan mentioned six key characteristics exhibited by many troubled veterans that he had seen. First, they experienced intense guilt about killing in Vietnam and about surviving the war, when so many of their fellow soldiers did not. These feelings sometimes motivated self-punishment, manifested in substance abuse, one-car accidents, and reckless, quasi-suicidal behavior. Second, they felt scapegoated and betrayed by their country. Third, they experienced rage at society and especially at those who they believed tried to manipulate them. Fourth, they experienced emotional numbing. Fifth, they felt disconnected from other people. Sixth, they experienced an inability to love or trust others or to accept love in return.

There are differences as well as similarities between the post-Vietnam syndrome and PTSD in the DSM-5 (APA 2013). Although guilt disappeared from the DSM in 1987, it reappeared in DSM-5. Irritability has replaced the rage at society and established authority, whereas psychic numbing and difficulty experiencing loving feelings for others remain in today's criteria. However, many symptoms are missing from Shatan's list, including sleep disturbance, flashbacks, exaggerated startle, intrusive recollections, nightmares, physiological reactions to reminders of the trauma, and avoidance of these reminders. The failure of Shatan to mention these symptoms does not mean that troubled veterans did not experience them, but it does imply that they were not especially salient to Shatan.

Conceptual Challenges to Identifying PTSD Throughout History

Answering questions about the transhistorical character of PTSD presents challenges to scholars seeking to answer them. One might consult medical records throughout history, armed with the DSM-5 PTSD criteria checklist, and note whether people exposed to traumatic events throughout history would have qualified for PTSD today.

Problems immediately arise, however. According to the descriptive, atheoretical approach to diagnosis that has held sway since DSM-III, PTSD is defined exhaustively by its symptoms, plus its course. This "operational" approach means that each revision of the DSM creates a new PTSD, and because the disorder is defined by its symptoms, it makes no sense to say that one version is any more or less valid than another one. Operational definitions are stipulative; standards of correctness or truth do not apply to them.

Despite lip service to operational definitions, most psychopathologists are not operationists. They are philosophical realists whose implicit concept of disorder or disease holds that symptoms reflect an underlying, latent entity. Hence, symptoms do not define the disorder; they are manifestations of it. This intuition motivates claims that despite the symptomatic variability among shell shock, battle fatigue, and PTSD, these syndromes are actually variant presentations of the same timeless, trauma-induced psychobiological disorder.

This intuition also motivates the diagnostic revision process. Revision presupposes that successive versions of a diagnosis come progressively closer to capturing the underlying reality of the disorder. Diagnostic revisions are nonsensical under an operationist construal of mental disorder because a disorder is nothing but its symptoms. But under a realist construal, revisions can approximate truths about how the world really is.

Yet even this realist interpretation of PTSD encounters problems. Because the latent cause of the symptomatic variation is unobservable, we can never be sure that it is the source of symptomatic diversity. That is, if wildly different presentations occur throughout history, as Jones et al. (2002) found, how can we justify bracketing them under the same PTSD rubric? If headaches, "hysterical" paralysis, weakness, breathlessness, and so forth all count as manifestations of PTSD, does the diagnosis becomes nothing more than a conceptual placeholder for whatever reaction a person has following exposure to trauma? *Something* must connect these diverse presentations if we are to claim that each is a variant form of the same condition.

One option would be to designate exposure to a traumatic stressor as the unifying factor. Hence, PTSD would be any symptomatic profile arising in response to a traumatic stressor. This would justify grouping shell shock, battle fatigue, and PTSD under the same category as manifestations of the same timeless condition. Whatever results from traumatic exposure qualifies as PTSD.

Unfortunately, this approach encounters problems, too. First, only a minority of people who encounter traumatic stressors develops PTSD (Breslau et al. 1991), hence PTSD cannot be a "universal reaction to severe stressors" (Osterman and de Jong 2007:439). However, assuming that we can distinguish normal from abnormal stress reactions, we might label as PTSD any abnormal reaction to a trauma, resulting in a one (trauma) to many (diverse symptomatic presentations) mapping. This would entail a low threshold for affirming that PTSD is a transhistorical entity. Throughout history, PTSD would amount to any abnormal reaction to trauma, whatever the symptoms may be. PTSD, as we know it, would disintegrate as recognizable syndrome possessing core symptoms that occur across its instantiation across trauma victims throughout time.

Yet even this liberal approach to affirming the transhistorical character of PTSD produces problems. It assumes that the concept of trauma is temporally invariant. However, the definition of trauma, as embodied in criterion A of the PTSD diagnostic set, has undergone a conceptual bracket creep whereby the range of presumptively traumatic stressors has broadened considerably over the course of its revisions (McNally 2003a, 2009). Although DSM-III implied that PTSD could arise only following exposure to a circumscribed set of *traumatic* stressors, such as rape, combat, and torture, DSM-IV-TR allowed a broad range of events to qualify, many falling well within the bounds of ordinary life (e.g., unexpected death of a loved one). In fact, it did not even require that someone be physically present at the scene of the trauma to qualify as a trauma survivor, an implication discrepant from the original concept (McNally and Breslau 2008). Feeling helpless upon learning about threats to other people now certifies the recipient of such news as a survivor of trauma just as much as the people undergoing the threat itself. Hence, researchers have reported that 4 percent of Americans living far from the sites of the terrorist attacks of September 11, 2001, developed apparent PTSD (Schlenger et al. 2002), presumably by witnessing the violence on television.[1] In keeping with a very broad notion of trauma, giving birth to a healthy baby (Olde et al. 2006), undergoing extraction of a wisdom tooth (de Jongh et al. 2008), and encountering obnoxious jokes in the workplace (Mc-Donald 2003) are stressors that have allegedly produced PTSD symptoms or the complete syndrome itself. These reports have provoked skeptical reactions, including from historians of war trauma. For example, as Shephard (2004) remarked, "Any unit of classification that simultaneously encompasses the experience of surviving Auschwitz and that of being told rude jokes at work must, by any reasonable lay standard, be a nonsense, a patent absurdity" (57).

What, then, should we make of these reports? One interpretation is that people encountering subtraumatic stressors misconstrue normal reactions with pathological ones, especially when they complete checklists of PTSD symptoms rather than undergo diagnostic interviews. Another interpretation is that people who develop apparent PTSD following exposure to relatively mild stressors possess significant psychobiological vulnerabilities that amplify the impact of these stressors. That is, these cases may reflect a background/foreground inversion whereby the trauma recedes into the causal background, and the risk factors move into the causal foreground (McNally 2009). There is very limited evidence bearing directly on this hypothesis (Breslau 2011), and only mixed support has emerged for it (McNally and Robinaugh 2011). Indeed, inconsistent with this hypothesis, two epidemiological studies indicated that risk factors heighten the probability of PTSD irrespective of the severity of the stressor (Breslau, Chen, et al. 2013; Breslau, Troost, et al. 2013).

Further destabilizing our concept of trauma are studies showing that stressors falling short of criterion A can produce more PTSD symptoms or higher rates of the disorder than stressors that do meet criterion A (Gold et al. 2005; Long et al. 2008; Mol et al. 2005; van Hooff et al. 2009). Suffice it to say, the diversity of events that can cause PTSD symptoms or the full syndrome itself pose serious problems for scholars hoping to study the transhistoricity of PTSD. Clearly, a one-to-many approach to identifying PTSD throughout history will not work if what counts as a trauma can vary so dramatically.

Finally, consider vicarious trauma. Seeing other people being tortured or killed is an undeniably traumatic experience today. Yet witnessing the suffering of others has often been a form of entertainment throughout history. In ancient Rome, criminals, Christians, and others were tied to stakes in the amphitheaters to make it easy for ravenous lions to eat them alive before thousands of cheering spectators (Auguet 1972:93–96). As the poet Martial noted, even victims who remained alive after being mauled by lions no longer "had the semblance of a body" (Martial, quoted in Auguet 1972:95). Many people viewing such horrors today would develop PTSD. Yesterday's entertainment is today's trauma, surely a sign of moral progress. In fact, philosophers in classical antiquity regarded mercy and pity as pathological emotions (Stark 1997:212). Christianity celebrated these emotions, perhaps altering human psychology in the process.

Conclusions

Traumatologists encounter a puzzling paradox: the disorder appears to occur across cultures today, but its stability over time is unclear, even among war veterans in Western societies during the twentieth century. Hence, the evidence for cross-cultural validity appears stronger than for transhistorical validity. Is it possible that Western culture has so permeated non-Western societies throughout the developing world that PTSD as an idiom of distress has been absorbed as well, as some data suggest (Yeomans et al. 2008)?

Finally, understanding PTSD from a historical perspective may be especially challenging if what counts as traumatic varies as a function of context. For example, people whose understanding of trauma has been shaped by the horrors of World War II (Snyder 2010), including having survived Nazi death factories, such as Treblinka (Raichman 2011), which were far more horrific than the Nazi concentration camps (Grossman [1944] 2010), are unlikely to be much affected by the stressors not included in criterion A that can apparently cause PTSD today. Perhaps one unfortunate consequence of the otherwise undeniable benefits of modernity is diminished resilience. Our relatively greater comfort, safety, health, and well-being may have rendered us more vulnerable to stressors far less toxic than the ones occurring during World

War II, for example. If so, then the decline in violence occurring over the past thousand years, the mid-twentieth century notwithstanding (Pinker 2011), may have only broadened the kinds of stressors that can incite PTSD rather than diminishing its incidence over time.

Note

1. The DSM-5 (APA 2013) committee narrowed the definition of what counts as a qualifying traumatic stressor. For one to qualify for indirect exposure to trauma, a person must learn that a close friend or family member has died violently or accidentally or has survived a threat to his or her life. Moreover, exposure to trauma via television or other electronic media no longer qualifies the viewer as a trauma survivor unless the exposure concerns the viewer's occupation (e.g., viewing scenes of carnage for an emergency personnel worker).

References

American Psychiatric Association
    1980 Diagnostic and Statistical Manual of Mental Disorders. 3rd edition. Washington, D.C.: American Psychiatric Association.
    2000 Diagnostic and Statistical Manual of Mental Disorders. 4th edition, text rev. Washington, D.C.: American Psychiatric Association.
    2013 Diagnostic and Statistical Manual of Mental Disorders. 5th edition. Washington, D.C.: American Psychiatric Association.
Auguet, Roland
    1972 Cruelty and Civilization: The Roman Games. London: Routledge.
Breslau, Naomi
    2011 Causes of Posttraumatic Stress Disorder. In Causality and Psychopathology: Finding the Determinants of Disorders and Their Cures. P. E. Shrout, K. M. Keyes, and K. Ornstein, eds. Pp. 297–320. Oxford: Oxford University Press.
Breslau, Naomi, Qiaoling Chen, and Zhehui Luo
    2013 The Role of Intelligence in Posttraumatic Stress Disorder: Does It Vary by Trauma Severity? PLos ONE 8:e65391.
Breslau, Naomi, Glenn C. Davis, Patricia Andreski, and Edward Peterson
    1991 Traumatic Events and Posttraumatic Stress Disorder in an Urban Population of Young Adults. Archives of General Psychiatry 48:216–22.
Breslau, Naomi, John P. Troost, Kipling Bohnert, and Zhehui Luo
    2013 Influence of Predispositions on Post-Traumatic Stress Disorder: Does It Vary by Trauma Severity? Psychological Medicine 43:381–90.

Brewin, Chris R.

2003 Post-Traumatic Stress Disorder: Malady or Myth? New Haven, Conn.: Yale University Press.

2011 The Nature and Significance of Memory Disturbance in Posttraumatic Stress Disorder. Annual Review of Clinical Psychology 7:203–27.

Dean, Eric T., Jr.

1997 Shook over Hell: Post-Traumatic Stress, Vietnam, and the Civil War. Cambridge, Mass.: Harvard University Press.

de Jongh, Ad, Miranda Olff, Hans van Hoolwerff, Irene H. A. Aarman, Birit Broekman, Ramon Lindaur, and Frits Boer

2008 Anxiety and Post-Traumatic Stress Symptoms Following Wisdom Tooth Removal. Behaviour Research and Therapy 46:1305–10.

Evans, Katie, J. McGrath, and R. Milns

2003 Searching for Schizophrenia in Ancient Greek and Roman Literature: A Systematic Review. Acta Psychiatrica Scandinavica 107:323–30.

Gold, Sari D., Brian P. Marx, Jose M. Soler-Baillo, and Denise Sloan

2005 Is Life Stress More Traumatic Than Traumatic Stress? Journal of Anxiety Disorders 19:687–98.

Grossman, Vassily

(1944) 2010 The Hell of Treblinka. In The Road: Stories, Journalism, and Essays. R. Chandler, ed. Pp. 116–62. New York: New York Review of Books.

Hare, Edward

1988 Schizophrenia as a Recent Disease. British Journal of Psychiatry 153:521–31.

Hayek, Friedrich A.

1978 Law, Legislation and Liberty. Vol. 2, The Mirage of Social Justice. Chicago: University of Chicago Press.

Hinton, Devon E., Vuth Pich, Dara Chhean, Mark H. Pollack, and Richard J. McNally

2005 Sleep Paralysis Among Cambodian Refugees: Association with PTSD Diagnosis and Severity. Depression and Anxiety 22:47–51.

Hufford, David J.

1982 The Terror That Comes in the Night: An Experience-Centered Study of Supernatural Assault Traditions. Philadelphia: University of Pennsylvania Press.

Jones, Edgar, Robert Hodgins-Vermaas, Helen McCartney, Brian Everitt, Charlotte Beech, Denise Poynter, Ian Palmer, Kenneth Hyams, and Simon Wessely

2002 Post-Combat Syndromes from the Boer War to the Gulf War: A Cluster Analysis of Their Nature and Attribution. British Medical Journal 324 (February 9, 2002):1–7.

Jones, Edgar, Robert H. Vermaas, Helen McCartney, Charlotte Beech, Ian Palmer, Kenneth Hyams, and Simon Wessely

2003 Flashbacks and Post-Traumatic Stress Disorder: The Genesis of a Twentieth-Century Diagnosis. British Journal of Psychiatry 182:158–63.

Jones, Edgar, and Simon Wessely
    2005 Shell Shock to PTSD: Military Psychiatry from 1900 to the Gulf War. Hove,
        UK: Psychology Press.
Kulka, Richard A., William E. Schlenger, John A. Fairbank, Richard L. Hough, B.
        Kathleen Jordan, Charles R. Marmar, and Daniel S. Weiss
    1990 Trauma and the Vietnam War Generation: Report of Findings from the Na-
        tional Vietnam Veterans Readjustment Study. New York: Brunner/Mazel.
Lifton, Robert J.
    1973 Home from the War: Vietnam Veterans; Neither Victims nor Executioners.
        New York: Touchstone.
Long, Mary E, Jon D. Elhai, Amy Schweinle, Matt J. Gray, Anouk L. Grubaugh, and B.
        Christopher Frueh
    2008 Differences in Posttraumatic Stress Disorder Diagnostic Rates and Symptom
        Severity Between Criterion A1 and Non-Criterion A1 Stressors. Journal of Anxi-
        ety Disorders 22:1255–63.
Marlowe, David H.
    2001 Psychological and Psychosocial Consequences of Combat and Deployment:
        With Special Emphasis on the Gulf War. Santa Monica, Calif.: RAND.
McDonald, James J., Jr.
    2003 Posttraumatic Stress Dishonesty. Employee Relations Law Journal 28:93–111.
McNally, Richard J.
    2003a Progress and Controversy in the Study of Posttraumatic Stress Disorder.
        Annual Review of Psychology 54:229–52.
    2003b Remembering Trauma. Cambridge, Mass.: Belknap Press of Harvard University
        Press.
    2009 Can We Fix PTSD in DSM-V? Depression and Anxiety 26:597–600.
    2011 What Is Mental Illness? Cambridge, Mass.: Belknap Press of Harvard Univer-
        sity Press.
McNally, Richard J., and Naomi Breslau
    2008 Does Virtual Trauma Cause Posttraumatic Stress Disorder? American Psy-
        chologist 62:282–83.
McNally, Richard J., and Susan A. Clancy
    2005a Sleep Paralysis, Sexual Abuse, and Space Alien Abduction. Transcultural
        Psychiatry 42:113–22.
    2005b Sleep Paralysis in Adults Reporting Repressed, Recovered, or Continuous
        Memories of Childhood Sexual Abuse. Journal of Anxiety Disorders 19:595–602.
McNally, Richard J., and Donald J. Robinaugh
    2011 Risk Factors and Posttraumatic Stress Disorder: Are They Especially Predictive
        Following Exposure to Less Severe Stressors? Depression and Anxiety 28:1091–96.
Mol, Saskia S. L., Arnoud Arntz, Job F. M. Metsemakers, Geert-Jan Dinant, Pauline A. P.
        Vilters-van Montfort, and J. Andre Knottnerus

2005 Symptoms of Post-Traumatic Stress Disorder After Non-Traumatic Events: Evidence from an Open Population Study. British Journal of Psychiatry 186:494–99.

Nicosia, Gerald
2001 Home to War: A History of the Vietnam Veterans' Movement. New York: Crown.

Olde, Eelco, Onno van der Hart, Rolf Kleber, and Maarten van Son
2006 Posttraumatic Stress Disorder Following Childbirth: A Review. Clinical Psychology Review 26:1–16.

Osterman, Janet E., and Joop T. V. M. de Jong
2007 Cultural Issues and Trauma. In Handbook of PTSD: Science and Practice. Matthew J. Friedman, Terence M. Keane, and Patricia A. Resick, eds. Pp. 425–46. New York: Guilford.

Otto, Michael W., Naomi M. Simon, Mark Powers, Devon Hinton, Alyson Zalta, and Mark H. Pollack
2006 Rates of Isolated Sleep Paralysis in Outpatients with Anxiety Disorders. Journal of Anxiety Disorders 20:687–93.

Pinker, Steven
2011 The Better Angels of Our Nature: Why Violence Has Declined. New York: Viking.

Rajchman, Chil
2011 The Last Jew of Treblinka: A Survivor's Memory 1942–1943. Solon Beinfeld, trans. New York: Pegasus Books.

Schlenger, William E., Juesta M. Caddell, Lori Ebert, B. Kathleen Jordan, Kathryn M. Rourke, David Wilson, Lisa Thalji, L. Michael Dennis, John A. Fairbank, and Richard A Kulka
2002 Psychological Reactions to Terrorist Attacks: Findings from the National Study of Americans' Reactions to September 11. Journal of the American Medical Association 288:581–88.

Searle, John R.
1992 The Rediscovery of Mind. Cambridge, Mass.: MIT Press.

Shatan, Chaim F.
1972 Post-Vietnam Syndrome. New York Times, May 6.
1973 The Grief of Soldiers: Vietnam Combat Veterans' Self-Help Movement. American Journal of Orthopsychiatry 43:640–53.

Shay, Jonathan
1994 Achilles in Vietnam: Combat Trauma and the Undoing of Character. New York: Atheneum.

Shephard, Ben
2004 Risk Factors and PTSD: A Historian's Perspective. In Posttraumatic Stress Disorder: Issues and Controversies, Gerald M. Rosen, ed. Pp. 39–61. Chichester, UK: Wiley.

Snyder, Timothy
2010 Bloodlands: Europe Between Hitler and Stalin. New York: Basic.
Sparr, Landy F., and R. K. Pitman
2007 PTSD and the Law. *In* Handbook of PTSD: Science and Practice. Matthew J. Friedman, Terence M. Keane, and Patricia A. Resick, eds. Pp. 449–68. New York: Guilford.
Stark, Rodney
1997 The Rise of Christianity. New York: Harper Collins.
Summerfield, Derek
2001 The Invention of Post-Traumatic Stress Disorder and the Social Usefulness of a Psychiatric Category. British Medical Journal 322:95–98.
Van Hooff, Miranda, Alexander C. McFarlane, Jenelle Baur, Maria Abraham, and Daniel J. Barnes
2009 The Stressor Criterion A-1 and PTSD: A Matter of Opinion? Journal of Anxiety Disorders 23:77-86.
Watters, Ethan
2010 Crazy Like Us: The Globalization of the American Psyche. New York: Free Press.
Wessely, Simon
2005 Risk, Psychiatry and the Military. British Journal of Psychiatry 186:459–66.
Yehuda, Rachel, and Alexander C. McFarlane
1997 Introduction. *In* Psychobiology of Posttraumatic Stress Disorder. Rachel Yehuda and Alexander C. McFarlane, eds. Pp. xi–xv. New York: New York Academy of Sciences.
Yeomans, Peter D., James D. Herbert, and Evan M. Forman
2008 Symptom Comparison Across Multiple Solicitation Methods Among Burundians with Traumatic Event Histories. Journal of Traumatic Stress 21:231–34.
Young, Allan
1995 The Harmony of Illusions: Inventing Post-Traumatic Stress Disorder. Princeton, N.J.: Princeton University Press.

CHAPTER 3

What Is "PTSD"? The Heterogeneity Thesis

Allan Young and Naomi Breslau

The diagnostic validity of posttraumatic stress disorder (PTSD) presumes that the DSM symptom list represents a disorder that exists independently of the language and technology employed in diagnosis. These symptoms are manifestly ambiguous but derive their distinctiveness and diagnostic utility via their connection to PTSD's trauma etiology. Differential diagnosis is impossible without a traumatic etiology. However, the unifying etiology is intrinsically heterogeneous. Heterogeneity does not challenge the disorder's validity, the idea that PTSD is, in some sense, universal. In this chapter, we advance a framework for investigating (1) the heterogeneous character of PTSD and (2) the culturally pervasive rhetoric of "trauma," exemplified by PTSD.

Sources of Heterogeneity

"Heterogeneity" refers to disunity within an apparent unity. PTSD researchers mention two sources of heterogeneity. The first source is *structural heterogeneity*, a matter of moving between levels of abstraction, descending from a type to the subtypes that compose the type. Multiple kinds of traumatic events are listed on the DSM-5 checklist (under diagnostic criterion A). These include the threat of imminent death, the threat or experience of serious injury or sexual violation, witnessing such events happening to others, and learning about the violent death of a close relative or friend. (The previous edition specified that traumatic experiences must include strong negative emotions—fear, helplessness, or horror, but DSM-5 removed this requirement.) The A criterion generates many subtypes, keyed to the distinctive characteristics of particular kinds of traumatic events (e.g., combat, rape) and the demographic features of the victims—their gender, age, intelligence, and so on. The diagnostic criteria identifying PTSD are polythetic, and this is a further source of structural heterogeneity. For example, criterion D identifies cognitive changes (thoughts, mood); diagnosis requires a victim to manifest at least three symptoms from a list of seven symptoms (e.g., self-blame, a negative emotion [shame, anger], inability to express positive emotions). In this way, the criterion creates a variety of overlapping diagnostic profiles.

Structural heterogeneity is an overt feature of PTSD: it guides research programs and is a stimulus for debate. *Perspectival heterogeneity* is a covert feature of PTSD—real but generally unacknowledged. It comprises *parallel* versions of PTSD rather than subtypes. Before proceeding further with the subject of perspectival heterogeneity, it will be useful to compare it with "bracket creep," a term coined by Richard McNally (2003, 2009).

PTSD began life in DSM-III (1980). Diagnostic features were revised in subsequent editions, but the changes were generally minor with two notable exceptions. First, DSM-III presumed that victims would have one psychiatric diagnosis at a time, while later editions allowed the possibility of coexisting disorders. The change was significant because interest, then and now, focuses on "chronic PTSD" subtype, where the syndrome persist longer than six months, and is generally accompanied comorbid diagnoses, notably depression and anxiety. Juxtaposing PTSD with mood disorders created suspicions about causality. Were depression and anxiety reactions to trauma, or were these people predisposed to react to distressful experiences in a pathological way? Second, DSM-III had defined traumatic events as falling "outside the range of usual human experience" and likely to "evoke significant symptoms of distress in almost anyone." The events mentioned in the DSM—combat, rape, bombing, torture, death camps—encouraged the idea that PTSD would be a *normal response* to extraordinary events. The following edition (DSM-IIIR, 1987) revised this definition. As in DSM-III, traumatic events would include "serious threats to one's life or physical integrity" and similar threats to close relatives and friends. But these events now included less devastating events, such as the sudden destruction of one's home or community, *witnessing* someone seriously injured or killed in an accident or through physical violence, and seeing victims soon after the events. In this manner, the syndrome was reframed as a *pathological response* to experiences that are uncommon but not necessarily extraordinary, and are successfully managed by most people.

These changes undermined the idea that traumatic events are objective phenomena, possessing an intrinsic potency. Events *become* traumatic because they are consciously or unconsciously *perceived* as being horrendous, ontologically destabilizing, and so on. Thus the subjective contribution to trauma explained why 20 percent of U.S. soldiers engaged in combat in Vietnam developed chronic PTSD and also why 80 percent did not. The bracket creep problem, according to McNally, is that the two changes to the DSM-III concept of trauma opened the diagnostic door to trivial events that could be regarded as subjectively traumatic. Bracket creep introduced a form of heterogeneity, comprising parallel conceptions of PTSD, divided by their respective interpretations of the stressor criterion. On the other hand, the two versions are epistemologically unequal. The DSM-III version provides a standard for judging whether events are plausibly traumatic. Without denying the utility of McNally's distinction, we will be proposing something quite different.

What Is "PTSD"?

We begin by offering an ostensive answer—pointing to the places where PTSD is found, and the things in which PTSD is presumed to manifest itself. There are five primary locations:

1. *A DSM or ICD text* listing symptomatic features, grouped according to diagnostic criteria.
2. *Exemplars*: clinical cases whose symptoms are visible (not merely inferred) and unambiguous (not plausibly attributed to alternative classifications). In practice, exemplars are limited to cases with documented traumatic stressors and with no comorbid depression or anxiety disorder.
3. *Clinical cases*: people diagnosed with the PTSD syndrome as described in the DSM and ICD texts. Exemplars are clinical cases, but a majority of clinical cases are not exemplars.
4. *Epidemiological populations*: aggregates of people transformed into "composite individuals," to provide platforms for testing hypotheses, delineating puzzles, mapping distributions, and the like.

5. A *disorder*, equivalent to the biological and cognitive mechanisms that are believed to drive this syndrome. While no reliable biomarker is available for diagnosing clinical cases of PTSD, evidence of a distinctive disorder based in the hypothalamic-pituitary-adrenal axis (HPA axis) has been demonstrated in epidemiological populations.

Thus "PTSD" is encountered as a text, a disorder, exemplars, clinical cases, and epidemiological populations. These manifestations are connected to one another by family resemblances: their features overlap rather than converge, but they are perceived as sharing an essence or core identity. However the concept of PTSD is more realistically identified as a "form of life," shaped by culture and historical contingency, and therefore incorrectly perceived as timeless.

This pervasive misperception (timelessness) is grounded on a false dichotomy that divides psychiatric science from psychiatric culture. Our term "culture" refers to a system of tacit meanings, dispositions (values, sentiments), and pragmatics (ways of knowing what to do or say next). Researchers understand that culture is connected to psychiatry in two ways. There is culture *and* psychiatry, as when it is presumed that the posttraumatic syndrome can be expressed in superficially different ways in different cultures. There is likewise the possibility of culture *in* psychiatry, for example the idea that the social phobia syndrome and anorexia nervosa are distinctively Western phenomena. In the following pages, we argue that there is a third possibility that is generally ignored, a culture *of* psychiatry—culture intrinsic to the operations of psychiatric science. Researchers have generally ignored this possibility, believing that science and culture are incompatible ways of knowing and doing.

PTSD's Memory Logic

The structure of PTSD has remained unchanged from DSM-III onward. The disorder's diagnostic criteria comprise two main elements: the etiological event (the A criterion) and a posttraumatic syndrome (criteria B, C, and D in DSM-III and -IIIR, plus criterion E in DSM-IV). The elements are connected by an iconic pathway or "memory logic":

$$(A) \rightarrow (B) \rightarrow (C + D)$$

In plain English, a traumatic event creates a memory that is distressful, repetitive, and intrusive (involuntary). The traumatic memory provokes the autonomic nervous system and the survival response (fight, flight, freeze), causing difficulty sleeping, irritability, an exaggerated startle response, hypervigilance, difficulty concentrating, and motor restlessness. The victim adapts to the distressful memory and consequent arousal through symptomatic forms of avoidance and numbing.

DSM-III portrayed traumatic stressors (the A criterion) as categorically or universally distressful, making it unnecessary to distinguish between traumatic *events* and traumatic *experiences*. Subsequent epidemiological research indicated that a minority of people exposed to presumably traumatic events develops PTSD. Thus it is useful to distinguish between traumatic events and experiences: events become experiences in the presence of additional factors or vulnerabilities (X), particular to the affected individuals:

$$(A + X) \to (B) \to (C + D)$$

This understanding is implicit, rather than stated, in later editions of the DSM.

Prior to publication of DSM-5 in 2013, the PTSD working group posted a set of diagnostic criteria online, allowing researchers and clinicians to review and respond to the proposed list. The stated goal was to improve the classification's diagnostic validity by recalibrating the range of events that qualify for the A criterion. Proposed changes included downgrading the diagnostic significance of emotional numbing, and moving PTSD from its present place among the anxiety disorders a new category, to be called "trauma and stressor-related disorders." Perhaps the most controversial proposal was to eliminate the A criterion. At first glance, the proposal seems counterintuitive, a rejection of the memory logic that glues the disorder's features together. This was not the advocates' position though; in effect, they were arguing that PTSD's memory logic can be taken for granted:

The A-criterion is not valid [because] it is not an independent feature and therefore [it is] tautologic. The information . . . is already given through the presence or absence of the core symptoms of PTSD. (Maier 2009:105)

The full PTSD syndrome hardly ever occurs in the absence of an event that reasonably be described as traumatic: In other words, Criterion A simply describes the usual context of PTSD without contributing itself to diagnostic precision. (Brewin, Lanius, et al. 2009:369)

[Once the A criterion is eliminated,] PTSD will immediately come into alignment with all other psychiatric disorders, [leaving *clinicians*] free to focus on the symptomatic presentation and on the most appropriate treatment. (Brewin, Lanius, et al. 2009:370)

The proposal would limit the role of the working group to fine-tuning PTSD's remaining criteria. The rule of thumb would be that when B, C, and D co-occur, diagnosis will assume that the syndrome is a consequence of the trauma-level experience inscribed on the patient's other symptoms. For instance, a patient's phobic avoidance behavior will mirror or enact features of the traumatic event. Because treatment of the PTSD syndrome is generally nonspecific, the validity of the presumed traumatic event would be clinically unimportant, and a clinician would treat false positives and true cases in the same way. If the treatment proves efficacious, it would be advisable to continue with the present treatment. If the intervention is ineffective, then the practitioner should move on to an alternative treatment, proceeding in an empirical manner, familiar in psychiatry.

The deletion of the A criterion might have reduced PTSD's heterogeneity and the problems that heterogeneity creates for researchers and clinicians. At the same time, the proposal ignores the *forensic value* of the A criterion. PTSD serves multiple institutional interests: the A criterion works as a gatekeeper for determining eligibility for compensation and care of U.S. military veterans, and for the granting of refugee status (and privilege of residence) in several Western countries, including the United States, Canada, Denmark, and the Netherlands. These military veterans constitute the largest population diagnosed with PTSD, and the U.S. Veterans Administration Medical System continues to be the most significant sponsor of funded research on the disorder. The elimination of the A criterion would prohibitively increase the economic costs of serving and compensating claimants and might conceivably compromise efforts to identify and develop therapeutic interventions specific for PTSD.

Refining the A criterion, improving its diagnostic validity, means finding a way to simultaneously reduce false positives (people incorrectly diagnosed with PTSD) and false negatives (people incorrectly denied a PTSD diagnosis). The challenge is to accomplish both goals simultaneously, since efforts to make one standard more sensitive generally mean making the other weaker (less selective). Furthermore, influential stakeholders have conflicting interests: government agencies are bent on reducing illegitimate claimants, while patient advocacy groups are opposed to standards that will victimize the victims.

In PTSD, and unlike most diagnostic classifications, there is an additional kind of validity, attaching to its singular etiology and pathogenesis. It is this second kind of validity that justifies the disorder's inclusion in the DSMs. The publications of DSM-III marked a turning point in the history of American psychiatry. In principle, DSM-III excluded diagnostic classifications defined in whole or part by their etiology. The diagnosis of any disorder was to be based on a list of descriptive criteria; individual symptoms could be shared among disorders, but each disorder would be defined by its unique combination of symptoms. The PTSD classification violated both requirements: the list incorporates an etiology (the memory logic) and its descriptive symptoms coincide with the symptom lists for major depression and generalized anxiety disorder. Moreover, a high proportion of people diagnosed with PTSD are diagnosed with comorbid depression and generalized anxiety disorder. Thus the diagnostic validity of PTSD hinges on evidence of what can be called its "etiological validity." Questions concerning PTSD's etiological validity were raised around the time of its inclusion in DSM-III, and occasionally attract attention now. Concern focuses on the phenomenon of "bracket creep," the progressive expansion of situations qualifying as traumatic stressors.

Heterogeneous Memories

The earliest descriptions of memory-driven posttraumatic disorders date to the 1880s, and refer to cases involving supposedly neurological symptoms (Young 1995, ch. 1). Jean-Martin Charcot referred to these memories as "mental parasites," and his notion recurs in the writing of Pierre Janet and Sigmund Freud on traumatic neurosis and traumatic neurasthenia. A Parisian, described as "Le-log," is Charcot's iconic case. The man is knocked to the street by a runaway horse and wagon, and the wheels roll over his thighs, causing livid bruises. Le-log loses consciousness and on awakening discovers that his legs are paralyzed. He is brought to Charcot, a celebrated neurologist, who diagnoses Le-log's condition as psychogenic. As the story is retold in potted histories of PTSD, it stops at this point. But there is more to the story, for onlookers informed Charcot that Le-log collapsed *before* the wagon reached him and that its wheels never rolled over his legs. Charcot concluded that Le-log's recollection is not a memory of the past but rather a memory of the future, anticipating an event he believed was going to happen. When Le-log caught sight of the bruising, his fears were confirmed. Charcot's conclusion was, in effect, that traumatic memories come in these two forms, and mimicry (memories of the future) can be as toxic as the real thing (memories of the past). When reliable eyewitnesses are available, there is no problem in telling them apart. Otherwise, the physician must depend on his intuition; Janet and Freud famously developed methods for investigating this phenomenon.

There are multiple forms of traumatic memory: these include the iconic pathway

$$(A) \rightarrow (B) \rightarrow (C + D)$$

plus five forms of mimicry; all been known to psychiatry for over a century. The first of these kinds follows the pattern of Le-log. During World War I, prominent German army physicians, such as Fritz Kaufmann, claimed that most cases of traumatic hysteria affecting frontline soldiers could be assumed to be memories of the future. A second kind is constructed around a real event that was not markedly distressful when it was originally experienced. Only in retrospect, sometimes years after the original occasion, the event becomes ominous and its memory troubling. The characteristic chronology turns the iconic pathway on its head. The sequence starts with C and D: the presenting complaints are symptoms ordinarily associated with depression, generalized anxiety, and alcohol and substance abuse. The patient and his (her) therapist now proceed to discover a plausible precipitating event buried in a dormant memory. The sequence can end here: the discovery of a serviceable memory provides the patient with a socially and psychologically respectable etiology for stigmatized behavior.

$$(C + D) \rightarrow (B) \rightarrow (A)$$

On the other hand, the sequence of events can proceed beyond this point, so that the remembered experience is not simply recalled, but actively reexperienced in intrusive thoughts, images, and dreams, and it is transformed into something disturbing and traumatic. During this process, the event is recontextualized—that is, it is understood in an entirely new way—and acquires an emotional power and psychological salience that it did not originally possess but now duplicates, rather than simply mimicking, iconic traumatic memories. The sequence, which is similar to Freud's conception of *Nachträglichkeit* (belatedness), is conventionally and mistakenly diagnosed as delayed onset PTSD:

$$(C + D) \rightarrow (B) \rightarrow (A) \; becomes \; (B) \rightarrow (C + D)$$

There are two final ways in which iconic traumatic memory is imitated. One is *factitious* memory, the case where someone develops an intense psychological identification with a borrowed or imagined etiological event, or, more commonly, identification with a grossly distorted representation of an autobiographical event. Factitious memory is often described as a form of self-deception, but the phenomenon equally betokens efforts aimed at salvaging or rebuilding the individual's sense of self (French et al. 2009). Number two is *fictitious* traumatic memory or malingering. By definition, a malingerer is aware of dissimulating, and there is no self-deception; in practice, the boundary between fictitious and factitious memories is porous, and easily transgressed via autosuggestion—a subject of intense interest to trauma doctors a century ago, but for the wrong reasons no longer considered interesting (Chrobak and Zaragoza 2009).

In summary, psychiatry is familiar with multiple kinds of traumatic memory for more than a century. They include iconic traumatic memories, memories of the future, retrospective memories, belated memories, factitious memories, and fictitious memories.

Now recall the distinctions made in the previous section. PTSD manifests itself to researchers and clinicians in four ways:

1. *A text*: the DSM symptom list.
2. *Exemplars*: share the distinctive disorder (etiology) encoded in the text.
3. *Clinical cases and populations*: people who conform to the symptom list but do not necessarily share the disorder.
4. *Epidemiological populations*: aggregates and composite people based on clinical populations.

Put these manifestations and memories together:

1. Exemplars include only iconic memory.
2. Clinical populations include all six kinds of memory.

The majority of clinical cases of PTSD correspond to the "chronic" type, meaning that symptoms have persisted for six months or longer. The great majority of chronic cases are associated with comorbid diagnoses; exemplars are rare. Most PTSD research is devoted to the chronic type. The cultural importance of exemplars is largely rhetorical: deflecting doubts about PTSD's intrinsic validity. Thus our conclusion: because PTSD is defined by its memory logic, and it comprises several kinds of memories, PTSD must be considered an inherently heterogeneous phenomenon. But this conclusion rests on a key assumption, namely that there is no effective means of differentiating the different kinds of traumatic memory—nothing equivalent to the onlookers who helped Charcot diagnose the case of Le-log. In the following section, we wish to argue that this is indeed the case: there are no means adequate for performing this task.

Malleable Memories

Traumatic memories are conventionally represented as if they were object-like things, stored in a library-like mental location, waiting to be retrieved. An idea still popular among PTSD researchers is that traumatic memories are also uniquely "indelible," analogous to videotapes and DVDs. There is no compelling evidence that traumatic memories are unlike other memories in this respect (McNally 2005). *All episodic memories are intrinsically malleable.* In his famous 1932 monograph, *Remembering,* Fredrick Bartlett described memories penetrating consciousness through a *process,* in which mnemonic traces of an experience are reassembled, recalibrated, updated, and reschematized. Reassembly draws on semantic memory (substantive knowledge) and fragments of other, associated episodic memories and is affected, to a greater or less degree, by the individual's current state and life situation. Thus memories—the product that enters consciousness—are intrinsically malleable. This process has been intensively studied during the intervening years (Conway and Playdell-Pearce 2000; Hardt et al. 2010; Hassabis and Maguire

2007; Schacter et al.1998; Schacter and Addis 2007). Cognitive neuroscience portrays malleability as evidence of memory's evolutionary origin and function. Memories of the past are simultaneously memories for the future: a means of enhancing the organism's ability to respond to new situations, rather than a medium for providing faithful photocopies of the past (Dudai 2009 and 2006). Memories provide the templates we depend on for interpreting novel and ambiguous events, but the templates are themselves reshaped for each occasion.

The malleability of memory is illustrated in a pivotal study of American veterans (n = 59) of the First Gulf War (Southwick et al. 1997). The men were interviewed one month after returning from the theater of operations, and reinterviewed two years later. On both occasions, they completed a nineteen-item questionnaire concerning their combat experiences. In the second interview, 70 percent of the men reported experiencing at least one combat event that had not been reported in the initial interview. The most commonly reported newly remembered events were "bizarre disfiguration of bodies as a result of wounds," "seeing others killed or wounded," and "extreme threat to your personal safety." The researchers emphasize that the majority of newly remembered experiences concern "objectively described severe events," rather than "subjectively evaluated experiences." (The second interview also provided evidence of forgetting: 46 percent of the respondents failed to report one or more of the events that they had reported one month after returning home.)

The researchers traced the new experiences to two sources. First, during the interval between interviews, the men typically viewed media accounts of the military actions in which they had participated and had conversations with fellow veterans about their Gulf War experiences. It is presumed that the images and narratives that the veterans absorbed during this interim period would, in some cases, be a source of factitious memories. Southwick and colleagues suggest an additional possibility, corresponding to the "retrospective memory" process. "Individuals who became increasingly symptomatic over time unknowingly exaggerated their memory for trauma events as a way to understand or explain their emerging psychopathology" (Southwick et al. 1997:176). In support of this hypothesis, the researchers point to a positive correlation between number of PTSD symptoms and number of new events reported by the participants in the study. Analogous findings are reported in study of U.S. soldiers (n = 460) who served in a peacekeeping mission in Somalia (Roemer et al. 1998, Orsillo et al. 1998); research on a second

sample of veterans of the First Gulf War (King et al. 2000); and an epidemiological study of civilians (Hepp et al. 2006).

The malleability of memory is the outward manifestation of the process
that produces the different kinds of memories that are represented in PTSD.
It is likewise a manifestation of the relationship among these six kinds. The
six kinds can be thought of as positions along a continuum, each kind capable of metamorphizing into another kind: transiting from retrospective
traumatic memory or factitious memory into iconic memory (see Trivers
2011, ch. 3, on "self-deception"):

$$(C+D) \rightarrow (B) \rightarrow (A) \text{ transits to } (B) \rightarrow (C+D)$$

Contrast this perspective with Chris Brewin's position on traumatic memory. In Brewin's account, the phenomenology of reexperiencing (the B criterion) is the output of a dual memory system, comprising "verbally accessible
memory" (VAM) and "situationally accessible memory" (SAM) (Brewin 2003;
see Brewin and Holmes 2003 for a genealogy). In more recent publications,
VAM and SAM have been revised and relabeled, as "contextual memory"
(C-memory) and "sensation-based memory" (S-memory) (Brewin, Gregory,
et al. 2010). C-memory is verbally accessible (meaning that it can be put into
words) and can be voluntary or involuntary (intrusive). The corresponding
mental representations (called C-reps) include "meaningful interpretations
of events," trauma narratives, schematized representations, and "novel images that combine object and conceptual information in flexible ways."
S-memory is involuntary, and its representations involve autonomic arousal
and response. Retrieval is a form of reenactment, cued to the individual's current situation. "Long-lasting S-reps, formed by emotionally salient experiences, may be retrieved by corresponding emotional states or by sensory cues
in the external environment, with this sensory reliving component given a
context and modulated by activation of the corresponding C-reps." *Flashbacks* are prototypical S-reps: "an adaptive process in which stored information is re-presented and processed once the danger is passed." They persist
because the victim fails to align the traumatic S-rep with efficacious C-reps.
Failure to process these S-reps is typically a consequence of avoidance behavior (a C criterion symptom) and the victim's inability to progress beyond
the fragmentary C-reps that are symptomatic of his condition (Brewin, Gregory, et al. 2010:221, 222, 225).

Brewin's account reflects the prevailing, conventional understanding of PTSD. It conflates two empirically distinct manifestations of PTSD: the exemplar, in which PTSD is identified with an iconic traumatic memory, and a population-based manifestation, which encapsulates six kinds of malleable memory. In Brewin's account, belatedness is understood quite literally, as a traumatic experience waiting to be represented, rather than a process in which representations (reconsolidation) are being produced (Andrews et al. 2007). Further, the ability of diagnosis to differentiate iconic traumatic memories from mimicry is taken for granted, rather than examined and vindicated.

Heterogeneity and History

Posttraumatic syndromes have attracted the interest of clinical medicine for 150 years. Over time, the characteristic symptoms—patients' self-reports and clinical expectations—change. Landmark research based on British army clinical records from the Boer War to the Gulf War, conducted by Edgar Jones, Simon Wessely, and their associates, identified four symptom clusters: cardiac, epigastric, sensory-motor, and psychological. All four clusters are reported throughout this period, but their relative significance waxes and wanes. Likewise, putative causal mechanisms fall in and out of fashion (Jones et al. 2002). Change is partly explained by developments in psychiatric theories, empirical knowledge, and technologies. Developments internal to psychiatry are only part of the explanation, however. The proposal to eliminate the A criterion in DSM-5, discussed above, went nowhere even though it made good sense from a psychiatric perspective. It failed because it was oblivious to the social, political, and forensic utility of identifiable traumatic stressors—a mechanism for determining culpability and awarding compensation for war-related posttraumatic disability and for regulating eligibility for asylum-seeker status.

The connection between trauma and history is unique, and it is an additional source of heterogeneity. Every diagnostic classification has a history; however the posttraumatic syndromes, including PTSD, are historical in an additional sense. One can describe the engagement between trauma and history as multiple episodes that follow a regular pattern. Each episode starts with an event of encompassing violence and an epidemic of posttraumatic casualties. The epidemic is a source of controversy over its scope: the numbers affected, their etiology, impairment, and differential diagnosis; the distribution of culpability and obligation; the economic and social costs; and the appropriate intervention strategies—including treatment and prevention. Resources are mobilized (manpower, technologies, facilities) for managing casualties and claimants and conducting research. A distinctive *assemblage* emerges, colored by national medical traditions, institutional cultures, and popular attitudes. The posttraumatic syndromes—shell shock, PTSD, mild traumatic brain injury (mTBI), Gulf War syndrome, second-generation Holocaust trauma, and so on—and corresponding *subjectivities*, the patient's self-awareness of his or her situation, are products of their respective assemblages.

For example, during World War II, large numbers of British soldiers were diagnosed with "non-ulcer dyspepsia." According to Jones and Wessely (2004), the soldiers' presenting symptoms were psychosomatic and precipitated by stress: they were elective symptoms, essentially an idiom of distress that needs be understood in cultural and historical context. Their prominent place in soldiers' complaints and anxieties originated in the public's perception of an epidemic of peptic ulceration, and their factual knowledge of the deadly consequences of intestinal perforations. The bacterial origins of peptic ulcers were subsequently discovered, patients successfully treated with newly discovered antibacterial drugs, and the epidemic of non-ulcer dyspepsia disappeared from the ranks. Hotopf and Wessely (2005) account for the recrudescence of stress-related somatic symptoms after the 1990–91 Gulf War in a similar way, by tracing the onset of the symptoms to a widespread fear in the general population of environmental toxins on the one hand, and the veterans' belief that they had been exposed to dangerous toxic agents (including nerve gas) while in the Middle East and also prior to deployment (via vaccination).

We can identify a string of fairly discrete episodes, each conforming to the indicated pattern: a World War I episode, a post–Vietnam War episode, a post-Holocaust episode, a Gulf War episode, a post-9/11 episode, a humanitarian crisis episode, and an Iraq and Afghanistan incursion episode. There may be compelling reasons for expanding the list—for example, by adding a recovered memory and dissociation episode—but this one will do for the time being. The list is roughly chronological. The chronology is occasionally counterintuitive—the post-Holocaust episode begins after the post–Vietnam

War episode, World War I is included in the episodes but World War II and the Korean conflict are not—but the sequence is historically accurate. With the exception of the World War I episode, these episodes continue to roll on into our own time.

We have space for just one illustration. Following the 9/11 attack on the World Trade Center, researchers published epidemiological data indicating, they claimed, a nationwide epidemic of PTSD attributable to "distant PTSD." A relatively small number of reported victims had been in lower Manhattan at the time of the attack and were directly exposed to traumatic stressors. Many thousands of others, living all over the United States, were diagnosed at a distance as victims of distant PTSD—the result of a traumatogenic witnessing mediated by television. In addition, the publications provide evidence of a dose-response effect, indicating that risk of symptoms increased with the number of exposures.

DSM-IV includes pathogenic witnessing in the A criterion but makes no reference to distant PTSD. The PTSD committee for DSM-5 was preparing to exclude this possibility from the A criterion, but this skepticism is a recent development. Peer reviewers and editors for the major journals that published this epidemiological research—*JAMA* (*Journal of the American Medical Association*), *American Journal of Psychiatry*, and *Archives of General Psychiatry*—found the etiology unproblematic. In the publications, the victims of distant PTSD are assessed with a variety of conditions, including "PTSD" or "probable PTSD," (a small minority of victims meeting all DSM-IV criteria), "partial PTSD," "PTSD symptoms," and "PTSD reactions." The majority of victims are assessed with the last three phenomena. The symptoms are indistinguishable from depression, generalized anxiety, and generic folk diagnoses such as "being stressed out." The *aggregate effect* of reading these publications is to model PTSD as a unitary phenomenon expressed along a continuum, with full-blown cases at one end and cases comprising isolated and ordinarily innocuous experiences, such as problems sleeping, at the other end.

Unlike previous episodes, the epidemic that followed 9/11 had no matching clinical population. Distant trauma produced no casualties, but rather an appreciable at-risk population. The researchers emphasized the clinical and public policy implications of the epidemic, and the need to develop and deploy effective prophylactic measures. Researchers identified a second population, composed of respondents who reported no symptoms. These individuals were not simply "normal," but possessed a distinctive, psycho-biological trait, referred to as "resilience." These populations constituted a previously ignored object of inquiry, a researchable and fundable counter-part of a pathologized population (comprising people diagnosed with PTSD, partial PTSD, etc.). Thus it would be mistaken to conclude that research on distant PTSD had left no bodies behind. (See Young 2007 for an analysis of the epidemiological data, and a comprehensive history of resilience follow-ing 9/11.)

Conclusion

Each of these episodes is a distinctive historical-cultural configuration and needs to be understood in its own terms. There are similarities: shell shock, as originally understood, shares features with mild traumatic brain injury. Both syndromes were (are) understood to result from the effects on the brain of shock waves created by high explosives. In both instances, medical experts were generally unable to detect physical evidence of brain damage. There were also shared symptoms, and it is tempting to believe that they are a single dis-order described in different ways. Yet this conclusion ignores the essential difference between abstractions (diagnostic codes), prototypes (unambig-uous cases), and clinical populations, and it ignores likewise the histori-cally situated social and cultural factors that contribute to the production of codes, prototypes, and populations. PTSD—the signature creation of the post–Vietnam War episode—flaunts this generalization. The term is routinely used retrospectively to diagnose the past, and as the living lan-guage of epidemiology and clinical research from the Gulf War onward. But there is no real contradiction here: the language of PTSD represents a kind of cultural hegemony and lingua franca and not a refutation of heterogeneity.

Our intention in this chapter has been to provide a new way to look at PTSD, giving attention to its complexity and heterogeneity. This analysis should not be misconstrued as an effort to undermine PTSD's etiological va-lidity, but rather it is an effort to put PTSD in context. PTSD's etiology is bound to the nature of what we have called the iconic memory, and appar-ently intractable difficulties. The continuing search for biomarkers, the de-tection of risk factors, and calculations of heritability are efforts to sidestep this problem by recasting PTSD as a biological disorder. While the biological solution may be an effective response to many psychiatric disorders, this is not true of PTSD.

References

American Psychiatric Association

1980 Diagnostic and Statistical Manual of Mental Disorder. 3rd edition. Washington, D.C.: American Psychiatric Association.

1987 Diagnostic and Statistical Manual of Mental Disorder. 3rd edition. Text revision. Washington, D.C.: American Psychiatric Association.

1994 Diagnostic and Statistical Manual of Mental Disorder. 4th edition. Washington, D.C.: American Psychiatric Association.

2000 Diagnostic and Statistical Manual of Mental Disorder. 4th edition. Text revision. Washington, D.C.: American Psychiatric Association.

2013 Diagnostic and Statistical Manual of Mental Disorder. 5th edition. Washington, D.C.: American Psychiatric Association.

Andrews, Bernice, Chris Brewin, Rosanna Philpott, and Lorna Stewart

2007 Delayed-Onset Posttraumatic Stress Disorder: A Systematic Review of the Evidence. American Journal of Psychiatry 164(9):1319–26.

Bramsen, Inge, Anja J. E. Dirkzwager, Suzanne C. M. van Esch, and Henk M. van der Ploeg

2001 Consistency of Self-Reports of Traumatic Events in a Population of Dutch Peacekeepers. Journal of Traumatic Stress 14(4):733–40.

Brewin, Chris R.

2003 Posttraumatic Stress Disorder: Malady or Myth? New Haven, Conn.: Yale University Press.

Brewin, Chris R., James D. Gregory, Michelle Lipton, and Neil Burgess

2010 Intrusive Images in Psychological Disorders: Characteristics, Neural Mechanisms, and Treatment Implications. Psychological Review 117(1):210–32.

Brewin, Chris R., and Emily A. Holmes

2003 Psychological Theories of Posttraumatic Stress Disorder. Clinical Psychology Review 23(3):339–76.

Brewin Chris R., Ruth A. Lanius, Andrei Novac, Ulrich Schnyder, and Sandro Galea

2009 Reformulating PTSD for DSM-V: Life After Criterion A. Journal of Traumatic Stress 22(5):366–73.

Breslau, Naomi, Kipling M. Bohnert, and Karestan C. Koenen

2010 The 9/11 Terrorist Attack and Posttraumatic Stress Disorder Revisited. Journal of Nervous and Mental Disease 198(8):539–43.

Chrobak, Quin M., and Maria S. Zaragoza

2009 The Cognitive Consequences of Forced Fabrication: Evidence from Studies of Eyewitness Suggestibility. In Confabulation: Views from Neuroscience, Psychiatry,

Psychology, and Philosophy. William Hirstein, ed. Pp. 67–90. Oxford: Oxford University Press.

Clancy, Susan

2010 The Trauma Myth: The Truth About the Sexual Abuse of Children—and Its Aftermath. New York: Basic.

Conway, Martin A., and Christopher W. Playdell-Pearce

2000 The Construction of Autobiographical Memories in the Self-Memory System. Psychological Review 107(2):261–88.

Dudai, Yadin

2006 Reconsolidation: The Advantage of Being Refocused. Current Opinion in Neurobiology 16(2):174–78.

2009 Predicting Not to Predict Too Much: How the Cellular Machinery of Memory Anticipates the Uncertain Future. Philosophical Transactions of the Royal Society of London B: Biological Sciences 364(1521):1255–62.

French, Lauren, Maryanne Garry, and Elizabeth Loftus

2009 False Memories: A Kind of Confabulation in Non-Clinical Subjects. *In* Confabulation: Views from Neuroscience, Psychiatry, Psychology, and Philosophy. William Hirstein, ed. Pp. 33–66. Oxford: Oxford University Press.

Hardt, Oliver, Einar Örn Einarsson, and Karim Nader

2010 A Bridge over Troubled Water: Reconsolidation as a Link Between Cognitive and Neuroscientific Memory Research Traditions. Annual Review of Psychology 61:141–67.

Hassabis, Demis and Eleanor A. Maguire

2007 Deconstructing Episodic Memory with Construction. Trends in Cognitive Sciences 11: 299–306.

Hepp, Urs, Alex Gamma, Gabriella Milos, Dominique Eich, Vladeta Ajdacic-Gross, Wulf Rössler, Jules Angst, Ulrich Schnyder

2006 Inconsistency in Reporting Potentially Traumatic Events. British Journal of Psychiatry 188: 278–83.

Hotopf, Matthew, and Simon Wessely

2005 Can Epidemiology Clear the Fog of War? Lessons from the 1990–91 Gulf War. International Journal of Epidemiology 34(4):791–800.

Jones, Edgar, Robert Hodgins-Vermaas, Helen McCartney, Brian Everitt, Charlotte Beech, Denise Poynter, Ian Palmer, Kenneth Hyams, and Simon Wessely

2002 Post-Combat Syndromes from the Boer War to the Gulf War: A Cluster Analysis of Their Nature and Attribution. British Medical Journal 324:321–24.

Jones, Edgar, and Simon Wessely

2004 Hearts, Guts and Minds: Somatization in the Military from 1900. Journal of Psychosomatic Research 56(4):425–29.

King, Daniel W., Lynda A. King, Darin J. Erickson, Mina T. Huang, Erica J. Sharkansky, and Jessica Wolf

2000 Posttraumatic Stress Disorder and Retrospectively Reported Stressor Exposure: A Longitudinal Prediction Model. Journal of Abnormal Psychology 109: 624–33.

Maier, Thomas
2006 Post-Traumatic Stress Disorder Revisited: Deconstructing the A-Criterion. Medical Hypotheses 66(1):103–6.

McNally, Richard J.
2003 Progress and Controversy in the Study of Posttraumatic Stress Disorder. Annual Review of Psychology 54(1):229–52.
2005 Debunking Myths About Trauma and Memory. Canadian Journal of Psychiatry 50(13):817–22.
2009 Can We Fix PTSD in DSM-V? Depression and Anxiety 26(7):597–600.

Orsillo, Susan M., Lizabeth Roemer, Brett T. Litz, Pete Ehlich, and Matthew J. Friedman
1998 Psychiatric Symptomatology Associated with Contemporary Peacekeeping: An Examination of Post-Mission Functioning Among Peacekeepers in Somalia. Journal of Traumatic Stress 11:611–25.

Roemer, Lizabeth, Susan M. Orsillo, T. D. Borkovec, and Brett T. Litz
1998 Emotional Response at the Time of a Potentially Traumatizing Event and PTSD Symptomatology: A Preliminary Retrospective Analysis of the DSM-IV Criterion A-2. Journal of Behavior Therapy and Experimental Psychiatry 29:123–30.

Schacter, Daniel L., and Donna R. Addis
2007 The Cognitive Neuroscience of Constructive Memory: Remembering the Past and Imagining the Future. Philosophical Transactions of the Royal Society B: Biological Sciences 356(1481):1493–1403.

Schacter, Daniel L., Donna R. Addis, and Randy L. Buckner
2007 Remembering the Past to Imagine the Future: The Prospective Brain. Nature Reviews, Neuroscience 8: 657–61.

Schacter, Daniel, Kenneth A. Norman, and Wilma Koutstaal
1998 The Cognitive Neuroscience of Constructive Memory. Annual Review of Psychology 49:289–318.

Southwick, Steven M., C. Andrew Morgan III, Andreas L. Nicolaou, and Dennis S. Charney
1997 Consistency of Memory for Combat-Related Traumatic Events in Veterans of Operation Desert Storm. American Journal of Psychiatry 154(2):173–77.

Trivers, Robert
2011 The Folly of Fools: The Logic of Deceit and Self-Deception in Human Life. New York: Basic.

Wessely, Simon, Catherine Unwin, Matthew Hotopf, Lisa Hull, Khalida Ismail, V. Nicolaou, and A. David
2003 Stability of Recall of Military Hazards over Time: Evidence from the Persian Gulf War of 1991. British Journal of Psychiatry 183:314–22.

Young, Allan

　　1995 The Harmony of Illusions: Inventing Posttraumatic Stress Disorder. Princeton: Princeton University Press.

　　2004 When Traumatic Memory Was a Problem: On the Antecedents of PTSD. *In* Posttraumatic Stress Disorder: Issues and Controversies. Gerald M. Rosen, ed. Pp. 127–46. London: Wiley.

　　2007a PTSD of the Virtual Kind—Trauma and Resilience in Post 9/11 America. *In* Trauma and Memory: Reading, Healing, and Making Law. Austin Sarat, Nadav Davidovitch, and Michal Alberstein, eds. Pp. 21–48. Palo Alto, Calif.: Stanford University Press.

　　2007b 9/11: In the Wake of the Terrorist Attacks. Journal of Nervous and Mental Disease 195(12):1030–32.

CHAPTER 4

From Shell Shock to PTSD and Traumatic Brain Injury: A Historical Perspective on Responses to Combat Trauma

James K. Boehnlein and Devon E. Hinton

Mr. TR is a twenty-eight-year-old single combat veteran who was wounded by a roadside bomb while driving in a convoy several weeks before the conclusion of his second deployment in Iraq. Several members of his unit riding just ahead of his vehicle were killed, but his vehicle was spared from the direct force of the intense blast. He hit his head on the roof of his vehicle but did not lose consciousness. He and other members of his unit immediately attended to those who were killed and seriously wounded. He vaguely remembers general sounds and images of the event but does not remember specific details of what he did to help before the dead and wounded were evacuated. When he returned to base that night he began to experience an intense headache that continued through the following days and weeks. In addition he developed marked sensitivity to light and sound, and occasional nausea, and sometimes would become dizzy when going about his daily routine. Even though the dizziness disappeared and the headache and sensitivity to light and sound improved over the following months after he returned to the United States, he noticed it was more difficult for him to focus and concentrate on his daily tasks, and to remember what he had read in his community college classes. Friends and family told him that he had become more irritable and difficult to live with, as opposed to the first few homecoming weeks after his return from Iraq. He had not noticed the irritability himself, but he had noticed being tired and very anxious most of the time. He had not been sleeping well, and several times a week he was awakening in a sweat from intense dreams of the bombing, with graphic images of the carnage that had occurred.

Since initial nineteenth-century descriptions in the scientific literature of conditions that resemble what is now called posttraumatic stress disorder (PTSD), there has been controversy about PTSD's validity as a psychiatric condition, and continuing debate over 150 years about its core symptoms and behavioral manifestations. Moreover, there has been ongoing debate within the scientific community and in the society at large about whether PTSD and its associated symptoms are psychological or neurological, and whether or not PTSD and mild traumatic brain injury (mTBI) are distinct entities or overlapping conditions. Each condition, PTSD and mTBI, or some overlapping entity, has carried a variety of labels such as irritable heart (Civil War), shell shock (World War I), and battle fatigue (World War II). These various labels each have had implications for diagnosis and treatment, and also they have had broader social implications in regard to disability, along with the social perception of disability and associated stigma (Kugelmann 2009). The World Health Organization (WHO) currently defines mTBI as an acute brain injury resulting from mechanical energy to the head from external physical forces (Table 4.1). The most common symptoms of mTBI include headache, dizziness, fatigue, insomnia, vision problems, sensitivity to noise and light, memory problems, difficulties with focus and concentration, impulsivity, depression, irritability, anxiety, and personality changes (U.S. Department of Veterans Affairs 2011).

In this chapter we will focus on the historical medical/psychiatric perceptions of clinicians, researchers, and others in the scientific community regarding assessment and treatment of mTBI/PTSD; individual and social perceptions of the PTSD/mTBI interface and their implications for personal and social identity; and the understanding of symptoms, behavior, and associated disability among combat veterans, their families, and the society at large. We also will describe the implications of these complex and overlapping conceptualizations of PTSD and mTBI for effective treatment, rehabilitation, recovery, and functioning in work and interpersonal relationships (Verfaellie et al. 2014).

Although PTSD and mTBI are encountered outside of the military in all sectors of civilian life, in this chapter we will be focusing primarily on PTSD/mTBI in the context of military service. To provide an important historical perspective we will review the evolution of PTSD/mTBI terminology, including

Table 4.1. Operational Criteria for Mild Traumatic Brain Injury (mTBI)

(1) One or more of the following:
   A. Confusion or disorientation
   B. Loss of consciousness for 30 minutes or less
   C. Posttraumatic amnesia for less than 24 hours
   D. Other transient neurological abnormalities such as focal signs, seizure, and intracranial lesion not requiring surgery
(2) Glasgow Coma Scale score of 13–15 after 30 minutes postinjury or later upon presentation for health care [Note: Glasgow Coma Scale is a 15-point clinical scale for assessing level of consciousness after acute traumatic brain injury.]
(3) Manifestations of mTBI must not be due to drugs, alcohol, or medications; caused by other injuries or by treatment for other injuries (e.g., systemic injuries, facial injuries, or intubation); caused by other problems (e.g., psychological trauma, language barrier, or coexisting medical conditions); or caused by penetrating craniocerebral injury.

Source: Holm et al. 2005:140

the contributions of science, politics, and the sociocultural environment to the evolution of how combat trauma has been understood and perceived. Since even now there is confusion and controversy about scientific conceptualizations of combat trauma, we will describe the relevance of the veteran's own understanding of his/her distress, how that affects the search for help and assistance, and how health care providers themselves view symptoms, behavior, and treatment. Also, how do the views of veterans, families, care providers and the society at large affect self-perception, help seeking, and ultimately, recovery? Also we will try to show how disorders attributed to the trauma of head injury or other physical injury overlapped and differed in each period and how the conceptualization of the PTSD syndrome emerged apart from physical trauma. The theories of each disorder influenced each other, and those persons with an injury thought capable of bringing about a physically caused trauma syndrome (e.g., exposure to an explosion) became hypervigilant to its symptoms. There emerged a certain trauma episteme based on theories of the effects of psychological and physical trauma.

Some theorists (Breslau 2004; Young 1995) have argued that trauma disorder is also shaped to a large extent by society and culture. They argue that cultural and social factors can be important determinants of susceptibility to PTSD by shaping ideas of what constitutes a trauma, and what constitutes abnormal and normal responses to trauma (Stein et al. 2007). Most historians suggest that changes in collective sensibilities, for example, the way in which trauma and the victims of trauma are depicted, come about as a result of scientific developments, but in fact the direction of the causal relationship is far from being unidirectional as there also is a collective process by which a society defines its values and norms, and embodies them in individual subjects (Fassin and Rechtman 2009). In the following sections we will examine several theories of psychological and physical trauma and the syndromes they were thought to cause in their specific historical periods and then will focus on the example of TBI in recent wars in Afghanistan and Iraq.

A Historical Perspective of the PTSD/TBI Interface

In the mid-nineteenth century clinical descriptions of the survivors of train accidents began to appear in the British literature, with accounts of physical and emotional distress such as insomnia, distressing dreams, memory and concentration disturbances, irritability, and multiple somatic symptoms labeled as railroad spine syndrome (Erichsen 1867). At around the same time, irritable heart was described among Civil War veterans who had palpitations, chest pain, rapid pulse, headache, dizziness, insomnia, and unpleasant dreams: "Holding at the time the common belief that functional and organic affections are widely separate, I failed at first to seize the fact that the apparently dissimilar states were in reality one, or rather, that one grew out of the other. But as patients multiplied I began to trace the connection; and observation showed me what I trust to demonstrate in this paper, the links connecting the disorders" (Da Costa 1871:21). It is interesting to note that Da Costa's description included symptoms that we now describe as core symptoms of TBI (headache and dizziness). He believed that "strains and blows," "rheumatism," "scurvy," tobacco, and even pressure from a waist belt or knapsack could have been aggravating factors, and "hard field service" was identified as a cause in 38.5 percent of cases (Da Costa 1871; also see Kugelmann 2009).

In describing the phenomenon of railway spine, Erichsen did not present any anatomical or pathological evidence supporting the diagnosis but argued through clinical observations that, like the brain, the spinal cord was susceptible to concussions that could induce molecular changes (Caplan 1995). He described several clinical cases in detail (Erichsen 1867), one striking example being a man whom he examined for the first time fifteen months after the man had sustained a relatively minor injury without loss of consciousness.

His symptoms included sensitivity to noise and light; seeing flashes of light; numbing, tingling, and burning in the right arm and leg; unusual gait; frightening dreams; irritability; and poor memory. On physical exam, Erichsen noted three tender points with both superficial and deep pressure on the spine. Erichsen also was very much aware of the social context of his theories, including the developing controversy in medicine and the courts regarding the often tenuous connection between seemingly minor injuries and the disturbed behavior of survivors: "That discrepancy of opinion as to the relations between apparent cause and alleged affect; as to the significance and value of particular symptoms, and as to the probable result in any given case, must always exist, there can be no doubt, more especially where the assigned cause of the evil appears to be trivial, where the secondary phenomena develop themselves so slowly and so insidiously that it is often difficult to establish a connecting link between them and the accident" (Erichsen 1867:18).

It was impossible to document molecular derangement of the spinal cord. But much was at stake. If the train wreck was thought to have caused changes in the nervous system, namely, the spinal cord, then much compensation was thought to be due to those victims. However, if it was rather a psychological response that resulted in the various symptoms of railroad spine, then it was thought that much less money—if any—need be paid by the railroad companies. Debates raged on this issue. Increasingly, though, the symptoms of Erichsen's so-called spinal concussion patients were attributed to simulation or hysteria; nonorganic explanations of railroad spine disability became dominant in the last quarter of the nineteenth century (Keller and Chappell 1996). Arguments from diverse segments of the medical community converged, including influential opinions from Herbert Page and other railway surgeons who were highly skeptical of any physiological or anatomical basis for injuries, and from Charcot and other neurologists on both sides of the Atlantic. By 1885, Charcot had come to accept Page's opinion that psychological factors were responsible for traumatic hysteria, but he still speculated that mental trauma in some manner induced an indiscernible physiological disturbance in the nervous system (Caplan 1995). This evolution over several decades of arguments regarding the etiology of railway spine, with a provocative mix of medical, legal, and political perspectives, provides an important sociocultural template for similar debates over the past century, including those regarding shell shock, postconcussive syndrome, and mTBI/PTSD.

In the late nineteenth and early twentieth centuries, between the American Civil War and World War I, psychoanalysis was in its ascendency, and reactions to war were viewed as a traumatic neurosis. Pierre Janet described dissociation as a reaction to overwhelming stress. As noted recently by van der Kolk and van der Hart (1989), Janet's considerable contributions to contemporary trauma theories include his notion that memories can be stored on various levels—as narratives, sensory perceptions, visual images such as nightmares and hallucinations, and visceral sensations such as anxiety reactions and psychosomatic symptoms. Kraepelin and Freud both described traumatic neuroses (Kinzie and Goetz 1996), with Freud ([1919] 1955) defining the traumatic neurosis of war as a conflict in which the ego is defending itself against mortal danger. Yet, throughout his career Freud had a difficult time reconciling his theories of intrapsychic conflict and child development with the effects of war violence on the adult psyche.

All modern wars have been associated with some type of syndrome characterized by unexplained medical symptoms (Jones et al. 2002). The medical community's response to injured soldiers during and after WWI provides a fascinating example of how etiological theories of neuropsychiatric conditions are influenced not only by the state of science in any historical era, but also by the sociocultural and political environment. The medical and psychiatric literature of shell shock among World War I combatants, particularly in Britain, is especially relevant to the mTBI/PTSD debate in the contemporary Iraq/Afghanistan psychiatry research literature.

Most medical historians are in agreement that prior to World War I hysteria and neurasthenia were the two main nervous disorders recognized by British psychiatry, and the diagnosis of shell shock was comprised of these two categories; in fact, they were connected by an etiological role attributed to heredity, emphasizing a dialogue between the individual body and the social and political environment of family and nation (Loughran 2008). Additionally, a weakened nervous system common to both hysteria and neurasthenia was considered to be either inborn or acquired in the environment from an unexpected shock or an illness.

In the World War I literature a wide range of symptoms that are now, in the early twenty-first century, attributed to either mTBI or PTSD were attributed to shell shock. These symptoms include confusion, memory loss, dizziness, nightmares, cyclic and intense mood disturbances, and many others that have both physiological and psychological manifestations. A soldier might be diagnosed with either of two different subcategories of shell shock in World War I, which determined where he was sent for treatment (at the front or to England), the type of treatment he received (intense intervention or rest/rehabilitation), and the ease or difficulty of being awarded compensation and pension. The general "shell shock" term could be understood as a mix of different disorders ranging from a psychological reaction to war (a PTSD-like syndrome), a physiological response to prolonged fear (a mix of anxiety and PTSD symptoms), and cases of actual concussion (Loughran 2012).

During and after World War I, explanations of the etiology and pathology of shell shock varied widely among organic and nonorganic psychological and behavioral factors, but any soldier in the war zone with fatigue, memory loss, or dizziness was considered a potential shell shock case (Jones et al. 2007). Mott (1916:iii) described typical symptoms of shell shock as including slow reaction times, mental dullness, confusion, headache and fatigue with prolonged mental effort, amnesia, hyperacusis, startle, and terrifying dreams, and he noted that nearly all cases of shell shock were associated with a disturbance or loss of consciousness of variable duration. He also believed that psychic trauma played a considerable part in the production of symptoms of shell shock without visible injury, occurring "in individuals of a neuropathic or psychopathic predisposition, or of a timorous or nervous disposition." Salmon (1917:513) prefigured the contemporary debate on the differential diagnosis of PTSD and mTBI by describing cases of soldiers exposed to shell explosions that include "patients in whom, while there may or may not be damage to the central nervous system, the symptoms are those of neuroses familiar in civil practice . . . in which there is possibility but no proof of damage to the central nervous system, the symptoms present which might be attributable to such damage are quite overshadowed by the characteristic of the neuroses." Salmon also noted (1917:514), "But many hundreds of soldiers who have not been exposed to battle conditions at all develop symptoms almost identical with those in men whose nervous disorders are attributed to shell fire." There was much debate in the postwar years about what were legitimate or illegitimate sequelae of war trauma, and only those men who broke down in socioculturally acceptable ways could be labeled as honorably wounded and be eligible for state assistance in Canada, Britain, or the United States (Humphries 2010).

Myers (1915) eloquently described three case studies of temporary loss of memory, vision, smell, and taste, along with insomnia and startle, after proximal shell explosions. Prominent in these cases were the soldiers' fixation on the intense combat prior to the shell explosions, and Myers believed there was some component of hysteria in the three cases. Mott (1916) described traumatic combat reactions within the context of hysteria (paralysis, tremors) and neurasthenia (fatigue, headache), and he included terrifying dreams as an example of how intense fear of death or horror of seeing comrades killed could adversely affect mental functioning. At initial clinical presentation, soldiers appeared depressed, anxious, or as though they "were losing their minds" (Rhein 1919:10).

In the interwar period and at the beginning of World War II the debate about the etiology of shell shock did not disappear but instead evolved into debates about "the post-traumatic concussion state" (Schaller 1939) or other terms centered on the term "concussion." Russell (1942) described a chronic postconcussion syndrome as the persistence of headache, dizziness, loss of concentration, nervousness, and anxiety that persists indefinitely after an often slight head injury. He believed that in these cases the physical symptoms were grossly aggravated and exaggerated by psychological factors such as anxiety. Fulton (1942) expanded on the initial World War I blast-injury literature by attempting to integrate more recent research on the cerebral physiological effects of blast waves into evolving, but still perplexing, understandings of combat blast injuries. Before the development of neuroimaging, Wittenbrook (1941) accurately noted that the severity of head injury often is of no value in determining postconcussive functioning. And some writers began to show impatience with dichotomous views of combat-related dysfunction that reinforced discreet organic/functional or physiological/psychological etiological constructs. For example, Denny-Brown (1943:429–30) noted in discussing the postconcussion syndrome that "whatever the mechanism of production of these symptoms which make up the syndrome, the underlying failure may be psychoneurotic or an organic remainder from the injury or a combination of the two. . . . The underlying cause may be any or all of three factors—severe general damage to the brain having intellectual impairment, constitutional liability to psychoneurotic reactions, and undue physical or mental stress in the post-traumatic period." Symonds (1942:604) echoed much of the emerging literature of the time: "As to the distinction between physiogenic and the psychogenic factors in a given case, they appear in most cases so closely intertwined that to separate them is unnatural. . . . That a man with a hurt brain should have a disturbed mind is to be expected [and] it is equally to be expected that this disturbance will affect his capacity for adjustment as a whole."

In the immediate post-World War II era, there was some focus on sequelae of combat stress, but a good deal of the trauma literature focused on the "concentration camp syndrome" among Holocaust survivors, which included depression, anxiety, and multiple somatic symptoms. During the 1950s organic factors were considered to be the major contributors to the concentration camp syndrome (Hoppe 1971). Eitinger (1961, 1980) believed that physical trauma, starvation, and infection caused damage to the brain, and he believed that both physical and psychological factors contributed to the syndrome.

The return of soldiers from the Vietnam War spurred another distinct era of trauma literature in the 1980s and 1990s, but much of that literature focused on psychological, sociocultural, and political factors that may be contributors to postcombat symptoms, behavior, and disability. Physical trauma had little role in these theories. A major part of this literature argues that PTSD symptoms result from both classical conditioning of emotional responses to extreme traumatic stimuli and operant conditioning of avoidance of traumatic stimuli, resulting in the traumatic experience overwhelming the emotional and cognitive system and promoting excessive sensitivity to threatening stimuli and impairing fear extinction processes (Dayan and Oliac 2010). Vulnerability factors are thought to be childhood experiences, comorbidity, or social supports (Stein et al. 2007).

Current PTSD/mTBI Perspectives

In the last ten years the trauma literature has entered yet a new era with the return of soldiers from Iraq and Afghanistan. More emphasis has been placed on the convergence of physiological, anatomical, psychological, and sociocultural factors that may contribute to postcombat dysfunction and disability. In some ways the literature has come full circle to more closely resemble the WWI trauma literature and its descriptions of shell shock. In the contemporary literature it is hypothesized that traumatic brain injury, even mild physiological and anatomical disruption, contributes to postcombat dysfunction and disability. Advances in neuroimaging reveal that previously unseen temporary or permanent brain damage is a major factor in contributing to current reconceptualizations of trauma. Recent evidence suggests that both TBI and PTSD are associated with overlapping neuropathological changes, neurochemical dysregulation, and deficits in neural structure and function, one example being that in both TBI and PTSD inadequate frontal inhibition of the limbic structures results in exaggerated amygdala responses and resultant heightened responsivity to potential threat; chronic stress can impair prefrontal cortical and hippocampal functioning by producing dendritic retraction, restructuring, and disconnection (Kaplan et al. 2010). Another factor in the contemporary reconceptualization of combat trauma is the sheer accumulation of the twentieth- and twenty-first-century scientific literature that points to a more comprehensive model of trauma's effects on the human body, mind, and behavior. Comparing current mTBI and PTSD literature to the WWI shell shock and WWII postconcussion syndrome literature reveals key insights into these trauma syndromes, particularly when one takes into account the current sociocultural views of combat and its effects. This may lead to a more realistic view of the challenges facing combatants as they attempt to reintegrate with their families, jobs, and communities.

Early studies of the prevalence of mental health problems such as PTSD, depression, and generalized anxiety among soldiers returning from Iraq showed rates of about 15 percent to 19 percent (Hoge et al. 2004, 2006). Although not mentioned in these early studies, it became clear as the Iraq war continued that a large number of returning soldiers were presenting with symptoms of mTBI and postconcussive syndrome as the result of deployment-related head injuries from blast explosions, the prevalence ranging from 10 percent to 12 percent (Hoge et al. 2008; Schneiderman et al. 2008).

The picture is more complex when it is recognized that an actual physical trauma to the brain may cause not only brain injury but also PTSD. Physical trauma may change the brain in ways that make it more likely that PTSD-type syndromes may develop. Conversely, Kolb's hypothesis that excessive stimulation in PTSD leads to neuronal changes with impairment of learning habituation and stimulus discrimination (Kolb 1987; Lamprecht and Sack 2002) indicates that PTSD may contribute to structural brain injury. PTSD has been strongly associated with mTBI, and in one study 43.9 percent of soldiers who reported loss of consciousness and 27.3 percent with altered mental states met criteria for PTSD, compared to only 9.1 percent of those with no injuries (Hoge et al. 2008). In the same study, soldiers with mTBI reported significantly higher rates of physical and mental health problems than did soldiers with other injuries. Schneiderman et al. (2008) found that the strongest factor associated with postconcussive symptoms was PTSD; they postulated that the association of mTBI with PTSD may be due to life-threatening combat experiences that can result in mTBI or PTSD or, in some cases, symptoms associated with PTSD may be a manifestation of brain injury. Besides mediating the relationships between mTBI and physical symptoms, PTSD may also mediate the relationship between mTBI and psychosocial difficulty (Pietrzak et al. 2009).

The current lack of precision in research and clinical care related to PTSD/mTBI is partially rooted in the fact that the two conditions share a number of overlapping symptoms such as impaired concentration and memory, fatigue, irritability, impulsivity, depression, and anxiety. Although headache, dizziness, nausea, and photosensitivity are commonly seen in mTBI and less so in PTSD (but somatic symptoms like headache and dizziness are highly associated with anxiety and PTSD), the symptom pattern is certainly not universal, and many combat veterans do not have those specific symptoms; and yet still, a veteran who fears having such symptoms may easily notice them upon hypervigantly seeking them in the body. Moreover, it is often difficult to identify and quantify the details of a blast injury in regard to its strength and duration because of the intensity and confusion of combat. Immediate postconcussion recovery even from relatively mild stimuli can be complicated by repetitive and cumulative concussions and by the emotional stress of combat. In a study of UK soldiers returning from deployment in Iraq, postconcussive symptoms were indeed associated with self-reported exposure to blasts while in combat, but the exact same symptoms were also associated with other in-theater exposures such as potential exposure to depleted uranium and aiding the wounded, suggesting that postconcussive symptoms were a nonspecific indication of distress (Fear et al. 2009). Overall, it remains very difficult to determine whether TBI symptoms in any specific individual are due to physical injury to the brain or to a mix of TBI and PTSD symptoms, or are communicated as an idiom of distress to describe intense physical, psychological, and emotional suffering. It is difficult to disentangle the knot of brain injury, PTSD, and idioms of distress.

Scientific research on blast injuries is still in its beginning stage, making yet more complicated the PTSD/mTBI distinction. Kennedy et al. (2010) note that there are well-studied effects of blast waves on air-filled organs of the body such as the ear canal, lungs, and intestines, but the effects on the brain, particularly in cases of mTBI, have yet to be clearly identified. In attempting to integrate biologically based explanations of PTSD and mTBI, they propose that elevated reexperiencing symptoms after blast mTBI arise from the neurological overactivation of brain areas underlying memory and arousal, and when the traumatic injury occurs during a prolonged period of chronic stress in the context of combat, exaggeration of biological dysregulation may occur. In blast injuries there may be unique neurological effects on the brain from changes in physiological function during exposure to compressive/decompressive changes. A recent study among twelve Iraq war veterans with persistent postconcussive symptoms revealed that, compared to controls, veterans with mTBI (with or without PTSD) exhibited a decreased cerebral metabolic rate of glucose in the cerebellum, vermis, pons, and medial temporal lobe, suggesting that regional brain hypometabolism may constitute a neurobiological substrate for chronic postconcussive symptoms in repetitive blast-trauma mTBI (Peskind et al. 2011). The mechanism of injury in individual cases could be the result of the complex propagation and reflection of the primary blast wave, and effects from acceleration and rotation, fragment impact, heating, emitted gases, or electromagnetic waves (Risling 2010). Cellular structural reorganization in frontal and temporal regions of the brain as a result of concussive brain injury are occurring in the same brain region where PTSD also is provoking neuronal reorganization (Kennedy et al. 2007). Cognitive impairment and emotional dyscontrol associated with TBI can impair resilience that is essential for recovery from PTSD (Lew et al. 2008). Given the possible range of biological effects that result from concussive events and other brain traumas, it may be that TBI is not a unitary disorder. It may well be that concussion events so common in Afghanistan and Iraq, the result of the paradigmatic trauma of these wars—the explosion of improvised explosive devices, mines, and other ordinances—may result in specific and discernable effects that interact with the psychological impact of trauma.

The Social Context of Diagnostic Perception and Treatment

In considering the complexity of the interface between PTSD and mTBI, the ultimate issue is the cumulative impact of cognitive dysfunction (memory, attention, sensory-motor integration), neurobehavioral disorders (mood, anxiety, sleep), and somatosensory disruptions on social dysfunction and overall quality of life (Halbauer et al. 2009). At the same time, how cognitive and behavioral limitations are perceived by patients, families, and society can affect personal identity and confidence, family relationships, and society's acceptance of the person and his or her limitations. Generally speaking, in most societies around the world, including the United States, theories of causation of behavioral disorders linked to physical or physiological factors, such as structural brain injury, are more easily accepted than those linked to psychological factors. This perception influences acceptance of the individual in personal, familial, and social spheres, and it also influences how symptoms and disability are presented to health and social systems. During historical eras such as after WWI and in our own, in which there is such controversy about the physiological and psychological nexus of combat injury and postcombat behavioral and social dysfunction, there can be added confusion for all parties that makes it difficult to maximize treatment, rehabilitation, and functioning.

For the individual soldier there is great pride in self-reliance, and a fear of loss of control or autonomy if diagnosed with a neurological or psychiatric condition. There is avoidance of seeking help because treatment is for those who are weak or "crazy." There is real concern that family members or health professionals will not understand or believe accounts of traumatic events and will not appreciate the shame that the soldier experiences. Additionally, there is the fear of rejection from family, society, and the military, with implications not only for a favorable individual and social identity, but for career retention and advancement.

Stigma itself is a frequent impediment to self-acceptance, seeking help, and acceptance of treatment (Stecker et al. 2007). Labeling of neuropsychiatric dysfunction and the use of diagnostic terms, as shell shock was used in World War I, have implications for the assessment and treatment of Iraq and Afghanistan war veterans in the current era. Jones et al. (2007) note that shell shock was largely free from stigma when used in the early phase of World War I because it was perceived as a neurological lesion, but later it became a more controversial diagnosis when the military discouraged its use and suggested an association with malingering.

In referencing a contemporary study of postconcussive syndrome by Whittaker, Kemp, and House (2007) that suggested that subjects who believed that their symptoms have lasting effects were at higher risk of experiencing an enduring disorder, Jones et al. (2007) discuss the importance of labels in affecting prognosis and conclude that strongly held negative beliefs play a part in maintaining symptoms and functioning, and that for this reason the British army banned the use of the term "shell shock" in 1917. In the current era labeling remains controversial because of implications for such diverse social factors as stigma, hope for recovery, and disability determination. The term "concussion" is sometimes preferred instead of "brain injury" or "mTBI" because it may promote more hope in recovery, but concussion could also be construed as a euphemism; patients may prefer a diagnosis of TBI instead of PTSD because of the stigma associated with PTSD (Sayer et al. 2009). When there are so many overlapping presenting symptoms among conditions whose etiology and pathology are vague and imprecise, the decision to label a patient with one specific diagnosis as opposed to multiple comorbid diagnoses also is fraught with controversy. Kennedy et al. (2007) note that multiple diagnoses are more likely to qualify the patient for disability benefits, which is justifiable if the diagnoses cause cumulative rather than overlapping disability, but at the same time the presence of multiple diagnoses can convince the patient that he or she is more disabled, thereby unconsciously or deliberately fostering secondary gain.

More generally, there can be profoundly different interpersonal and social courses of disorder when symptoms such as rage and startle are attributed to brain hemorrhages or neurophysiological dysfunction than when they are attributed to the psychological effects of war traumas. These create profoundly different self-images and result in very different reactions from others and very different ideas about how and when recovery will occur. At present, given the difficulty of discerning the true origin of disorder (brain injury, PTSD, a combination), there remain different narrative lines that can be chosen by a war trauma survivor during recovery in order to create his or her identity and also meaning for the traumatic experience.

Coming Full Circle: Shell Shock, PTSD, and mTBI

As we have detailed, the medical community, the military, and society at large have had shifting views of the psychological and physical wounds of war over the past century. In certain times actual physical damage to the nervous system and brain have been thought to play a major role in producing a trauma syndrome. The collision of trains; the explosion of fired projectiles into

trenches; the explosion of ordnance under a Humvee: these are different instances of the traumatic event.

Current science now is better able to visualize the effects of physical
trauma on the brain, but the linking of these injuries to actual TBI symptoms is far from settled. It is a nascent science. In the future, studies of brain
injury and PTSD hopefully will inform one another, allowing an analysis of
the effects of each and their interaction with an individual having both disorders.

TBI confers additional risk of PTSD and associated psychological
symptoms above and beyond that associated with psychological trauma
(Vasterling et al. 2009). Mild TBI and PTSD can be associated with mild
neuropsychological impairment, so that there can be significant overlap in
the neuropsychological domains of each disorder, and the effects of mTBI and
PTSD on postconcussive symptoms may be additive; if deficits in executive
functioning are associated with both mTBI and PTSD, the individual's control over the recall of emotionally charged trauma memories would be less
amenable to effective self-management of emotional response to memories,
and the loss of cognitive efficiency would adversely affect occupational performance or overall psychosocial functioning (Vasterling et al. 2009). One
can envision a science in which the specific neuropsychological deficits caused
by PTSD can be examined in relationship to specific damage caused to the
brain by externally caused trauma. Furthermore, that same science might reveal specific neuropsychological functioning and brain activity when TBI or
PTSD symptoms are endorsed as an idiom of distress. Furthermore, a combination of qualitative and quantitative research methods may yield a neurobiological and universal core at the biological end of a continuum, with a
large variety of culturally induced phenomena at the sociopsychological end
of the continuum (de Jong 2005).

Diagnoses may be historical constructions, but the struggle of the human
mind to deal with blows to the brain, the body, and the integrity of the self
during and after combat trauma endures over time, as eloquently described
by Lewis (1942:608) even before contemporary advances in neuroscience and
neuroimaging:

> I believe we have no unequivocal criteria; no final distinction, between
> physiogenic and psychogenic because the search implies a dualism
> which is not there. . . . The patient, as a wholly integrated human be-
> ing, deals with what happens to him in ways that are determined by

his hereditary endowment and previous experiences; if he sustains an injury to his head, his behavior at any subsequent stage cannot be thought of as simply the sum of his normal functions plus the reduced or altered functions due to this destructive lesion. This behavior at every stage is a reaction to an existing situation in which his symptoms at the time, his financial, social, domestic and other difficulties are elements; the form of the reaction will obviously be determined by what has happened to him up to now. It is therefore in principle a plastic response, not a fixed one.

Psychopathology of trauma is not static, and culture has an impact on the expression of distressing memories (Jones et al. 2003). Most important, how the patient, the family, the medical team, and society view and interpret symptoms and behavior will influence not only how the condition is assessed, labeled, and treated; it also will affect the self-concept of the injured person and how others view and treat the person's suffering and disability. And it can shape the interpersonal course of the disorder and can pattern help seeking (Hinton and Lewis-Fernández 2010).

In treatment, the overlap of mTBI and PTSD needs to be addressed. To optimize treatment adherence, boost self-confidence, and mobilize the support network, patient and family education during recovery can reinforce the fact that the diagnoses of PTSD and mTBI are not mutually exclusive and can be complementary ways of understanding the complex and interlocking effects of combat injury. For example, it can be explained that PTSD reexperiencing symptoms after blast-related mTBI arise from neurological overactivation of brain areas underlying memory and arousal in an environment of chronic combat stress (Kennedy et al. 2010). The clinician can appreciate and empathetically explain the overlapping cognitive effects of blast injury and hyperarousal and also explain subsequent effects on the soldier's perception of personal safety, personal somatic and cognitive integrity, and ability to succeed in work, school, and personal relationships. Even though there are overall schema for understanding and treating comorbid PTSD and mTBI that have been enhanced by advances in contemporary medicine, it is important to recognize, particularly in a clinical area in which there are still so many questions, that each patient presents with a different combination of limitations and strengths that result from the convergence of life history, combat trauma, and the person's unique cognitive and somatic nature. This recognition can enhance the effectiveness of patient care, and the survivor's optimal recovery and social reintegration.

References

Breslau, Joshua
    2004 Cultures of Trauma: Anthropological Views of Posttraumatic Stress Disorder in International Health. Culture, Medicine, and Psychiatry 28:113–26.
Caplan, Eric M.
    1995 Trains, Brains, and Sprains: Railway Spine and the Origins of Psychoneuroses. Bulletin of the History of Medicine 69:387–419.
Da Costa, Jacob Mendes
    1871 On Irritable Heart: A Clinical Study of a Form of Functional Cardiac Disorder and Its Consequence. American Journal of Medical Science 16:17–52.
Dayan, Jacques, and Bertrand Oliac
    2010 From Hysteria and Shell Shock to Posttraumatic Stress Disorder: Comments on Psychoanalytic and Neuropsychological Approaches. Journal of Physiology—Paris 104:296–302.
De Jong, Joop T.
    2005 Commentary: Deconstructing Critiques on the Internationalization of PTSD. Culture, Medicine and Psychiatry 29:361–70.
Denny-Brown, Derek
    1943 Post-Concussion Syndrome: A Critique. Annals of Internal Medicine 19:427–32.
Eitinger, Leo
    1961 Pathology of the Concentration Camp Syndrome: Preliminary Report. Archives of General Psychiatry 5:371–79.
    1980 The Concentration Camp Syndrome and Its Late Sequelae. In Survivors, Victims and Perpetrators: Essays on the Nazi Holocaust. Joel E. Dimsdale, ed. Pp. 127–60. Washington, D.C.: Hemisphere.
Erichsen, John Eric
    1867 On Railway and Other Injuries of the Nervous System. Philadelphia: Henry C. Lea.
Fassin, Didier, and Richard Rechtman
    2009 The Empire of Trauma: An Inquiry into the Condition of Victimhood. Princeton, N.J.: Princeton University Press.
Fear, Nicola T., Edgar Jones, M. Groom, Neil Greenberg, Lisa Hull, T. J. Hodgetts, and Simon Wessely
    2009 Symptoms of Post-Concussional Syndrome Are Non-Specifically Related to Mild Traumatic Brain Injury in UK Armed Forces Personnel on Return from

Deployment in Iraq: An Analysis of Self-Reported Data. Psychological Medicine 39:1379–87.

Freud, Sigmund
(1919) 1955 Introduction to Psycho-Analysis and the War Neuroses. *In* An Infantile Neurosis and Other Works, 17. J. Strachey, ed. Pp. 207–10. London: Hogarth.

Fulton, John F.
1942 Blast and Concussion in the Present War. New England Journal of Medicine 226:1–8.

Halbauer, Joshua D., J. Wesson Ashford, Jamie M. Zeitzer, Maheen M. Adamson, Henry L. Lew, and Jerome A. Yesavage
2009 Neuropsychiatric Diagnosis and Management of Chronic Sequelae of War-Related Mild to Moderate Traumatic Brain Injury. Journal of Rehabilitation Research and Development 46:757–96.

Hinton, Devon E., and Roberto Lewis-Fernández
2010 Idioms of Distress Among Trauma Survivors: Subtypes and Clinical Utility. Culture, Medicine, and Psychiatry 34:209–18.

Hoge, Charles W., Jennifer L. Auchterlonie, and Charles S. Milliken
2006 Mental Health Problems, Use of Mental Health Services, and Attrition from Military Service After Returning from Deployment to Iraq or Afghanistan. Journal of the American Medical Association 295:1023–32.

Hoge, Charles W., Carl A. Castro, Stephen C. Messer, Dennis McGurk, Dave I. Cotting, and Robert L. Koffman
2004 Combat Duty in Iraq and Afghanistan, Mental Health Problems, and Barriers to Care. New England Journal of Medicine 351:13–22.

Hoge, Charles W., Dennis McGurk, Jeffrey L. Thomas, Anthony L. Cox, Charles C. Engel, and Carl A. Castro,
2008 Mild Traumatic Brain Injury in U.S. Soldiers Returning from Iraq. New England Journal of Medicine 358:453–63.

Holm, Lena, J. David Cassidy, Linda J. Carroll, and Jorgen Borg
2005 Summary of the WHO Collaborative Centre for Neurotrauma Task Force on Mild Traumatic Brain Injury. Journal of Rehabilitation Medicine 37:137–41.

Hoppe, Klaus D.
1971 The Aftermath of Nazi Persecution Reflected in Recent Psychiatric Literature. International Psychiatric Clinics 8:169–204.

Humphries, Mark
2010 War's Long Shadow: Masculinity, Medicine, and the Gendered Politics of Trauma, 1914–1939. Canadian Historical Review 91:503–31.

Jones, Edgar, Nicola T. Fear, and Simon Wessely
2007 Shell Shock and Mild Traumatic Brain Injury: A Historical Review. American Journal of Psychiatry 164:1641–45.

Jones, Edgar, Robert Hodgins-Vermaas, Helen McCartney, Charlotte Beech, Ian Palmer, Kenneth Hyams, and Simon Wessely

2003 Flashbacks and Post-Traumatic Stress Disorder: The Genesis of a 20th Century Diagnosis. British Journal of Psychiatry 182:158–63.

Jones, Edgar, Robert Hodgins-Vermaas, Helen McCartney, Brian Everitt, Charlotte Beech, Denise Poynter, Ian Palmer, Kenneth Hyams, and Simon Wessely
2002 Post-Combat Syndromes from the Boer War to the Gulf War: A Cluster Analysis of Their Nature and Attribution. British Medical Journal 324:1–7.

Kaplan, Gary B., Jennifer J. Vasterling, and Priyanka C. Vedak
2010 Brain-Derived Neurotrophic Factor in Traumatic Brain Injury, Post-Traumatic Stress Disorder, and Their Comorbid Conditions: Role in Pathogenesis and Treatment. Behavioural Pharmacology 21:427–37.

Keller, Thomas, and Thomas Chappell
1996 The Rise and Fall of Erichsen's Disease. Spine 21:1597–1601.

Kennedy, Jan E., Michael S. Jaffee, Gregory A. Leskin, James W. Stokes, Felix O. Leal, and Pamela J. Fitzpatrick
2007 Posttraumatic Stress Disorder and Posttraumatic Stress Disorder-Like Symptoms and Mild Traumatic Brain Injury. Journal of Rehabilitation Research and Development 44:895–920.

Kennedy, Jan E., Felix O. Leal, Jeffrey D. Lewis, Maren A. Cullen, and Ricardo R. Amador
2010 Posttraumatic Stress Symptoms in OIF/OEF Service Members with Blast-Related and Non-Blast-Related Mild TBI. Neurorehabilitation 26:223–31.

Kinzie, J. David, and Rupert R. Goetz
1996 A Century of Controversy Surrounding Posttraumatic Stress-Spectrum Syndromes: The Impact on DSM-III and DSM-IV. Journal of Traumatic Stress 9:159–79.

Kolb, Lawrence C.
1987 A Neuropsychological Hypothesis Explaining Posttraumatic Stress Disorders. American Journal of Psychiatry 144:989–95.

Kugelmann, Robert
2009 The Irritable Heart Syndrome in the American Civil War. In Culture and Panic Disorder, Devon E. Hinton and Byron J. Good, eds. Pp. 57–85. Palo Alto, Calif.: Stanford University Press.

Lamprecht, Friedhelm, and Martin Sack
2002 Post-Traumatic Stress Disorder Revisited. Psychosomatic Medicine 64:222–37.

Lew, Henry L., Rodney D. Vanderploeg, David F. Moore, Karen Schwab, Leah Friedman, Jerome Yesavage, Terence M. Keane, Deborah L. Warden, and Barbara J. Sigford
2008 Overlap of Mild TBI and Mental Health Conditions in Returning OIF/OEF Service Members and Veterans. Journal of Rehabilitation Research and Development 45:xi–xvi.

Lewis, A.
1942 Discussion on Differential Diagnosis and Treatment of Post-Contusional States. Proceedings of the Royal Society of Medicine 35:601–14.

Loughran, Tracey

2008 Hysteria and Neurasthenia in Pre-1914 British Medical Discourse and in Histories of Shell-Shock. History of Psychiatry 19:25–46.

2012 Shell Shock, Trauma, and the First World War: The Making of a Diagnosis and Its Histories. Journal of the History of Medicine and Allied Sciences 67: 94–119.

Mott, F. W.

1916 Special Discussion on Shell Shock Without Visible Signs of Injury. Proceedings of the Royal Society of Medicine 9:i–xxxii.

Myers, Charles S.

1915 A Contribution to the Study of Shell Shock. Lancet 1:316–20.

Peskind, Elaine R., Eric C. Petrie, Donna J. Cross, Kathleen Pagulayan, Kathleen McCraw, David Hoff, Kim Hart, Chang-En Yu, Murray A. Raskind, David G. Cook, and Satoshi Minoshima

2011 Cerebrocerebellar Hypometabolism Associated with Repetitive Blast Exposure Mild Traumatic Brain Injury in 12 Iraq War Veterans with Persistent Post-Concussive Symptoms. Neuroimage 54 (Suppl 1):S76–82.

Pietrzak, Robert H., Douglas C. Johnson, Marc B. Goldstein, James C. Malley, and Steven M. Southwick

2009 Posttraumatic Stress Disorder Mediates the Relationship Between Mild Traumatic Brain Injury and Health and Psychosocial Functioning in Veterans of Operations Enduring Freedom and Iraqi Freedom. Journal of Nervous and Mental Disease 197:748–53.

Rhein, John H. W.

1919 Neuropsychiatric Problems at the Front During Combat. Journal of Abnormal Psychology 14:9–14.

Risling, Marten

2010 Blast Induced Brain Injuries—A Grand Challenge in TBI Research. Frontiers in Neurology 1:1–2.

Russell, W. Ritchie

1942 Medical Aspects of Head Injury. British Medical Journal 2:521–23.

Salmon, Thomas W.

1917 The Care and Treatment of Mental Diseases and War Neuroses ("Shell Shock") in the British Army. Mental Hygiene 1:509–47.

Sayer, Nina A., Nancy A. Rettmann, Kathleen F. Carlson, Nancy Bernardy, Barbara J. Sigford, Jessica L. Hamblen, and Matthew J. Friedman

2009 Veterans with History of Mild Traumatic Brain Injury and Posttraumatic Stress Disorder: Challenges from Provider Perspective. Journal of Rehabilitation Research and Development 46:703–16.

Schaller, Walter F.

1939 After-Effects of Head Injury. Journal of the American Medical Association 113:1779–85.

Schneiderman, Aaron I., Elisa R. Braver, and Han K. Kang

2008 Understanding Sequelae of Injury Mechanisms and Mild Traumatic Brain Injury Incurred During the Conflicts in Iraq and Afghanistan: Persistent Postconcussive Symptoms and Posttraumatic Stress Disorder. American Journal of
Epidemiology 167:1446–52.

Stecker, Tracy, John C. Fortney, Francis Hamilton, and Icek Ajzen

2007 An Assessment of Beliefs About Mental Health Care Among Veterans Who
Served in Iraq. Psychiatric Services 58:1358–61.

Stein, Dan J., Soraya Seedat, Amy Iversen, and Simon Wessely

2007 Post-Traumatic Stress Disorder: Medicine and Politics. Lancet 369:139–44.

Symonds, C. P.

1942 Discussion on Differential Diagnosis and Treatment of Post-Contusional States.
Proceedings of the Royal Society of Medicine 35:601–14.

U.S. Department of Veterans Affairs, National Center for PTSD

2011 Traumatic Brain Injury and PTSD. http://www.ptsd.va.gov/public/pages/trau
matic_brain_injury_and_ptsd.asp, accessed May 11.

van der Kolk, Bessel, and Onno van der Hart

1989 Pierre Janet and the Breakdown of Adaptation in Psychological Trauma.
American Journal of Psychiatry 146:1530–40.

Vasterling Jennifer J., Mieke Verfaellie, and Karen D. Sullivan

2009 Mild Traumatic Brain Injury and Posttraumatic Stress Disorder in Returning
Veterans: Perspectives from Cognitive Neuroscience. Clinical Psychology Review 29:674–84.

Verfaellie, Mieke, Ginette Lafleche, Avron Spiro, and Kathryn Bousquet

2014 Neuropsychological Outcomes in OEF/OIF Veterans with Self-Report of Blast
Exposure: Associations with Mental Health, but Not mTBI. Neuropsychology
28:337–46.

Whittaker Robert, Steven Kemp, and Allan House

2007 Illness Perceptions and Outcome in Mild Head Injury: A Longitudinal Study.
Journal of Neurology, Neurosurgery and Psychiatry 78:644–46.

Wittenbrook, J. M.

1941 The Post-Concussion Syndrome: A Clinical Entity. Journal of Nervous and
Mental Disease 94:170–76.

Young, Allan

1995 The Harmony of Illusions: Inventing Post-Traumatic Stress Disorder. Princeton, N.J.: Princeton University Press.

PART III

Cross-Cultural Perspectives

CHAPTER 5

Trauma in the Lifeworlds of Adolescents: Hard Luck and Trouble in the Land of Enchantment

Janis H. Jenkins and Bridget M. Haas

In this chapter, we argue that the diagnosis of posttraumatic stress disorder (PTSD) requires substantial elaboration when applied to adolescents living under conditions of structural violence and cultural conflict. We make this claim on the basis of ethnographic and clinical research data collected for a study of forty-seven adolescents in the American Southwest funded by the National Institute of Mental Health (NIMH).[1] To take a step toward understanding the social and psychological nexus of trauma, our analysis is grounded in case studies that illustrate the primacy and insistence of lived experience. This analysis reveals that problems faced by these youths cannot be apprehended apart from both the historical circumstances of their production and the sheer density of traumatic life events. The events consist of violence, loss, and betrayal that biographically reverberate. When these events are recurrent or unrelenting, it should be obvious that conceptualizations of trauma must come to incorporate social and developmental trajectories that unsurprisingly complicate and supersede the rudimentary diagnostic descriptor of PTSD. Indeed, our research with New Mexican youths lays bare the raw quality of trauma not as circumscribed events of acuity but as recurrent events and inexorable conditions of acuity. There is no "habituation." There is no "adaptation." Insecurity and strain delineate lives through a pattern we have identified as precarious. Our analysis draws on the formulation by Jenkins (2015a, b) of "extraordinary conditions" as matters of subjective experience and structural violence. Our analysis also draws on the notion of precarity as advanced by Anne Lovell (2013) when applied to experience of near-danger and life-threatening circumstances. In the present ethnographic case, precarity prominently includes social abandonment and indifference (Jenkins 2015a). These conditions of existential vulnerability and harm are deeply rooted in regional legacies of geopolitical conflict and oppression that are centuries in the making (Sanchez [1940] 1996; Chávez 2006). These conditions supply the breeding grounds for recurrent cycles of trauma and rupture in the social relations of kin and community.

We wish to point out that it is not our intention to conduct an inquiry into the status of the diagnosis of PTSD as a moral, ontological, or political category. In an account of the extensive geographic scale and application of the term, Fassin and Rechtman (2009) offer an historical analysis of trauma as "empire" instituted through uncontested claims of the veracity and moral worthiness of PTSD. This account of the institutional genealogy is useful to trace the contemporary circulation of the concept. In contrast, our interest is the lived experiences of adolescents and their families who have actually experienced major psychic trauma. Many of the families have extensive histories of trauma, the vastness and complexity of which simply cannot be captured by a clinical diagnostic perspective. This comes as no surprise to experienced clinicians. Our use of the term "psychic trauma" instead of "PTSD" is therefore not meant to portray these terms as diametric. We agree with the position articulated by Byron Good (1994) that anthropological research on mental illness does well to utilize psychiatric diagnostic categories as a starting point for analysis and comparison. This position is well taken as a counter to wholesale dismissal of DSM criteria as a priori of no use for the description or organization of particular kinds of illnesses. This point needs to be made explicit since it is an anthropological commonplace to dismiss diagnostic constructs as presumptively universal. Such a priori judgments are typically made in the absence of empirical research.

We take as our starting point the fact that the adolescents we discuss in this chapter met the criteria for PTSD (described more fully below). Our larger project, however, is to elaborate the structure of these youths' experiences. We see our approach as a stepwise one, in which we take diagnoses of PTSD as our point of departure for a fuller elaboration of our participants' lived experiences. Our intent in using the term "psychic trauma" is to move beyond clinical descriptions and to draw theoretical attention to the complicated cultural and psychological dimensions of these young people's lived realities. In this regard, our analysis is firmly grounded within an existential, phenomenological, and psychodynamic framework. At the same time, we emphasize that these considerations must be understood as critically connected to and reciprocally shaped by larger social and structural forces. Thus while we are primarily concerned with phenomenological aspects of adolescents experiencing psychic trauma, our contention is that these aspects of experience are always informed by broader forces and institutions, as we underscore throughout our discussion.

While our case studies in this chapter, as with our larger research sample, come from a particular geographic region—the American Southwest— comprised predominantly of Hispanic, Native American, and Anglo-American adolescents and their families, we do not purport to describe a homogenous or space- and time-bound way of experiencing or understanding trauma. Rather, the cultural analysis presented here adopts a broader conceptualization of culture as a way of being-in-the-world in which local, shared symbolic forms articulate with intrapersonal and psychic processes. Hence, from the outset, our analysis assumes the important connection between culture and psyche, as well as the inseparability of subjectivity and intersubjectivity (Jenkins and Barrett 2004).

Study Background and Methods

This chapter draws on data from a longitudinal study, "Southwest Youth and the Experience of Psychiatric Treatment" (SWYEPT), in which we investigated the experiences of adolescents in psychiatric residential treatment in the Southwest United States, namely New Mexico. Our interest here, as with the larger project, is in elucidating the sociocultural dimensions of psychic trauma and mental illness among these youths. Methods of data collection included ethnographic interviews with adolescents and their families; interviews with clinicians and social workers; clinical observations; and observations of homes and communities. In addition, study participants were administered the Structured Clinical Interview for DSM Disorders (for children it is known as KID-SCID), a semistructured interview used for making the major DSM Axis I diagnoses. The KID-SCID was administered by one of two study team members (a child psychiatrist and clinical psychologist both trained specifically to reliably administer this research diagnostic interview). Adolescents were approached and recruited in psychiatric facilities, although much of our follow-up interviews and observations occurred within homes. Adolescents and their caregivers were interviewed at various intervals over a period of one to two years.

In the last decade, New Mexico has experienced a 13.2 percent increase in growth, with the 2010 U.S. Census reporting a population of just over two million. The primary sites of our study were the two most populous cities in the state, Albuquerque and Las Cruces. However, New Mexico maintains a largely rural character, and, indeed, a good portion of our fieldwork entailed traveling to much less populated areas within the state. According to census data, the population of New Mexico is predominantly Hispanic (46.3 percent), followed by Anglo-Americans (40.5 percent) and Native Americans (9.4 percent). New Mexico has a notably high rate of child poverty at 30 percent, one of the highest in the country (Macartney 2011:6).

The majority of adolescents in our study came from low-income households, and many lived in neighborhoods or communities addled with drug use and gang activity. Housing instability and transience as well as familial fragmentation largely marked the lives of these adolescents. For example, it was not uncommon to find an adolescent living with another family member at the time of a follow-up interview, or to discover that the family had abruptly fled (from violence or eviction) their previous home. Overall, the lives of the families in our study unfolded in contexts of structural violence (Farmer 2004), marked by the presence of drugs, violent crime, and high unemployment, and a lack of access to educational, health, and social services.

Street drugs were plentiful and near ubiquitous in many of the neighborhoods where our study participants lived. Albuquerque and Las Cruces are major points of transmission of heroin and other drugs for the Southwest, Midwest, and Pacific Northwest. New Mexico has the inauspicious distinction of the highest per capita rate of heroin-related deaths in the nation. Overall, drug-related overdose in New Mexico was recently reported as the leading cause of unintentional death (New Mexico Department of Health 2011). Drug use, including use of alcohol, cannabis, methamphetamines, and cocaine, was common among adolescents in our study.

The existence of trauma in the lives of many of these adolescents emerged as a key finding in this study. Adolescents and their families cited a range of traumatic events and life conditions including, but not limited to, physical, sexual, and emotional abuse and assault; witnessing of deaths, physical violence, or suicide attempts of family or friends; exposure to gang-related activities, including sexual and physical assault and drug abuse; contact with police or the juvenile justice system; neglect or abandonment; and housing instability (family being evicted and/or adolescents being removed from the home).

Adolescents in our study were primarily recruited from a large, university-based psychiatric hospital for children in Albuquerque. Our study of adolescents in residential psychiatric treatment centers included a comparison sample of nonhospitalized adolescents recruited from a public school district. However, this chapter focuses solely on data collected among the hospitalized sample. Children were referred here from all over the state. Over time, with the retrenchment of health care services, the average stay for patients had declined from one year to thirty days for residential patients. During the six-year period of the study (2005–11) we saw that time eroded even further. This restriction of services was the source of great dismay for clinicians, patients, and families. Under pressure from a health care management company that had received the state contract within a year prior to our study's beginning, payment for both residential treatment and day treatment was approved with decreasing frequency, and more beds had to be allocated to acute care for the institution to remain financially viable. At the time of our work, a day hospital program had recently been eliminated, and one of the inpatient cottages had switched from residential to acute care. Of the six units, each with a capacity for approximately nine patients, one was dedicated to girls who were in legal trouble, one was for residential treatment of adolescents, two were primarily for acute care of adolescents, and two were for acute care of younger children. Simultaneous to the downsizing of health services during the course of the study, Value Options, the largest privately held health care corporation in the country at that time, began the process of centralizing all mental and behavioral services. Through what was said to be competitive bidding in 2005, the state of New Mexico selected Value Options to oversee public funding and delivery of health care throughout the state. Value Options operated as the state's single managed care entity for the delivery of mental and behavioral health care.

Participants in the study included forty-seven adolescents, twenty-five boys, and twenty-two girls between the ages of thirteen and seventeen. The ethnicity of study participants included a fairly equal distribution of Hispanic, Anglo-American, and Native American groups, although there were other combinations of ethnicity to include African American and Southeast Asian ancestry. The average age of the teens was fourteen. Close to 75 percent of our study participants had been previously hospitalized on multiple occasions. Data from the KID-SCID are remarkable with regard to the co-occurrence of psychiatric diagnoses.

Thirteen adolescents (28 percent) met full diagnostic criteria for PTSD. Girls were nearly twice as likely to meet full diagnostic criteria for PTSD compared to boys in our study (eight or 36.4 percent and five or 20 percent, respectively). This does not include several more who were clinically subsyndromal for PTSD. For research and clinical practice alike, the diagnosis of PTSD is complicated in ways that are not entirely comparable to other conditions such as depression or psychosis. Assuming validity of the information provided by the patient, that is, that they are willing to offer actual accounts of their experience to the diagnostician, posing a series of questions may lead to a diagnosis on the basis of specific criteria. In the case of PTSD, however, diagnosis can be considerably more difficult. Since the disorder can be characterized by avoidance or profound disturbances of memory, for example, direct questions in these realms can be fruitless. Given this, it is possible that the percentages of identified cases underestimate the problem.

Diagnostic criteria aside, however, these youths commonly had committed violent acts, had attempted suicide, had experienced recent deaths of loved ones, had made heavy use of drugs and alcohol, had had legal troubles, were the object physical and/or sexual abuse (an alarming number of girls were raped multiple times), and engaged in routine self-cutting. These existential dimensions of psychic trauma, which is our theoretical focus, are highlighted in the following cases of two study participants, Danielle and Luis.[2] Both Danielle and Luis met the research diagnostic criteria for PTSD. Yet, it is by investigating the phenomenological features of their experiences of psychic trauma that we make a critical move toward elaborating the meaning and experience of their diagnoses.

Case Studies

Danielle Ramirez

At the time that we met Danielle, a chubby, attractive, and pleasant Hispanic girl who was just days from her fifteenth birthday, she was living with her mother, stepfather, grandfather, and three siblings in a working-class neighborhood that she described as fairly safe and comfortable. However, the relatively stability of her living situation at that time belied Danielle's extensive history of housing instability, familial fragmentation, violence, abuse, and related mental health struggles.

Danielle had recently been discharged from the children's psychiatric hospital, having been there for close to six months. This hospitalization, her second, had been prompted by an incident at school in which Danielle had confided to a male classmate that she had thought about choking people with a shoelace. This boy subsequently took a shoelace and attempted to choke several students claiming, when caught by school officials, that Danielle forced him to do it. School officials and police officers confiscated several of Danielle's notebooks from her backpack, in which she had written "awful stuff," such as her desire to harm and choke people, including her mother. In lieu of being taken to juvenile detention, Danielle was admitted to the hospital for psychiatric treatment. In addition to PTSD, Danielle was also diagnosed with psychosis, major depressive disorder, separation anxiety disorder, and oppositional defiant disorder.

Danielle's history of mental health challenges started in her childhood. Danielle grew up in a poor town just east of Albuquerque with her siblings, her mother, and her mother's husband, Donny, until she was ten years old. Having been led to believe that Donny was her biological father, Danielle was devastated when, at age seven, Donny told Danielle to "get out of my face . . . 'cause you ain't my daughter." Danielle recalled her reaction: "I felt like I was worthless, like, I didn't have no purpose in life."

Throughout Danielle's childhood, her mother, Victoria, was a heroin dealer and active gang member. Though Victoria claimed not to use any drugs other than alcohol or marijuana, there was frequent "partying" (including heavy drug use and sexual encounters) that took place at the family's home(s), and Danielle and her siblings were exposed to egregious acts of violence, including murder. For example, Danielle noted a particularly horrifying incident in which her uncle was shot and killed in the family's front yard in a gang fight. Furthermore, domestic violence permeated family life, and Danielle would often witness her mother and Donny in "knock-down, drag-out" physical altercations.

When Danielle was nine years old, Victoria was arrested for aggravated assault with a deadly weapon and was sentenced to two and a half years in prison. Danielle was sent to live with her maternal grandmother, who was a heroin-addicted gang member. It was at this time that Danielle began to experience frightening auditory hallucinations. As she told interviewers, Danielle had, from a very young age, had an imaginary friend with whom she conversed called "the Man." She insisted that "the Man was not that scary when I was little, but whenever I turned nine, he started being really mean to me." Asked to elaborate, she explained: "He started yelling at me. He started screaming at me. He would tell me I was no good. He would tell me that I should just kill myself."

After Victoria was released from prison, in an attempt to stay out of gang life, the family moved to Albuquerque, where they lived in an area referred to as "the war zone," given the neighborhood's prevalence of drug and gang-related violence. By this time, Victoria had divorced Donny. Fed up with the violence in the neighborhood, the family moved back to a town east of Albuquerque, where they remained for close to two years. While Victoria still did not return to gang life, she remained friends with gang members, with whom she partied and engaged in promiscuous behavior. Additionally, Victoria's siblings and parents, who lived in the area, were all active gang members. Thus, violence remained a salient part of Danielle's life, and she continued to be haunted by the Man. After another brutal physical altercation and fearing legal repercussions, Victoria fled back to Albuquerque, leaving Danielle to live with Donny and his girlfriend. Donny was emotionally and sexually abusive, raping Danielle on two occasions. Danielle was also expelled from school for attacking a classmate who was making fun of her and her mother, reporting that "the voices told me to get a knife and stab him." Feeling angry and hopeless, Danielle attempted to commit suicide by hanging, but the rope broke. Danielle demanded that Donny take her to her mother in Albuquerque.

After returning to Albuquerque, Danielle disclosed the sexual assaults to her mother and older sister. Danielle's hallucinations increased: "The voices were getting louder and louder." She was hospitalized and spent two months at a residential psychiatric treatment center. While she found this treatment center to be a "bad experience"—primarily due to the fact that she was constantly restrained to the point where she had bruises on her arms—she did credit the hospitalization for getting her on medication that helped mitigate her symptoms. The voices, Danielle reported, did not disappear but "got quieter."

Danielle was discharged from psychiatric treatment and spent the next year at home with her family: her mother, her three siblings, her grandfather, and her mother's new husband, Mark. Danielle liked Mark, describing him as a "real understanding person," and quickly began to refer to him as "Dad." Victoria had been attending weekly counseling sessions and had been making attempts to "turn [her] life around."

Victoria, in her interviews, talked at length about her familial history of gang-related violence, drug and alcohol addiction, and neglect and abuse. She recounted: "You know, I grew up watching my mom abuse herself. You know, she got shot, she almost died. . . . drinking, partying. Everybody doing drugs. They didn't care if we [she and her siblings] were sitting there. . . . So as far back as I remember, I remember people using needles." After witnessing her uncle's murder when she was nine years old, Victoria recounts: "I stopped talking. I just started hurting myself. And my mom was in her addiction. She didn't want to deal with me, so she just put me in the [psychiatric] hospital. For a year and a half."

Determined to stop the cycle of violence and abuse that had character-ized her family legacy for generations, Victoria boasted to research staff that in addition to quitting gang life, drugs, and alcohol, she also no longer yelled at her children and was trying to improve communication among everyone in the family. Danielle saw an improvement in her own life at this time. She did continue to see the Man and hear voices, but these were kept to a mini-mum with psychiatric medication.

Danielle's struggles were far from over, however. Only months after be-ing discharged from her first hospitalization, Danielle was feeling unloved and again attempted suicide, this time by taking "a whole bunch of Seroquel." Danielle was extremely sick for several days, with severe abdominal pains and vomiting. Yet she did not reveal to anyone that she had attempted to kill her-self by overdosing on Seroquel. In fact, Danielle said, "nobody really paid attention to me, so they couldn't even tell if I was sick or not." Her suicide attempt and profound feelings of loneliness and neglect did not come to light until she was hospitalized for the second time, following the school incident with the shoelace described earlier.

Danielle understood her diagnosis of PTSD to mean "something tragic has happened to you while you were young and it messes up your chemicals in your brain or something like that." Given that the Man became menacing at the time that Victoria went to prison and the auditory hallucinations and suicide attempts occurred during and after periods of intense sexual and emotional abuse, Danielle framed these as main factors in the development of her PTSD: "When my mom went to jail that's when it [hallucinations] started, like, getting really bad. And then whenever I went with my stepdad it got really, really bad."

While Danielle pointed to specific incidents of her mother's imprison-ment and to sexual abuse perpetrated by her stepfather as possible origins of her PTSD diagnosis, Victoria was much more ambivalent regarding this matter. When asked her thoughts on what may have accounted for Danielle's PTSD symptoms, Victoria offered multiple, if sometimes conflicting, speculations. At first, Victoria offered that Danielle's mental health issues may have been prompted by the crowded apartment with few amenities that the family shared at the time: "I think maybe the living situation was too much." Yet Victoria later revealed more ambivalence about the source of Danielle's symptoms, particularly her auditory hallucinations: "Um, at first I, I thought it was because of everything that I had, um—going to prison, um, all the things they witnessed me do. I mean, 'cause the first time my son seen me shoot someone he was like seven. . . . And I can imagine what these kids seen." Victoria even speculated that the origin(s) of Danielle's trauma could be located even earlier, as she wondered, "Was it something that I did when I was pregnant, the behaviors or—'cause I did drink and my husband used to beat me up a lot when I was pregnant with her." Yet, these perspectives of self-blame were also tempered by her statement that ultimately Danielle's mental health issues are "not all me, but maybe a little bit is me."

If Danielle and, especially, Victoria seemed ambivalent about the etiology of Danielle's mental health struggles, they also had doubts about the veracity of the PTSD diagnosis itself. Both Danielle and Victoria wondered to interviewers if what Danielle "really [had]" was PTSD or something else, namely schizophrenia. Danielle noted: "Well, I think I have schizophrenia because I seen the Man way before . . . way before the rape and, um, [before] bad things happened to me." Danielle noted that "schizophrenia is the same thing as PTSD but schizophrenia is when something has never happened to you but you still see things [hallucinations]."

While Danielle noted to interviewers that clinicians never gave her a diagnosis of schizophrenia, Victoria recalled one of the children's psychiatric hospital clinicians suggesting that Danielle's symptoms "seem like schizophrenia." (We should note that according to our conversations with hospital clinicians and according to results of the psychiatrist-administered SCID, Danielle did not meet the diagnostic criteria for schizophrenia.) Victoria, however, dismissed the idea of a schizophrenia diagnosis, noting: "I did some research and schizophrenia doesn't happen to chicks."

At our last meeting with the family, Danielle reported doing much better. Victoria, who was still sober and attending counseling, was looking for a new neighborhood in which to live, primarily so that Danielle could resume school the following academic year. Danielle expressed hopes to get back into school so that she could eventually become an architect. She rarely experienced auditory or visual hallucinations anymore, a fact that she attributed to a change and increase in psychiatric medications during her second hospitalization. In his clinical notes following the SCID interview, our research psychiatrist expressed his sense that "a more settled environment will be supportive" for Danielle but simultaneously underscored the enduring effects of the "significant exposure to instability, insecurity, neglect and abuse in [Danielle's] early years."

Luis Gonzales

Upon enrolling in our study, Luis, a lanky, slightly awkward, and quiet but affable Hispanic sixteen-year-old, had just moved to a residential treatment center after spending two weeks in an acute psychiatric inpatient unit. By both his own account and that of his family's, Luis struggled with issues of depression, anxiety, paranoia, and intense anger. Requests to clean his room at home or drives to the grocery store with his grandmother would evoke panic and anger in Luis for reasons that he could not quite explain: "I just get nervous around, like, when things start to happen—I don't know what to do anymore. I just get nervous and start freaking out." Luis also used alcohol and marijuana, which he described as a way of coping with his emotional difficulties.

Luis vacillated between self-isolation and highly destructive behavior. Though he had never harmed another person, he did sometimes harm himself, either by cutting himself or choking himself with a belt. More often, when he felt angry or anxious, he would violently destroy property. At the time of enrollment in the study, Luis had been admitted to the acute psychiatric unit following a violent episode in which he took a sledgehammer to his grandmother's small trailer, where he and his mother were also living at the time. After he had put a "couch-sized hole" in the external wall of the trailer, his mother called the police, who escorted Luis to the children's psychiatric hospital. Luis was diagnosed with PTSD as well as depression and separation anxiety disorder.

Growing up, Luis moved frequently: by his own account, he had moved nine times by the time he was twelve. Luis had not had contact with his biological father since he was three years old. His mother remarried when Luis was a toddler, and Luis had a younger half sister, who was six years his junior (ten years old at the time we enrolled Luis in the study). Luis's mother, Paula, who was a drug addict, was in and out of jail throughout Luis's life. During his mother's episodes of incarceration, Luis sometimes lived with his stepfather (his younger sister's biological father), Kevin, though he was usually sent to live with his aunt Linda, who was also a drug addict, or his grandmother, both of whom lived in areas of poverty rife with drug users and gang members. Kevin was emotionally and physically abusive. Luis recalled, for example, Kevin smashing his head with the lid of a washing machine. Luis also recounted times when he, at age eleven or twelve, was locked in a closet while his mother and stepfather used drugs and had sex.

In 2005, Luis's mother divorced Kevin. Their relationship had been increasingly difficult and destructive, and Paula had discovered that Kevin had slept with her sister Linda. At this time, Paula was heavily using drugs, primarily cocaine, and was, as she put it, "in a crisis situation." She attempted suicide by cutting her wrists and a vein in her neck. Luis witnessed his mother's suicide attempt and subsequently became very agitated and upset, claiming, "I couldn't take it." Luis's grandmother Manuela took him to the psychiatric unit of a local hospital, where he was admitted for two weeks for inpatient care.

While both Paula and Luis were hospitalized, Kevin reported Paula to the local child and family services, and, following an investigation, Paula was charged with child endangerment and neglect, and Luis was sent to foster care for two years, which Luis described as the worst time of his life. Manuela was made Luis's legal guardian following his release from foster care, and he moved into the small trailer that Manuela shared with her partner of twenty-five years, Roberto. The trailer was small and crowded and located in a poor, drug-addled neighborhood. Paula had also been living with Manuela and Roberto at this time, though the state denied her custody of Luis. Moreover, in the years preceding Paula's suicide attempt, Kevin had secured a restraining order against Paula, and Paula was allowed only minimal contact with her daughter. On the evening prior to our first interview with the family, Linda had been arrested and imprisoned on drug charges, which Manuela had described as "a blessing" given Linda's history of "terrorizing this family." Indeed, Linda, a crack cocaine addict had been visiting Manuela's home at all hours of the night, begging for or stealing money, especially from Luis.

Luis articulated ambivalent and deeply fraught feelings regarding his family, particularly his mother. He expressed feeling "better when I'm with family" but also described anxious and angry feelings prompted by interactions with family members. When Luis was in treatment, he described feeling claustrophobic and angry at home, yet he also told interviewers that the hardest thing about being in residential treatment was that he wasn't able to be with his family or talk to his family when he wanted. Luis seemed to struggle the most in negotiating his desire for familial connection with his feelings of anger and abandonment toward his mother. Paula's sporadic attempts at reconnection with Luis were a particular point of contention for him: "She's always going to jail so I just—I don't like it when she goes to jail. . . . [Now] I'm talking to her but I'm still kind of mad at her and I don't like her touching me all the time 'cause sometimes she tries to give me hugs and kisses and stuff and I don't like that."

Paula likewise reflected ambivalent feelings regarding her relationship with Luis, reporting, "We really don't have good communication." Given her absences throughout Luis's life and her abdication of legal guardianship, both Paula and Luis struggled to define personal and relational expectations. Ultimately, Luis's grandmother emerged as the most stable figure in his life, though she struggled to balance taking care of Luis and caring not only for herself (she had serious health issues, including rheumatoid arthritis and diabetes), but also for her elderly father, who lived on his own. Manuela was nurturing and caring of Luis, but also reported feeling worn out by caring for him.

Luis and his family struggled to make sense of a diagnosis of PTSD, in that they expressed ambivalence over the origin of his emotional and psychological problems. Luis framed his grief, anger, anxiety, and paranoia as tied to his abuse by Kevin and his abandonment by his mother. Paula was more ambivalent regarding the impact of parental abuse and neglect on Luis. While she did cede that her episodes of neglect and abandonment added to Luis's struggles, Paula nonetheless conceived of the origin of Luis's problems, including PTSD symptomatology, as biologically based. More specifically, Luis's mother and grandmother—and to a much lesser extent Luis himself—cited brain surgery to correct a prematurely closed fontanel that Luis had undergone as an infant as a primary trauma from which his subsequent mental health issues stemmed. This surgery, Luis's caregivers stressed, was surely a "trauma" and caused a "brain injury" that resulted in Luis's psychiatric and emotional issues that developed in adolescence. Both Manuela and Paula were adamant about this despite the clinician's reassurance that such a surgery would not account for Luis's diagnoses of PTSD, depression, or anxiety.

In addition to viewing brain surgery as a key factor in the development of Luis's life struggles, Luis and his caregivers (mother and grandmother) also identified foster care as a key factor in his rage, anxiety, and paranoia. Luis asserted that it was when he went to foster care that his "life starting falling apart." Likewise, Manuela asserted that foster care "screwed [Luis] up really badly. To where's he's paranoid. [Luis] was *never* paranoid like that." She added: "If he has abandonment issues, I blame it on that." In addition to expressing ambivalence about the source of Luis's emotional and psychological issues, Luis's mother and grandmother expressed a struggle over finding the "right" diagnosis. Manuela, somewhat exasperatedly, described Luis's history of various psychiatric diagnoses, in addition to PTSD: "I've been told that [Luis] has anger-management problems. I've been told he's paranoid. And he suffers severe depression. Ok, and I've asked 'is there a possibility that he could be bipolar?' [Clinicians say,] No, no, no. It wasn't until now that [a hospital clinician] said that she thinks he's bipolar. And with something else, but they wouldn't know until he got older because he could outgrow it. I don't know if that's schizophrenic or, or what it is."

At the time of our second meeting with him, approximately five months following our initial interview, Luis had been feeling "less angry and paranoid," which he attributed to his medication regimen, though he also disliked taking medication and being prompted by his mother or grandmother to take his medication was a major trigger for his anger and anxiety. He and his mother were working on improving their relationship.

The attempts at rebuilding a relationship with his mother were curtailed shortly after our second meeting with Luis, however, as his mother was arrested and again put in jail following an automobile accident in which she was driving a stolen vehicle. She was in jail for six months and then put on one-year probation upon her release. In the eleven months between our second and third (and final) meeting with the family, Luis had been in and out of several psychiatric treatment centers as well as a juvenile detention home, each time following an episode of violent or destructive behavior. Luis had also begun abusing cocaine. At our research team's last contact with the family, Paula had been released from prison and was on probation. She had secured a part-time job as a security guard, was taking classes at a local community college, and was receiving counseling at her church. Linda had also been released from prison and was no longer using drugs. In contrast to this, Luis's problems had only seemed to increase during this same time period, and at the final research visit to the family, Luis had been hospitalized at a residential treatment center several hours away from Albuquerque. He had been there for three weeks and had six weeks left in the program. Both Manuela and Paula expressed concern about his anger, depression, and anxiety, as well as his newly developed cocaine habit. Underscoring the ambivalence that the family seemed to have toward Luis's future, Paula noted that Luis "was not proactive in his recovery," yet she also pointed the interviewer to a handmade Mother's Day card in which Luis had expressed his love for Paula and contrition for his past actions—something he never done previously and which Paula hoped was a sign of a more hopeful future.

Existential Vulnerability and Legacies of Harm

The cases of Danielle and Luis, like other research participants diagnosed with PTSD, reveal the ways in which the lives of the adolescents in our study are marked by what Jenkins (2015a) has identified as a "pattern of precarious conditions." These adolescents must often contend with social abandonment or neglect as they navigate their social worlds. The conditions of vulnerability in which these youths' lives unfold, and which are shaped by larger sociocultural, political, and economic forces, allow for repeated and pervasive acts of trauma to occur. Though the narratives presented here concern how symptoms that get identified as PTSD are negotiated within families, such familial dynamics must be understood as embedded in a larger set of histories, both intergenerational and regional.

Many parents discussed their own histories of abusive or violent childhoods and spoke of family legacies of drug abuse, gang activity, and social abandonment. Victoria's narrative painfully highlighted her own experiences of neglect and abandonment, as well as early exposure to violent crimes committed by her parents and other family members. While Victoria took to selling heroin at a young age, eleven, as a way to "get the hell out" of gang life and poverty, this only entrapped her further within these elements. Manuela summed up the family dynamics of Luis's extended family by stating: "We are a very dysfunctional family from the get-go. . . . At a time when people were nurturing their children, I was learning survival skills. . . . I was an abused person, I was an abused wife. I got my beatings. . . . [Paula] nearly drowned in the bathtub by her dad and that was just him." Within a context of economic and social marginalization, and subjected to multiple forms of violence, these women's agency took the form of survival. The lack of access to supportive social, economic, and health care resources that characterized the marginal positions of caregivers evoked an environment where self-preservation often trumped their ability to provide adequate protection or care for their children.

The intergenerational patterns of violence that were referenced across study participants' narratives must be seen within the broader framework of regional history, namely traced to the colonial history of New Mexico. An elaborated history of some five centuries of conflict among Native American, Spanish, Anglo-American, and Mexican populations is beyond the scope of this chapter (see Chávez 2006; Sanchez 1996). Yet, this historical context is critical to theorize how regional political and cultural instability gets reproduced within the intimate domain of the family in this setting (Garcia 2010; Jenkins 2015a).

Many of the families in our study, such as the families of Danielle and Luis, felt the constriction of social and economic disenfranchisement, drug and alcohol abuse, and various forms of violence. Against such a backdrop of vulnerable existence, where parental care is often altogether lacking or inadequate, multiple forms of child abuse and neglect are made possible. The configuration of the breakdown in human relations in turn fractures the psyches of those whose bodily and psychic dignity is violated. The rupture involved is profoundly disorganizing, so that symptoms of PTSD develop as sequelae of such patterned conditions.

Luis responded to the neglect and abandonment of his primary caregivers, namely his mother, with a self-system in which he would, at turns, isolate himself from the attention and care of others and be an explosive center of attention during dramatic episodes of material destruction. Such extreme behavior reflects the ambivalence and mistrust that Luis articulated regarding family relationships. His narratives reveal a desperate desire to connect with and be protected by family. Yet these narrative aspects are tempered by Luis's deep mistrust that such protection could even be a viable desire. For Luis, his childhood was characterized by shifting and ambiguous notions of not only *who* was there to care for him, but *if* anyone was there to care for him. In this way, mistrust and ambivalence about familial roles and connection are not just an understandable response to years of existential vulnerability and insecurity, but also emerge as an important system of self-protection. Resisting his mother's overtures at affection and her insistence that she's "not going anywhere," might have, for example, allowed Luis a measure of protection except that, in fact, she was back in jail months later. Seemingly lost in a world that consistently left him insecure and vulnerable, Luis engaged in behavior that both connected and alienated him from others; that repaired relationships and dismantled them; that protected him and harmed him.

Danielle also exhibited a sense of mistrust and ambivalence toward her family, particularly her mother. Her life story revealed a profound breakdown in the provision of parental protection as the ground for sustained and repetitive events that for her created deep and enduring psychic trauma. Danielle's history was marked by significant acts of abandonment and abdication of protection and care, starting with Donny's disavowal of her as his daughter, continuing with her mother's physical absences while in prison and with her leaving Danielle alone in Donny's care miles away from where she lived. Even Danielle's "nice" childhood imaginary friend became a menacing and haunting figure. Stripped of any sense of protection, care, or love, Danielle was awash in a lonely and hopeless world leading her to attempt suicide on two occasions. While Danielle expressed a sense of hope and excitement about her mother's newfound active parenting style, her narratives also revealed contradictory and ambivalent emotions surrounding family. This was made most clear after Danielle's confiscated notebooks revealed feelings of anger and even fantasy of harm toward her mother.

Family Struggles with Clinical Diagnoses

Both Luis and Danielle and their families struggled to make sense of these adolescents' psychiatric diagnoses, especially PTSD. The search for the cause of PTSD seemed to be a highly fraught endeavor for these families. Their attempts to map (their interpretation of) a diagnostic framework onto their life histories had conflicting and ambivalent results. Danielle's understanding of PTSD etiology as "something tragic [that] has happened to you while you were young" seems to echo others in our study. The issue at hand is identifying what the "something tragic" is, and how study participants identify it within this particular cultural context. As we have detailed, families in our study were subjected to "everyday violences," which in turn set the stage for social abdication of care and protection (Kleinman 2000). Part of what makes structural violence so trenchant in the lives of people on the margins is its routinization (Farmer 2003, 2004), its misrecognition as part of a social order that is taken for granted (Bourdieu 1977). Such routinization of violence(s) often obscures its force in shaping everyday lived experience and subjectivity. For example, in her narrative, Danielle identified her mother's imprisonment and the sexual assault by her stepfather as "tragic things that happened," productive of PTSD. Yet her narratives also recount a painful childhood in which she routinely witnessed violent crimes and drug abuse, and experienced parental neglect, though she identified none of these in her attempt to fit life experiences into her understanding of diagnostic categorization.

Yet our ethnographic data reveal that the lived experiences and circumstances of routinized violence and neglect, even if not overtly identified by participants as tragic or productive of psychiatric illness, are nonetheless productive of forms of psychic trauma. Experiences of housing instability and family rupture and witnessing drug abuse or violent crimes evoke anxious, fractured, and vulnerable subjective states of being. This is the case even if these experiences are not identified as specific etiologic factors of psychiatric illness.

In attempting to make sense of youths' psychic struggles, biomedical or biologically based explanatory frameworks seemed to have much more allure with parents than with adolescents themselves. Caregivers, as we have seen in the two cases presented above, often pointed to (or, rather, speculated on) potential biologically rooted causes of trauma. For instance, Paula and Manuela both stressed that Luis's brain surgery in infancy served as a "brain trauma" that at least partially, if not primarily, accounted for his behaviors in the present. Paula, when reflecting on the development of Luis's problems, underscored his compromised mental health as due to his brain surgery and suggested that her attempted suicide "was harder on him than I think a normal kid." This statement is striking in that it posits a biologically based etiology (brain injury/surgery) to Luis's anxiety, rage, and paranoia, and perceived "abnormal" personhood, while events of parental abuse and neglect are framed as exacerbating factors rather than primary sources of psychic trauma.

In further speculating on a biological genesis of Luis's behavior in adolescence, Manuela, rather offhandedly, noted: "I read in some medical record somewhere . . . that the lid to the washing machine hit [Luis] on the head and that he got a big egg [swelling on head] off of it. I don't ever remember that, OK, but from what [Luis] recalls, it was [Kevin] that slammed the lid on his head." She offered this to the interviewer as a way of providing further evidence of a "brain injury." Notably, Manuela's emphasis here is on the physical not the psychic effect of an act of abuse by a paternal figure. Luis, on the other hand, discussed this incident not in terms of its physicality but rather as an act of profound violation that provoked feelings of confusion and fear and a sense of existential vulnerability.

Ambivalence and contestation regarding youths' diagnoses occurred throughout families' narratives in our study. Indeed, the caregivers of both Luis and Danielle struggled over the right diagnosis. In the case of Danielle, the family questioned: PTSD or schizophrenia? For Luis, his grandmother cited various diagnoses ranging from PTSD to depression to bipolar disorder, ultimately concluding "I don't know . . . what it is." Both Luis and Danielle and their families struggled to locate the cause of their PTSD. Both of these young people highlighted specific episodes or relations of abuse and abandonment that undoubtedly informed their mental health. Yet both sets of families pointed to the existence of early symptoms of emotional problems: Luis had reportedly been "antisocial" as a toddler, and Danielle heard voices—albeit friendly ones—starting in early childhood. Such haziness regarding the locus or source of "the problem" for these families reflects the difficulty in identifying a singular—or even primary—source of psychic trauma in contexts of enduring and pervasive precarity. The lived experiences of the youth in our study suggest that psychic trauma is often diffuse and ambiguous in its origin and persistence in these young people's lifeworlds.

Concluding Remarks

The ethnographic data presented in this chapter underscore the necessity of cultural and psychological analyses of trauma to attend to both the personal and collective levels of experience. At the personal level, for adolescents subjected to psychic trauma, making meaning of everyday life and even of one's own existence can be a challenge. To be sure, the existential chaos of these adolescents' lives often evoked a sense of incomprehensibility or bafflement (Jenkins 2015a). Psychic trauma circumscribed these adolescents' very being-in-the-world, and these young people adapted their lives to respond to the chaos and existential threats that they continued to endure. At the collective level, our analyses reveal a pattern of conditions of neglect and abandonment that rendered many of the adolescents in our study vulnerable to repeated and sustained traumatic events. This pattern of neglect is rooted in family and regional histories of violence, loss, and struggle and occurs within a context of structural violence in which adolescents and their families often have few social resources to mitigate their sense of existential struggle.

Drawing on the case of warfare, Kardiner (1941) conceived of this type of reaction to trauma as a defensive move resulting from an individual's inability to adapt to the aftermath of the trauma. Indeed, there now are studies to show that adaptation following exposure to warfare is notoriously intricate (Jenkins 1991, 1996a, 1996b; Jenkins and Hollifield 2008; Jenkins and Valiente 1994). Extending this, recent studies have investigated the process of defense and adaptation of children who are repetitively exposed to traumatic events as the everyday conditions of their lives (Cook et al. 2005; Herman 1997; Holt et al. 2008; Margolin and Vickerman 2007; Patel 2000; van der Kolk 2005). Our work presented here aims to enrich our understanding of such defense and adaptation responses in children by ethnographically bringing into relief the contours of lives permeated by ongoing psychic trauma.

Taking our study participants' diagnoses of PTSD as a starting point, we have illustrated the theoretical importance of adopting a phenomenological, existential, and psychodynamic framework in elucidating psychic trauma. Our ethnographic investigation, reflected in the presentation of two case studies here, has underscored that profound experiences of violence and loss cannot be adequately described by diagnostic categories. There is a danger in reducing the complexity of lived experiences of chaos and fractured subjectivities wrought by violence to a diagnostic category of PTSD. Indeed, the struggles over making meaning of diagnoses among the families described here attest to the complexities of lived experiences of trauma. To begin to more fully comprehend experiences of trauma and loss, we must be more theoretically attuned to the contexts of psychological development and social historical structures from which they arise. While more substantial research on the primacy of lived experience is required, we believe that our analysis of precarious quality of life and suffering holds comparative relevance across a range of locales from London to Mumbai to Buenos Aires.

Notes

1. The authors were part of a collaborative research project (2005–11) funded by National Institute of Mental Health (Grant # RO1 MH071781-01, Thomas J. Csordas and Janis H. Jenkins, Co-Principal Investigators). Along with the PIs and Dr. Whitney Duncan, Dr. Bridget Haas carried out fieldwork for collection of adolescent and family interview and ethnographic observational data. The study entailed ethnographic interviews and observations based in Albuquerque but was carried out from all parts of the

state of New Mexico. Child psychiatrist Michael Stork, M.D., and clinical psychologist Mary Bancroft, Ph.D., accomplished the work of research diagnostic interviews. Data organization and analysis was with the assistance of Heather Hallman and Allen Tran, Eliza Dimas, Jessica Hsueh, Nofit Itzhak, Tara Maguire, Jessica Novak, and Celeste Padilla.

2. All names of study participants have been changed to protect confidentiality.

References

Bourdieu, Pierre
  1977 Outline of a Theory of Practice. Cambridge: Cambridge University Press.
Chávez, Thomas E.
  2006 New Mexico: Past and Future. Albuquerque: University of New Mexico Press.
Cook, Alexandra, Joseph Spinazzola, Julian Ford, Cheryl Lanktree, Margaret Blaustein, Marylene Cloitre, et al.
  2005 Complex Trauma in Children and Adolescents. Psychiatric Annals 35:390–98.
Farmer, Paul
  2003 Pathologies of Power: Health, Human Rights, and the New War on the Poor. Berkeley: University of California Press.
  2004 An Anthropology of Structural Violence. Current Anthropology 45(3):305–25.
Fassin, Didier, and Richard Rechtmann
  2009 The Empire of Trauma: An Inquiry into the Condition of Victimhood. Princeton, N.J.: Princeton University Press.
Garcia, Angela
  2010 The Pastoral Clinic: Addiction and Dispossession Along the Rio Grande. Berkeley: University of California Press.
Good, Byron J.
  1994 Culture and Psychopathology: Directions for Psychiatric Anthropology. In New Directions in Psychological Anthropology. Theodore Schwarz, Geoffrey White, and Catherine Lutz, eds. Pp. 181–205. Cambridge: Cambridge University Press.
Herman, Judith
  1997 Trauma and Recovery: The Aftermath of Violence—From Domestic Abuse to Political Terror. New York: Basic.
Hinton, Devon E., Alexander Hinton, Kok-Thay Eng, and Sophearith Choung
  2012 PTSD and Key Somatic Complaints and Cultural Syndromes Among Rural Cambodians: The Results of a Needs Assessment Survey. Medical Anthropology Quarterly 26(3):383–407.
Holt, Stephanie, Helen Buckley, and Sadhbh Whelan
  2008 The Impact of Exposure to Domestic Violence on Children and Young People: A Review of the Literature. Child Abuse and Neglect 32(8):797–810.

Jenkins, Janis H.

1991 The State Construction of Affect: Political Ethos and Mental Health Among Salvadoran Refugees. Culture, Medicine, and Psychiatry 15:139–65.

1996a Culture, Emotion, and Post-Traumatic Stress Disorder. In Ethnocultural Aspects of Post-Traumatic Stress Disorder. Anthony Marsella and Matthew J. Freedman, eds. Pp. 165–82. Washington, D.C.: American Psychological Association Press.

1996b The Impress of Extremity: Women's Experience of Trauma and Political Violence. In Gender and Health: An International Perspective. Carolyn Sargent and Caroline Brettel, eds. Upper Saddle River, N.J.: Prentice Hall.

2015a Strains of Psychic and Social Sinew: Trauma Among Youths in New Mexico. Medical Anthropology Quarterly 29:42–60.

2015b Extraordinary Conditions: Culture and Experience in Mental Illness. Berkeley: University of California Press.

Jenkins, Janis H., and Robert J. Barrett

2004 Introduction. In Schizophrenia, Culture, and Subjectivity. Janis H. Jenkins and Robert J. Barrett, eds. Pp. 1–25. Cambridge: Cambridge University Press.

Jenkins, Janis H., and Michael A. Hollifield

2008 Postcoloniality as the Aftermath of Terror Between Vietnamese Refugees. In Postcolonial Disorders. Mary-Jo DelVecchio Good, Sandra Teresa Hyde, Sarah Pinto, and Byron J. Good, eds. Pp. 378–96. Berkeley: University of California Press.

Jenkins, Janis H., and Martha Valiente.

1994 Bodily Transactions of the Passions: El Calor (The Heat) Among Salvadoran Women. In Embodiment and Experience: The Existential Ground of Culture and Self. Thomas J. Csordas, ed. Pp. 163–82. Cambridge: Cambridge University Press.

Kardiner, Abram

1941 The Traumatic Neuroses of War. New York: Paul B. Hoeber.

Kleinman, Arthur

2000 The Violences of Everyday Life: The Multiple Forms and Dynamics of Social Violence. In Violence and Subjectivity. Veena Das, Arthur Kleinman, Mamphela Ramphele, and Pamela Reynolds, eds. Pp. 226–41. Berkeley: University of California Press.

Lovell, Anne M.

2013 Tending to the Unseen in Extraordinary Circumstances: On Arendt's Natality and Severe Mental Illness After Hurricane Katrina. Iride: Filosofia e Discussione Pubblica 26:563–578.

Macartney, Suzanne

2011 Child Poverty in the United States 2009 and 2010: Selected Race Groups and Hispanic Origin. Washington, D.C.: U.S. Census Bureau.

Margolin, Gayla, and Katrina A. Vickerman

2007 Post-Traumatic Stress in Children and Adolescents Exposed to Family Violence: I. Overview and Issues. Professional Psychology: Research and Practice 38(6):613–19.

New Mexico Department of Health
2011 Indicator Report—Drug-Induced Deaths. State of New Mexico.
Patel, Vikram
2000 Culture and Mental Health Consequences of Trauma. Indian Journal of Social Work 61:619–30.
Sanchez, George
(1940) 1996 Forgotten People: A Study of New Mexicans. Albuquerque: University of New Mexico Press.
Van der Kolk, Bessel A.
2005 Developmental Trauma Disorder: Toward a Rational Diagnosis for Children with Complex Trauma Histories. Psychiatric Annals 35:401–8.

CHAPTER 6

Gendered Trauma and Its Effects: Domestic Violence and PTSD in Oaxaca

Whitney L. Duncan

Over the past two decades, the southern Mexican state of Oaxaca has seen dramatic increases in diagnosed mental illness, a spike in the availability of psychiatric and psychological services, and unprecedented demand for mental health care. Whereas in the early 1990s mental health practitioners were rare, now nearly every neighborhood in the state capital, Oaxaca City, has several, their practices ranging from biomedical psychiatry to gestalt therapy to hypnosis. Self-help options abound: among other member-run support groups, Oaxaca has thirty-eight centers for Neurotics Anonymous, an offshoot of Alcoholics Anonymous designed specifically to support those self-diagnosed with emotional and/or mental illness. Workshops on themes such as emotional intelligence, managing emotions, and living in peace take place nearly each week. Seeking institutional mental health care has become much more common as well; according to Oaxaca's Ministry of Health (Servicios de Salud de Oaxaca [or SSO] 2007), there was a threefold increase, from 2,551 to 7,433, in patients receiving first-time consultations at the public psychiatric hospital between 1993 and 2000 (Ramirez Almanza and Méndez Calderón 2007); in 2009, there were over 9,000 patients receiving them.

This growth in services has brought with it an increase in psychological and psychiatric discourse and a number of concerted efforts to promulgate psychological education—*psicoeducación*—throughout the state. As I will argue, global efforts to detect and deter domestic violence,[1] promote gender equality, and encourage women's empowerment dovetail with Oaxaca's burgeoning mental health sector to create a context in which violence and rights are increasingly spoken about and taught in the clinical setting. Such initiatives broadly circulate information around the necessity of treating not only the physical, but also the psychological and emotional effects of violence—and more and more people seem to be accessing psychological services to address these problems in therapy. If promoting awareness of domestic abuse as unacceptable is a relatively new phenomenon in Oaxaca, connecting it to psychological and emotional aftereffects—to trauma—is even more recent and represents an important shift of thought.

In this context concepts of trauma and posttraumatic stress disorder (PTSD) are emerging as salient means of interpreting social and political disturbances, albeit unevenly and in ways structured by cultural orientations toward particular types of violence. Curiously, while migration and political conflict are framed as both violent and extraordinary enough to occasion PTSD, domestic abuse is represented as a ubiquitous "cultural problem" too ingrained and ordinary to generate the disorder—despite the widespread campaigns against gender-based violence. Among mental health professionals, trauma resulting from domestic violence is thought to contribute to a spectrum of disorders, most commonly depression, anxiety, and personality disorders—but not PTSD.

The disparity between clinical practice and broader discourse on domestic and gender violence is surprising in light of the fact that diagnostic criteria for the types of trauma that may contribute to PTSD have broadened significantly in recent years. As McNally (2003, 2009) and others have pointed out, this diagnostic "bracket creep" has created a clinical ethos in which virtually any stressor is considered capable of generating the disorder.[2] No longer is PTSD particular to victims and witnesses of extreme violence (e.g., war veterans, sufferers of torture, and victims of rape); now, the diagnosis is applied to traumas resulting from events such as fender benders, overhearing sexual jokes in the workplace, and seeing violent events depicted on television (McNally 2003, 2009).[3] Domestic violence–related trauma has long been thought to contribute to PTSD; in fact, as Fassin and Rechtman (2009) and others have pointed out, the diagnosis came about through the convergence of social movements advocating for veterans and female victims of violence.[4] Given that domestic violence has been central to the development of PTSD as a diagnosis, that campaigns to eradicate domestic violence and emphasize the emotionally traumatic effects of abuse are widespread in Oaxaca, and that diagnoses for other disorders have been increasing rapidly in the state, the fact that PTSD is rarely applied in cases of domestic violence in this setting is especially striking.

Focusing on professional and lay understandings of trauma, this chapter examines several separate but interrelated processes. The first section shows how domestic and gender violence have come to the fore in Oaxaca through global and local campaigns and how they have become an important aspect of clinical psychological and psychiatric practice. I argue that particular notions of culture are mobilized in this process, contributing to representations of violence as culturally sanctioned and experientially mundane. The subsequent section examines how such representations contrast with representations of other types of violence and play into the local clinical ethos of PTSD. Rather than bracket creep, a "bracket narrowing" has taken place— one that highlights the roles of culture, gender, and structural violence in the experience and treatment of trauma-related disorder. The final section of the chapter presents case studies from the Oaxacan psychiatric hospital that illustrate the forgoing processes and highlight the role of trauma and the work of diagnoses in women's narratives. Put together, these processes show how, in the local incorporation of globalized discourses and psychiatric categories, cultural conceptions of violence and gender circumscribe professional and popular interpretations of distress.

Oaxaca in the Twenty-First Century

Oaxaca is one of Mexico's poorest·states: over 60 percent of its population lives in extreme or moderate poverty, and only a little over ten percent is *not* categorized as "poor or vulnerable" (CONEVAL 2012). Many residents lack basic necessities such as potable water, education, and health care, and its per capita income average is one of the lowest in the country. Oaxaca has a long history of migration, but economic reforms in Mexico over the past thirty years have by many accounts exacerbated rural poverty and contributed to outward migration flows.

Economic marginalization is most pervasive among Oaxaca's indigenous people, who, therefore, are the most likely to migrate to the United States in search of opportunity. The number of Oaxacans residing in the United States almost tripled between 1990 and 2005 (oaxaca.gob.mx). By 2009, over 1.2 million people—34 percent of Oaxaca's total population—lived outside of the state (Ruiz Quiróz and Cruz Vasquez 2009:33), the majority of these in the United States. Although migration has slowed over the past several years since the recession began, in many indigenous communities only a fraction of inhabitants remain, mostly women, children, and the elderly.

The state has extremely high indexes of domestic violence as well as childhood sexual assault, and in Oaxaca City, petty crime and random assaults are ever more prevalent. Although Oaxaca is safe compared to other states in Mexico suffering from drug cartel–related violence, Oaxacan residents regularly report increasing insecurity, instability, stress, tension, and anger—often directed toward the political apparatus, which is widely considered to be corrupt and rife with impunity. There is a pervasive nostalgia both in the city and in rural regions for the days in which one could walk the streets without fearing assault or robbery. One local psychologist went so far as to conjecture that the "social fabric in Oaxaca has come apart."

Some of this insecurity can be attributed to Oaxaca's 2006 conflicts, in which the former state governor Ulises Ruiz refused customary negotiations with the teachers' union during their annual demonstrations. Tensions escalated, tens of thousands of Oaxacans hoping for political and social change banded with the teachers to create a resistance movement, and both state and national police and military forces were called in to confront them. The clash between the two sides became violent, and an estimated thirty people were killed with many more injured over the course of the seven months the conflict lasted. Dozens of people are receiving psychological and medical care for the effects of torture they suffered during the conflict, and there are allegations of political prisoners still in captivity. The conflict continues to reverberate in Oaxaca City, both through a reduced tourist economy, which contributes to unemployment and a pervasive sense of mistrust and residual anger, which in turn flares up with every reminder of the corruption that characterizes state politics.

It is in this context of poverty, marginalization, political unrest, violence, and mass out-migration that Oaxaca's field of mental health services has thrived. Even with the recent boom in psychology, psychiatry, and alternative therapies (such as self-help groups, Reiki, yoga, and acupuncture), the mental health sector cannot keep up with demand (Duncan 2012). Psychologists and psychiatrists regularly mention that more and more Oaxacans suffer from emotional and psychological distress, that prevalence (along with detection) of psychiatric disorder has increased over the course of recent years, and that in general, life is increasingly stressful. These professionals frequently characterize their patients' lives as lacking in security and plagued by uncertainty and anxiety, which they attribute to factors ranging from lingering fears after the 2006 conflicts to migration to the more general consequences of urbanization, globalization, and economic crises. As one doctor and psychologist put it, "Well, we live in a more violent society; as opposed to twenty years ago Oaxaca is a more violent, more modern city; it's a city with more migration, which puts us in fashion with what's going on with the rest of the world, right? More violence, more anxiety, more depression, and more addiction. Anything new here?"

Gender and Domestic Violence in Oaxaca

"It Marks You"

A large part of the state's perceived violence problem stems from its extremely high indexes of domestic abuse and gender violence, a problem which has garnered a good deal of attention in recent years. Amapola, a fifty-six-year-old Oaxacan housekeeper and mother of three living in Oaxaca City, remembers when she began hearing talk about domestic violence in Oaxaca for the first time. Fifteen years ago, she assumed it was a normal aspect of life, that it was "a man's right . . . to hit me, to tell me I'm worthless, to be neglectful."[5] She elaborated:

> I never noticed I was living violence, you know? Because many times, for example, my father would say, "You have everything you need, don't you? You don't lack anything, you have food and a roof and—your husband, who cares? He doesn't show up? He'll show up sometime." When he disappeared or when my father knew that he was with some other woman—no, there's no problem. "You're his wife, you're in your house." These things traumatize you even if you think— you say everything is fine. You think things are fine, but throughout your life it marks you, and when you finally manage to understand the emotional damage it's caused, lives are completely destroyed. So

it's important what's happening now, that there are organizations and groups that can help.

Amapola's perception of gender inequality was formed long before she was married: her mother became pregnant with Amapola after being raped while her husband was in jail on false charges, and since Amapola was technically illegitimate, her mother did not insist that she have the same rights as her older half siblings. She worked from a young age and did not begin school until she was ten, then made it through the sixth grade before her parents could no longer afford her education. When she was sixteen, they insisted she marry a friend of hers with whom they thought she was carrying on. By eighteen she had her first daughter, and while her husband continued going out drinking and pursuing other women, Amapola assumed full responsibility for the home and family. "I started to see that I had a responsibility to take care of both my husband and my daughter. . . . I never thought I could leave and fight in my life for *me*, because I was told that this is what you have to do: live like this, raise a family."

Amapola did just that, until about ten years ago when her husband fell ill and was diagnosed with HIV. "They told me I had to take a test, too," Amapola said, "but I didn't know anything about the virus then. I said, 'No, not me! I'm religious—all I do is spend time with my children at home. I couldn't have it [the virus]." But her test was positive, as well. Now Amapola spends a great deal of her time and energy on her own treatment, which often requires full-day trips out to the HIV clinic. Despite her upbeat and energetic personality, she expresses feeling trapped in her marriage and stigmatized by many people in her church and community. Recently, Amapola has begun to think of these experiences as types of violence that have, through the years, traumatized her and contributed to feelings of isolation, anger, helplessness, vulnerability, and low self-esteem.

Amapola explained that there was very little attention paid to the problem of gender violence before, but as we drove by a billboard painted with the slogan "A Life Without Violence Against Women" advertising a 1-800 violence help line, she marveled at the changes she had seen in Oaxaca's recent history. Her understandings of violence have shifted dramatically over the years in conjunction with statewide and global efforts to detect and deter violence, promote gender equality and empowerment, and bolster development—efforts that have contributed to a profusion of initiatives and organizations focused on these objectives in Oaxaca (and Mexico more generally) during the last decade or so.[6] There, as in many other places, governmental public health efforts, NGOs, human rights and feminist organizations, churches, and mental health clinics explicitly attempt to define violence, educate the population about it, and encourage victims to seek services for support.

In this context, women's experience of both physical and psychological violence is increasingly talked about, dealt with in psychological therapy, and connected with traumatic emotional aftereffects. For Amapola, the explicit links between her own experience, violence, and trauma have emerged in the course of group and individual therapy at the HIV clinic. There, the psychologist focuses on identifying the traumas each woman has suffered and on "getting them out"—verbalizing, processing, and expressing them physically:

> [The psychologist] tells us that we need to work on these traumas; for example, there are exercises, there are therapies to get them out, get all of them out, talk about them. . . . She did one exercise where we hit something, to get it out, get out everything. . . . We have to first identify the problem . . . to be able to work on it, because a lot of the time we unconsciously carry this problem and therefore we don't overcome it, you know? And then you just keep living the same. . . . The doctor starts to say now that it's happened, there's no other solution, I can't stay in the same place, so the thing is working it to overcome it . . . to erase it so that we can be healthy, have a better quality of life, and to consider ourselves important . . . to build some self-esteem. To get it out, to clean the mind. . . . But it's not easy, it's not easy to do it. Rather, it's a long process.

The psychologist teaches women that traumas may be present whether or not they are identified or experienced as such; if gone unrecognized, they may cause emotional and psychological problems over the years. As Amapola put it, "living violence" can "mark you." Understood to be pathogenic in this way, the traumatic effects of violence must be brought to conscious awareness, expressed, and overcome in psychological therapy.

This understanding of violence and trauma is quite new for Oaxaca, where the general perception among both professionals and laypeople is that violence has historically been an assumed condition of women's existence that ought to be accepted with forbearance. The remainder of this section will discuss how gender violence and trauma have emerged as matters of both public and clinical concern, and how particular cultural tropes around *machismo* and women's experience have been employed in this process.

Local Gender Violence Initiatives

Although these changes have taken place gradually, in the past several years the issue of domestic and gender violence has become markedly more visible in the media, legislation, and political decision making. This is likely due to the growing national and international attention to the issue combined with improved detection and local increases in mental health services and psychological interventions, as discussed below. Mexico's National Institute of Statistics and Geography (Instituto Nacional de Estadística y Geografía, or INEGI) reports that over 43 percent of married women and women in domestic partnerships in Oaxaca have been victims of intimate partner violence (INEGI 2013:8). According to other national and statewide surveys and institutional staff members interviewed for the present study, anywhere between 40 to 80 percent of Oaxacan women have experienced some type of gender violence, including psychological/emotional violence, physical violence, sexual violence, property violence, and economic violence.[7]

Oaxaca's general institutional definition of "gender violence" as "any gender-based action or conduct that causes death, injury, or physical, sexual, or psychological suffering in the public or private sphere" originated at the 1994 Inter-American Convention on the Prevention, Punishment and Eradication of Violence Against Women—better known as the Convention of Belém do Pará—in Brazil, organized by the Organization of American States. Although in 1998 Mexico ratified the convention covenant and began enacting domestic violence–related reforms soon thereafter, Mexico did not pass the General Law on Women's Access to a Life Free of Violence, drawn up at the convention, until 2007, and Oaxaca did not pass it until February 2009, the penultimate Mexican state to do so. The passage seems to be contributing to increased attention to gender violence, equality, and human rights on an institutional level in the state.[8]

The Oaxacan Women's Institute (Instituto de la Mujer Oaxaqueña, hereafter referred to as the IMO) is one of the most visible of these establishments. Founded in 1998 as part of Mexico's National Women's Institute, the IMO seeks to eradicate discrimination against women, promote a gender perspective in all entities of public administration, and thus promote equality among men and women. As part of the General Law on Women's Access to a Life Free of Violence, the IMO founded its Center for Attention to Female Victims of Gender Violence in Oaxaca City in 2008. The center provides psychological, medical, and legal help for women who have suffered any type of gender violence, including a shelter for severely battered women. It has several doctors, psychologists, health promoters, social workers, and lawyers on staff, as well as a twenty-four-hour hotline.

Oaxaca's Ministry of Health (SSO) also has a number of departments and programs throughout the state aimed at prevention and treatment of violence. It recently created the Department of Prevention and Attention to Domestic Violence and Gender and the Specialized Center for Prevention and Attention to Domestic and Gender Violence, which offer educational sessions and staff hospitals and health clinics with people trained to deal with victims of violence. Oportunidades, Mexico's notorious cash-transfer development program that provides stipends to women who attend health sessions and checkups, also organizes talks on violence at public community health centers.

Creating Consciousness: The Cultural Trope of Violence

One of the main goals of these programs is to stimulate cultural change in Oaxaca. As Dr. Villareal, former director of the IMO's Center for Attention to Female Victims of Gender Violence, told me, the IMO is explicitly trying to alter the "cultural structure" of Oaxaca by bringing violence to public consciousness in all its forms "after so many years of cultural practices rendering it invisible, something normal, something commonplace, something acceptable." The theory that domestic violence is cultural is typical in both everyday talk and in the more pointed discourse of Oaxaca's antiviolence campaigns. This theory, or cultural trope of violence, as I will refer to it, maintains that abuse of women is a ubiquitous, natural, "invisibilized" (*invisibilizado*) aspect of the traditional ethos that must be unlearned. As such, Oaxacan—and often the larger Mexican or Latino—culture is characterized as male dominant and chauvinist, or *machista*.

One of the IMO's flyers explains how domestic violence is seen as part of a sociocultural system that says men are naturally superior to women: "Historically, beliefs, myths, customs, traditions, and values that society and culture have created around women and men, around the feminine and masculine worlds (duties, responsibilities, activities, roles, functions, behavior, dress, ways of being, living, and acting) have determined that men are 'naturally' superior and have given them power over women . . . who [are] considered naturally inferior." This flyer is typical of the educational materials disseminated throughout the state. Another distributed by the federal Special Prosecutor for Crimes of Violence Against Women and Human Trafficking (known as "FEVIMTRA"), tells women that

It's likely that you, like many women, are living in violence and you haven't noticed because you have learned that:

- A man is jealous because "he cares about his woman"
- He has a right to control us because "he takes care of us"
- It's "normal" that a man insult, threaten, or hit his partner when he's angry
- Women do things to deserve being hit or mistreated by their partners

These educational materials warn women that violence is not natural but a crime ("violence is a crime" or "*violencia es un delito*," is one of the most publicized slogans, printed on huge billboards, bus stops, and buildings); inform women they have a right to a life free of violence; and incite them to seek help immediately. Often such flyers include self-diagnostic quizzes asking questions whose answers indicate whether a woman is experiencing violence. "Do you feel that your partner is constantly controlling you 'out of love'?" "Does he criticize and humiliate you in public or in private, offer negative opinions about your appearance, the way you are, or the style of your clothing?" "Has he ever hit you with his hands, tugged you, or thrown things at you when angry or when you were discussing something?" A high score on the quiz tells a woman that she is "living violence" or that her relationship shows "signs of power abuse" (SSO educational materials 2011). Such quizzes are distributed at public clinics and, if a given clinic has staff members trained to detect and treat domestic violence, are often administered as part of female patients' standard appointment schedule.

Fleshed out, the cultural trope of violence maintains that machismo both sets the stage for domestic violence by tacitly approving of it or even encouraging it as a man's right, and also causes it to be perceived as a natural, taken-for-granted (thus invisibilized) aspect of female-male relations. Because violence is taken for granted, the trope posits that women do not know their rights, and so do not recognize that they are being violated; therefore, they do not speak out or have the tools to escape the abusive situations in which they find themselves. This model also suggests that violence is inherited and endemic, in the sense that mothers teach their daughters that violence (including infidelity) is something that cannot be helped and must be endured: "you are inculcated with the idea that the man rules the house, and if you choose to marry him you have to put up with him," as one psychologist put it. "It is a question of culture."[9]

"A Way of Life"

Although some professionals discuss domestic violence and mistreatment of women as a problem that affects rich and poor, mestizo and indigenous, and that spans education levels, many consider the problem to be worse in rural, indigenous regions, where customs and beliefs are thought to be stronger.[10] Dr. Cardozo, a psychiatrist who has practiced in Oaxaca since 1995, referred to domestic violence and mistreatment of women as "aspects of culture" that are "very, very common in our communities, in the interior regions of the state . . . and which I see as inadequate, but people from [rural regions] are so accustomed to that they see as a part of their lives, as a way of life."[11] This type of observation is characteristic of health practitioners who have treated patients in situations of violence. Dr. Sánchez, a psychiatrist, states: "We are talking about customs. Oaxaca still conforms to a basic family system in which the man is in charge. I have always said that in the pueblos they are crueler than in the city." Dr. Esquivel, another psychiatrist, claims that "in the Mixteca [a rural indigenous area] there is still the custom of hitting women—there is mistreatment but now they live it as a custom, it's normal to them, you know? They are behind in this sense. They don't defend their rights—they don't know what that means." Similarly, Noemi, a psychologist at IMO, stated:

> I always tell them, "you see, if you have [emotional problems] it's normal, because when you suffer violence you will have those types of symptoms. It's not that you are crazy, it's that you suffered from

violence." We throw out irrational ideas from the first session, try to pull them away from that. Because culturally, if you come from a village in the Sierra [a rural indigenous area], you don't even know what a psychologist is. . . . What's important is that [women] learn the concept of violence and that [they] see that violence is not normal. Because they think it is. Because they've lived it generation after generation, so it's hard for them to understand. I see the blockage, their resistance in the first ten minutes of the first session, but then from there they relax.

Because domestic violence is seen as an essential and invisible aspect of "culture," one of the main jobs of practitioners and anti–domestic violence campaigns is to define violence and make it visible such that women know they are suffering it. As indicated above, this involves nothing less than an attempt to effect broad cultural change by creating consciousness and changing everyday practices. Such a project is extraordinarily complex in a place like Oaxaca, with its sixteen indigenous groups, dizzying linguistic diversity, and daunting geography. The state is Mexico's fifth largest by area, and owing to its several large mountain ranges, it is quite difficult to navigate—many towns are almost completely isolated from major cities and highways. Furthermore, it is divided into eight regions and 571 municipalities—more than any other state in Mexico—most of which are structured according to the laws of "*usos y costumbres,*" in which each village elects its own municipal government through a traditional system of popular assembly. These factors combine to create an incredibly eclectic state, and one that includes quite independent populations and communities that often develop their own systems of health care and healing.

"Living Violence" and Healing Trauma

To reach Oaxaca's more remote regions, the IMO has a mobile clinic and boasts a visible media presence through billboards, flyers distributed throughout the state, and dozens of educational programs and commercials on women's rights that are aired on radio and television stations in Spanish, Zapotec, Mixtec, and Chinantec. One of their 2010 campaigns included a series of television and radio commercials depicting men not only physically attacking women, but also committing more subtle forms of violence like demeaning their partners, limiting their independence, or withholding money from them. "This too is violence," the commercials say. Dr. Villareal of the IMO maintained that their success in reaching women was mainly due to these media efforts:

> Many women just recently, through the media—through TV programs and other local diffusion that we are doing as well—they start to realize that what they are living is violence, what they thought was quotidian and normal. That your husband yells at you because the soup isn't hot enough, this is natural. That if the kids aren't bathed and they are crying because you didn't feed them and he hits you, when you're not getting any economic support so that you can feed them in the first place—they see this as something natural. But then violence becomes more visible [through the media] and many women open their eyes and say, "Ohhhhh, *I'm* living violence!" and they look for somewhere to seek help. They end up here . . . and I can't resolve their economic problems, but I can support them by offering psychological attention. Empower them so they are self-sufficient and self-determining. From there they start to work and make their own decisions to sustain themselves. They know then that they deserve a life free of violence.

It is here that the convergence between antiviolence gender equality campaigns and Oaxaca's burgeoning field of mental health services is most conspicuous. In addition to denormalizing, defining, preventing, and removing violence as a taken-for-granted assumption of daily existence, Oaxaca's antiviolence initiatives encourage victims to seek support—medical, legal, and, perhaps most prominently, psychological. As part of their more general work on violence, many of these initiatives explicitly attempt to promulgate understanding of emotional and psychological health: to spread psicoeducación. Talks and workshops, therefore, often teach the definitions of various psychiatric disorders and discuss topics such as expressing emotions, self-esteem and empowerment, and the function of psychologists and psychiatrists.

Anti–gender violence campaigns teach about and promote psychological treatment, and for their part, mental health practitioners themselves often either work in such campaigns or wind up confronting violence in their private practices. Most psychologists, psychiatrists, counselors, and others working in the context of mental health mention that whether or not patients initially come to their offices because of domestic violence or rape, it is often a part of patients' backgrounds, especially among women. Nearly every mental health practitioner and healer in the current study (N = 58) mentioned domestic violence as one of Oaxaca's main social and mental health problems and said they had routinely encountered the problem among patients in clinical practice. Although seeking psychological and psychiatric treatment still carries some stigma in Oaxaca, psicoeducación efforts—along with exposure to psychological practice and concepts in the media and an increase in practitioners in rural areas—are changing such perceptions. More and more, psychology is thought to be a necessary and helpful form of self-care (Duncan 2012).

In this vein, psychological violence is reportedly the most common type of violence in Oaxaca, and thousands of women have sought mental health care to deal with its effects. The local newspapers *El Imparcial* and *Diario Despertar* reported that in 2008 alone, twenty-five hundred women sought help for psychological violence at the IMO—and this number does not account for the many more who presumably sought help at community clinics, with private practitioners, and with alternative and traditional healers. The IMO's definition of psychological violence is slightly more encompassing than others', including "any action or omission that harms the emotional stability of women, which can consist of negligence, abandonment, repeated neglect, jealousy, insults, humiliations, devaluations, marginalization, indifference, destructive comparisons, rejection, blackmail, restriction of self-determination, and threats, which lead the victim to depression, isolation, devaluation, annulment of self-esteem, or even to suicide." As such, the meaning of violence itself expands to encompass not only physical abuse, rape, and aggression, but also nonphysical assaults on one's psyche or self. All forms of violence in this model—physical, sexual, psychological, economic—are considered capable of not only contributing to women's suffering, but also producing psychological and emotional sequelae, or trauma.[12]

Many psychologists and therapists explain that, because of the culture of machismo, women are not likely to connect emotional distress with violence, or even to realize that they are emotionally distressed to begin with (thus presenting with psychosomatic ailments). Therefore, therapy often focuses on making this connection explicit and on exploring what impacts the violence has had. This is part of *sensibilización* (sensitizing) and *concientización* (awareness building). Lidia, a psychologist from Spain who has also worked in El Salvador, said violence against women in Oaxaca is so normalized "it's often difficult to work . . . to make visible [to patients] that this is a situation of violence they are living, that it is affecting them . . . that it's not normal." Similarly, Roxana, a psychologist at a holistic mental health clinic who focuses on violence, has made concerted efforts to educate institutions (like SSO) and patients about detection, prevention, and treatment of violence, focusing especially on the emotional base of many physical problems and on the traumatic emotional impacts violence can have. Her perception is that state health services refuse to focus on domestic violence and continue to medicalize women's distress rather than acknowledge that their physical conditions "have to do with masked emotional suffering, at the bottom of which is domestic violence." Both Lidia and Roxana offer group therapy, individual therapy, and educational sessions in rural and urban settings.

Such discourse and practice is, as noted, quite new for Oaxaca, and goes hand in hand with more general changes in healing practices and orientations toward emotional experience in Oaxaca. As one local psychologist put it, "Fifteen years ago . . . we didn't associate the experience of domestic violence with the experience of trauma, you know? They were—they were worlds apart." In a very real sense, practitioners are both teaching and treating trauma and recovery in Oaxaca, and their project goes along with a broader mission to effect changes in Oaxacan culture more generally.

PTSD and the Meaning of Violence

"The Hand I've Been Dealt"

Given the growing attention to gender violence and emotional trauma as well as increasing rates of diagnosed mental disorder in Oaxaca, one might expect awareness and diagnosis of PTSD to have shot up considerably in recent years. PTSD's cachet has grown in Oaxacan clinical practice, but not in relation to domestic or gender violence, and not in popular awareness. Rather, PTSD has come into its own as a diagnosis in Oaxaca's clinical practice almost exclusively owing to the perceived traumas of political violence and migration, despite the fact that there are far fewer initiatives, organizations, and programs devoted to these types of violence.

This occurred to me only after interviewing over a dozen female outpatients at the public psychiatric hospital, Cruz del Sur.[13] Though various psychiatrists at the hospital had told me they increasingly diagnose PTSD in other contexts—suggesting that the diagnosis and its attendant symptoms were, indeed, salient there—during my first months at the outpatient unit I was struck by the fact that none of these women carried the diagnosis despite the violent experiences they had sustained. Rather, the majority were diagnosed with and treated for affective disorders, personality disorders, and mental delays (*retrasos mentales*). When I inquired as to whether PTSD was ever diagnosed in relation to domestic violence, psychiatrists and psychologists both in and outside of the hospital answered that because it is so chronic in Oaxaca, because it is a part of culture, women do not experience it as a traumatic event that occasions PTSD symptoms as defined by the DSM or the *International Classification of Diseases* (ICD). As one psychiatrist put it, "they don't live it as a posttraumatic stress, because it seems to me that they incorporate it as part of their life structure. They see it like, 'This is the hand I've been dealt.'"

Another psychiatrist explained that traumas generative of PTSD are always extremely violent and unexpected, not quotidian events like domestic violence. She said that PTSD-related trauma "has another meaning. For us, it's an unexpected event in which the person is normally affected in a sudden, violent way. . . . Violent not in the sense of physical violence precisely, but rather something intense that obviously one can't control. . . . Domestic violence isn't considered a traumatic event as such, and even less when it's chronic." Unsurprisingly, that psychiatrist, like many others, emphasized the necessity of patients presenting the specific characteristics of PTSD symptomatology in order for the diagnosis to be relevant. She explained that in the majority of domestic abuse, childhood rape, and sexual assault cases not treated immediately, the traumatic sequelae eventually translate to depression and anxiety.

Several factors are at play here. There are ongoing debates within the broader psychiatric community around what traumatic stressors are capable of causing PTSD, and thus what types of traumas and resultant symptoms make patients eligible for PTSD diagnoses according to the DSM. As the anthropological literature on PTSD has shown, in practice and according to the particular cultural setting, PTSD privileges some types of violence and traumatic experience while it excludes others (Breslau 2000; James 2004; Salis Gross 2004). This can be understood as a function of the interaction between professional preferences and perceptions, patient symptom reports and ease of expression, and more structural factors regarding what types of trauma merit resources, treatment, and professional attention. What is perceived as ordinary and bearable versus extraordinary and unbearable in a particular cultural setting affects both how individuals experience violence and express its emotional impacts as well as how professionals in that culture conceive of mental health and incorporate ideas about pathological conditions and treatments.

In many documented cases, the perception of a traumatized group of people leads to a huge growth in diagnoses of the disorder (James 2004; Stubbs 2005; Friedman-Peleg and Goodman 2010). Not so in Oaxaca. Rather than bracket creep, wherein the types of traumatic experience considered capable of causing PTSD expand to encompass any number of stressors (McNally 2003, 2009), PTSD in Oaxaca has undergone a type of bracket narrowing in relation to domestic violence. Has this happened because—as the ubiquitous cultural trope of violence suggests—women have actually normalized the experiences of violence, stress, and shock, such that these cannot be defined "outside the range of normal human experience"—as the DSM initially defined traumatic events—and thus would be unlikely to lead to PTSD symptomatology? Have women dissociated to protect themselves against symptoms? Have their traumatic experiences, often left undetected, transformed into other types of illness? Or are the symptoms of PTSD just not salient for Oaxacan women who have experienced situations of violence? These are possibilities, but I theorize that the discrepancy has as much, if not more, to do with local representations of violence and their resultant clinical ethos.

Framing Violence

In everyday discourse, quotidian talk, and the clinical context, political violence, migration, and gender violence are quite differently framed. As discussed above, domestic abuse is represented as a pervasive cultural problem so ingrained it could not possibly occasion PTSD. In contrast, the traumas and stresses of the 2006 conflicts and migration are represented as extraordinary, remarkable departures from the normal, moral order of things, which frequently result in posttraumatic stress. Numerous mental health practitioners said that not only had diagnoses of PTSD in relation to these social crises grown in recent years, but that the disorder is underdiagnosed and is likely much more prevalent than most people know.

This is perhaps an unsurprising characterization of the emotional impacts of the 2006 conflicts, which were quite historic and represented the most flagrant violence Oaxaca has seen in recent history. Migration, however, is quite commonplace: at least a quarter of Oaxacan families have one or more migrant family member, and in many towns the majority of males have left for the United States. This is not to downplay the emotional impact of migration, which can be quite severe for both migrants and their nonmigrating family members (see Duncan 2012, 2015 for additional discussion of migration and mental health in Oaxaca), but rather to point out that migration is—like domestic violence—quite a pervasive social phenomenon in Oaxaca, and one that has considerable history.

Interestingly, as in talk about gender violence, concepts of culture pervade talk around migration, but in quite a different sense. Mental health practitioners discuss migration as traumatic precisely because it represents an experience of extreme "culture shock." Dr. Sánchez, a psychiatrist, stated: "Migrants confront a culture that has nothing to do with what they know, and this is a trauma. It's a disorder that causes them stress and trauma and that confuses them, such that they arrive at a posttraumatic state. And this is in the sense of culture shock—we're not talking about rape, accidents, nothing like that; we're talking about a social phenomenon." Dr. Solis, another psychiatrist, asserted that "emigrants are a group that frequently get sick in the United States and they come back to Mexico ill. . . . These are people who go to the U.S. and experience an extreme clash of cultures—imagine, you come from a tiny village and you've never even gone to Oaxaca City or another big city of the type. . . . Suddenly you get to the U.S. and this causes huge culture shock. . . . And of course in addition, you live in constant stress, which adds to the problem of posttraumatic stress disorder."

Whereas gender violence is not considered a trauma capable of generating PTSD because it is experienced as a normal part of culture, then, migration is considered a trauma capable of generating PTSD because it is experienced as a cultural shock. (Psychiatrists also use "transcultural psychosis" as a diagnosis among former migrants.) Whether or not a migrant has a traumatic experience while away, that cultural shock in itself is, in the view of many mental health practitioners, enough to create the conditions necessary for PTSD.

Although people did not regularly discuss the cultural aspects of trauma in relation to the 2006 conflict—except to describe corruption and impunity as intrinsic aspects of Oaxaca's political culture—it is represented as an extraordinary and disturbing departure from the usual. "Panic," "stress," "fear," "instability," and "trauma" were frequently mentioned in reference to 2006, in addition to the various psychiatric disorders thought to have been generated or exacerbated by the conflicts, particularly PTSD.

Paulina, a psychologist, stated, "These are things that aren't spoken about, they're not said, but it impacted us emotionally a great deal, those of us who live in Oaxaca. The situation was so stressful that at six in the evening no one was on the streets because they were afraid of going home, afraid of the barricades.[14] There were moments in which . . . helicopters passed and when they did, people hid in their houses. Out of fear. It was a situation of panic, of fear, and no institution has dealt with it. So the emotional impacts have remained. That's where we are."

Jorge, a psychologist and activist, expressed similar views. According to him, "there is a lot of social violence in Oaxaca, and we have a repressive governor. It generates a totally unstable situation, a feeling of vulnerability. . . . It generates a situation of stress. Many people were tortured, disappeared, many people were assassinated, and this means that there are lots of women in processes of grief, of depression, of anxiety, of posttraumatic stress." Dr. Gutiérrez, a psychiatrist, pointed to the role of mental health practitioners in the conflict when he said that "2006 was something terrible and in some ways people have wanted to minimize it, but it was something that impacted the entire population. . . . It was terrible in various ways and was a watershed in the life of Oaxaca. More than anything it modified mental health. People see barricades and they get frightened, alarmed, they enter into panic, and, well, it's us [the mental health practitioners] who have treated it all."

Psychologists and psychiatrists say that circumstances recalling the 2006 conflicts regularly inspire panic, anxiety, and desperation in patients—mostly teachers—who were traumatized during those events. Oaxaca has a strong history and current tradition of social protest; sit-in demonstrations, called *plantones*, are frequent in the city center, and roadblocks set up by various protestors are a constant. Teachers' protests and plantones are required by the teachers' unions, and psychiatrists mentioned patients with PTSD diagnoses who experience flashbacks and panic attacks when they are called on to attend.

Dr. Cardozo, who has worked in both private and public psychiatric settings in Oaxaca for nearly two decades, mentioned PTSD caused by the 2006 conflicts as one of the most notable changes in Oaxacan mental health he has witnessed. "We have a psychiatric association and when we got together we saw that all of us had people with posttraumatic stress disorders and panic from the critical [2006] situation," he recalled. The violent events of 2006 account for almost all cases of PTSD Dr. Cardozo has treated, and he notes that since that year the disorder has become "much more notable, much more frequent." Dr. Álvaro, an outpatient psychiatrist at Cruz del Sur psychiatric hospital, echoed Dr. Cardozo's observations:

> I have seen it in consultations, sequelae of this movement in that many people present posttraumatic stress, you see that, or that they reach psychosis. . . . There were people in civilian brigades who were kidnapped, who were killed, police who detained you just out of suspicion. So yes, this has an impact, because the fact that someone can grab you out of suspicion, well this implies that you could just disappear, that you could be thrown in jail or that they could accuse you of any type of crime. This impacts the people here, and it's an impact in the sense that many are still in this situation. Therefore they should be in treatment, right? Now there are people who are frightened at the sight of a policeman. This is a sequelae of what happened since the movement—so yes, the movement altered mental health here.

Representations of both migration and 2006 often emphasize shock: the shock of a new culture in the case of migration, and the shock of unexpected, politically motivated brutality and conflict in the case of 2006. The victims of domestic violence, however, are considered to be beyond shock because such violence is expected and culturally sanctioned. Here, from practitioners' viewpoints, women's experience of violence is outside the "impress of extremity" (Jenkins 1996; see also Forché 1993).

Structural Violence in the Clinical Ethos

Overall, then, while migration and the 2006 conflicts are frequently portrayed as visible sources of shock, trauma, panic, transcultural psychosis, and PTSD, domestic violence is portrayed as a type of normalized traumatic stressor that contributes to a range of diffuse symptoms but *not* PTSD. In a sense, practitioners are calling attention to women's experience of structural violence: the historical, economic, political, social, and cultural means by which inequality is reproduced and by which particular groups become systematically marginalized, subjugated, and vulnerable to assaults on dignity, body, and psyche (see also Farmer 2003, 2004; Galtung 1969, 1990). Indeed, it could be argued that many Oaxacans' lives are constrained by structural violence; Oaxaca is a place characterized by widespread poverty that maps onto ethnicity and indigeneity, where the political process is frequently corrupt and exclusionary, and where women are particularly marginalized and at disproportionate risk for particular types of assault like rape and domestic abuse. Denouncing structural iniquities against women, some of which are culturally perpetuated, may indicate progressive movement away from such marginalization.

However, these representations have paradoxical consequences. It is precisely the theory that domestic violence is a normalized part of culture, so prevalent as to be invisible, that contributes to an understanding of the distress and trauma it causes as too ingrained to generate PTSD. This view in turn informs the local clinical ethos, in which the traumatic effects of domestic violence are almost uniformly diagnosed as affective and personality disorders. The paradox lies partially in the fact that unlike most diagnoses, PTSD is well known for its political resonance and ability to mobilize resources and draw attention to justice and inequality. Despite its flaws, the diagnosis could plausibly aid rather than impede local efforts to make visible, detect, prevent, and treat the emotional aftereffects of domestic violence. Instead, the cultural trope of violence contributes to a view of women as so accustomed to violence that they are almost inured to the most pernicious emotional impacts of the abuse they have sustained. However, as Judith Herman pointed out over two decades ago, "outside the range of usual human experience" is scarcely an accurate description of domestic violence, given its frightening prevalence. But "traumatic events are extraordinary, not because they occur rarely, but rather because they overwhelm the ordinary human adaptations to life" (Herman [1992] 1997:33).

Indeed, the only broad epidemiological study of PTSD in Oaxaca I have come across, conducted in four Mexican states and including over twenty-five hundred adults, found that the risk of PTSD was twice as high in Oaxaca as in the other states studied, and that 20 percent of Oaxacan women met the criteria for the disorder (Norris et al. 2003; Baker et al. 2005). Further, those who had experienced recurrent sexual, childhood, intimate partner, and family violence were *more* likely to meet the criteria than women reporting other types of violence. The authors note that the "routine stressors of poverty, discrimination, and oppression"—structural violence, essentially—"reduce women's capacities to cope with traumatic stressors" (Baker et al. 2005:526).

These findings are in line with other studies indicating that powerlessness, marginalization, and insecurity contribute to women's elevated risk of developing psychiatric symptoms and illnesses (Brown and Harris 1978; Desjarlais et al. 1995; Patel and Kleinman 2003; Kohrt and Worthman 2009). Overall, current research suggests that far from inuring women to the emotional and psychological sequelae of violence, chronic partner and family violence can put them at higher risk of PTSD—particularly when those women live in contexts of poverty, inequality, and discrimination, as so many Oaxacans do.

Gendered Trauma at the Psychiatric Hospital

This chapter has thus far examined several processes. First, I showed how gender violence and trauma have emerged as important areas of public and clinical concern in Oaxaca and how particular cultural tropes of violence are mobilized in that process. Second, I considered the differential use of PTSD in reference to particular types of violence, arguing that popular and professional representations of migration and political violence differ dramatically from representations of domestic violence, and in so doing circumscribe clinical interpretations of distress. Finally, I will examine how these processes manifest in the treatment of trauma at Oaxaca's public psychiatric hospital, Cruz del Sur, and how women themselves talk about the impacts of domestic violence.

Verónica: "I Have a Trauma"

Verónica is a thirty-five-year-old woman from a small rural village three hours south of the hospital. Shy and reserved, Verónica wore a threadbare polyester dress that looked as though it may have been her only one. She was accompanied by her husband, Emiliano, who asked permission to enter the room, bowing slightly and removing his large straw hat when he walked through the door. The couple described themselves as *campesinos*, or peasants, making a meager living off of a small bit of land they share with other relatives. Both Verónica and Emiliano could read but had not studied beyond primary school.

Verónica and Emiliano had been receiving treatment at the hospital for four months at the time of our interview, and both were taking fluoxetine

(Prozac). When I asked what type of problem had caused her to seek treatment, Verónica explained that she had a trauma resulting from domestic violence in her household when she was growing up: "I have a trauma (*yo tengo un trauma*) that I've carried since childhood, from when I was a little girl, from fear that my father was going to hit me or that he wanted to . . . what's it called? He wanted to . . . rape me. Attempted rape, that's how it was. And I grew up with this. With my family it was pure abuse (*puro golpe*). His drunkenness and the attempts [of rape], that's how I grew up, with this trauma all my childhood, up to the moment when I came to feel so horrible that I just couldn't go on."

The couple explained that most of Verónica's seven siblings also suffered from trauma, and that several had even migrated to the United States so as not to have to live near their abusive father. Verónica, however, continued to see her father regularly, and Emiliano explained that after these visits, Verónica's agitation and anger were at their worst. Whether or not she was in direct contact with her father, Verónica reported debilitating symptoms such as intense fear (*puro miedo*), sadness, excessive crying, desperation, suspicions that others were trying to harm her, and extreme "insecurity"—both in the sense of feeling unsafe and lacking confidence in herself. She also said her illness had led her to mistreat her children by screaming at them or punishing them unnecessarily because she always felt so desperate, angry, and impatient.

When Verónica told her sister-in-law about some of these experiences, the sister-in-law told her "it could that your mind is sick" (*puede ser que tu mente es la que está enferma*) and suggested that Verónica seek out a psychologist. At that point, Verónica did not yet know what "trauma" was, nor did she understand why she felt so badly all the time:

> *Verónica:* When I started getting treatment, they told me that I had a trauma. But before that, I just thought it was . . . it was my life . . . that that was my way of life, my way of being (*así era mi vida pues . . . así era mi forma de vivir, mi manera de ser*). I didn't know what I had . . .
> *Interviewer:* So who told you that?
> *V:* The doctor.
> *I:* The doctor in Miahuatlán.
> *V:* Yes.
> *I:* The psychologist?

V: Yes, [she said] "you have a trauma."

I: So what did you think when she told you that?

V: Well, I said—well, according to her that was a trauma, but that name for it—I didn't know about it. I didn't know the name "trauma."

Once she learned what it meant, "trauma" resonated with Verónica as an explanation for her distress. The idea that abuse—rather than personal short-comings or character defects—was to blame for her suffering provided a narrative to which Verónica could relate and around which she could fashion an understanding of herself and her social situation. She began taking Rivotril (clonazapam), which provided great relief. "It wasn't until then that I started to control myself," she said. "I went to a much better place. It was a life change. . . . I started being able to walk around talking with my neighbors and didn't feel badly, like I was bothering them. I started to feel more confident and to sense a change."

Once Verónica started to feel better, though, her doctor weaned her off the Rivotril, and her symptoms returned. She was told her treatment would be cheaper at the psychiatric hospital, so she went to Cruz del Sur. Meanwhile, Verónica and Emiliano both sought treatment from an herbalist and a *curandero,* but they said herbal and spiritual remedies were no help. The couple emphasized they needed psychiatric medicines, which go "straight to the central nerve" (*directo al nervio central*). At Cruz del Sur, the psychiatrist prescribed Prozac, which Verónica said was extremely effective, and diagnosed Verónica with depression and anxiety rather than trauma. Verónica said she did not have a clear understanding of what those diagnoses were, nor did she seem to identify with them (it was unclear whether she told the Cruz del Sur psychiatrist about her experience of childhood violence). She continued to attribute her problems to trauma caused by her father's abuse.

Flor: "I Feel I Have Wasted Away"

Flor is a forty-five-year-old woman who was born in Puebla and raised in Veracruz, but has lived in Oaxaca City for fourteen years. When I met her at the hospital, Flor was receiving psychiatric treatment in the outpatient unit with a diagnosis of severe depression. Her bearing was reserved, quiet, and sad, and she was quite thin. Unlike most patients, who are accompanied by a family member or partner, Flor waited for her appointment alone, standing rigidly in the waiting area in a leather jacket, clutching a black leather purse.

Though she spoke softly and seemed restrained, when Flor began to tell her story her sadness and desperation were evident. She explained that she had been depressed since she could remember and that she had attempted suicide numerous times throughout her life since the age of eighteen. Three months before we met, a final failed attempt led her to seek psychiatric attention for the first time, at which point she was hospitalized for a week. Flor had never heard of depression before her hospitalization, which was prompted by the Unit for Attention to Female Victims of Gender Violence at the Instituto de la Mujer Oaxaqueña (IMO). She went to them to seek help for the chronic domestic violence she has suffered since she was a child, and which she sees as the main contributing factor to her mental health problems: "The problem that has brought me to this strong depression is, my problem has been . . . family. Domestic violence . . . I suffered a lot of violence. Physical violence, emotional, I don't know what they call the violence that one suffers when you are harassed—sexual harassment. I suffered violence on the part of my stepfather when I was six, five—six years old. I spent my childhood with him, but with a lot of violence, a lot of aggression, physical, sexual, and emotional. Always—he was someone who made me afraid of many things."

When Flor was eighteen she began having convulsions, which her family blamed on hormonal changes but which she now believes were "nervous crises" (*crisis nerviosas*) caused by her intense desperation and anguish. After a childhood of abuse by her stepfather, Flor married a Oaxacan soldier, who was also abusive. She filed for a divorce over ten years earlier, but her husband still had not granted it at the time of my follow-up meeting with Flor in 2013. He was in and out of town for years because of his military obligations, and when he did find himself in Oaxaca with Flor and their two kids, Flor tried to distance herself to avoid his physical attacks and verbal abuse. He told her he would never be the one to leave and that if Flor wanted to separate, she would have to leave him. Finally, she did. At the time of our first interview, in 2010, she was living alone, not far from her kids (who were seventeen and twenty-three years old and living together), who Flor said were angry and disapproving of her illness and her decision to leave. Flor's isolation has been devastating. "So, recently I left my house and now I don't live with my kids. I am living alone because of the problems with my husband.

Yes, for threats and all that, I decided to leave my home. I filed a lawsuit against him, but it hasn't been heard. So, as a result of that I have a severe depression. I've tried to commit suicide several times. . . . I've gone way downhill. I have no value to myself or to others. There's no—I'm going through the motions now and I have no reason to be here (*no tengo un porqué por estar aquí*). I do things just to do them, nothing more, but I don't have a real reason to be here. This is why I come for psychological therapy and psychiatric consultations."

Flor had a negative experience as an inpatient at the hospital—she reported feeling trapped and bothered by the fact that the other women seemed so much sicker than she was; being there seemed an affirmation of the depths of illness she had reached. At the same time, she did not understand why she was discharged, since her symptoms were not controlled. Soon after going home, she had another crisis in which she stopped eating altogether. At the time we talked she reported that her eating patterns had gotten better, but overall she said she had not found "psychological or psychiatric control of any kind." Rather, she felt that she had "wasted away."

Much of Flor's story focused around her existential lack of purpose and her lack of self-worth. "Since I was a little girl I have not had an—any esteem for myself," she said. "No. I have really devalued myself as a woman, as a person. I don't feel as though I'm worth anything." This was a theme that Flor was working on with her psychologist at the hospital, who told her that she should value herself as a person and as a woman, and that it was lack of self-esteem and self-worth that has contributed to her depression. Both the psychologist and the psychiatrist emphasized that it would be a long road to recovery, and that Flor would have to work hard to get better by coming to her appointments and taking her medication.

Flor is not typical of outpatients in the sense that she is receiving regular therapy; because of time, distance, and lack of personnel in the hospital, most patients' treatment is confined to medication consultations with the psychiatrists. However, Flor said that the medication helps much more than the therapy—she takes Lexapro (a selective serotonin reuptake inhibitor [SSRI] for depression and anxiety) and Stilnox (for sleep problems), which she said help to calm and stabilize her. However, they are exorbitantly expensive (over US$300 a month) and have not assuaged many of her symptoms.

Flor endorsed having recently experienced every item on the Screen for Posttraumatic Stress Symptoms (SPTSS; Carlson 2001) except reliving her traumas, which she said usually happened only in nightmares.[15] She mentioned "thinking too much"; trouble sleeping and eating; nightmares of her husband attacking and hurting her; lack of desire to do anything; inability to keep herself from thinking about bad things that have happened to her; fear, discomfort, and the feeling of being "absent" when she is around others; anger and irritability; and excessive sweating and heart palpitations. She also mentioned being bothered by a new symptom of "forgetting things" and becoming disoriented; sometimes, she would find herself walking on the street and not know where she was or where she was going. She asked her psychiatrist if the medications could cause this, but the psychiatrist told her no, that this was a way to allow herself to leave her reality and to keep herself from processing her current and past experience. Flor described herself as feeling "closed, very deep in a hole, dark and where I can't find the exit." She had never heard of PTSD.

Although Flor tries to distract herself by embroidering, exercising, and doing chores (she stopped working as a vendor when her depression became too severe), she said "my head just keeps thinking, thinking things . . . even if I'm out in the street [doing things] my head just keeps on thinking."[16] Finally, Flor reported a profound sense of loneliness and solitude. "I feel like I have lost many things, I lost everything. . . . Family, kids, everything, no? I feel completely alone and this brings on my depressions. Sometimes I'm okay and sometimes I wake up with a depression that makes me want nothing to do with the outside world, nothing. I close up inside myself."

Several months after my interview with Flor, Dr. Villareal of the IMO mentioned her as a "success story"—she believed Flor's divorce had been granted, and she had become increasingly less isolated from her children. Dr. Villareal said that Flor's diagnosis had been changed by the Cruz del Sur psychiatrist, as well:

> The doctor told her that if she had noticed the violence she was living earlier, maybe her illness would not have become so extreme. She wouldn't have somatized so much and it wouldn't have become chronic—because now she has a personality disorder and bipolar disorder. They explained this to her and she was really angry, saying "Why? Why I am so sick? Because nobody told me before that the life I was living was going to make me sick? Now I'm going to have to take medicine for life, and now that I know I'm sick what makes me most angry is that I could have avoided this illness altogether." . . . Now she's

empowered, and though we're not going to be able to get rid of the illness, we can change her attitude.

When I met with Flor to follow up several years after our initial interview, however, she said the divorce still had not been granted and that it turned out she did not have bipolar disorder; her diagnosis had been reverted to depression. "I have really serious problems—I get sad and then the depression starts, the stress. I have a lot of stress, and it affects me too much. So I can never stop the medications. . . . I'm a depressive and it's pretty heavy, you know? Or I feel like I have some kind of attitude problem."

Discussion and Conclusions

Verónica's and Flor's stories illustrate several of the processes this chapter has described. Like Amapola, whose story I presented at the outset of the chapter, Verónica's and Flor's experiences have been shaped by highly visible anti-gender violence campaigns, which seek to draw attention to violence in all its manifestations and to reshape Oaxacans' thinking about gender relations more generally. Only recently have these women begun to explicitly define their experiences of domestic abuse as "violence," and the resultant emotional effects as "traumas." Additionally, both Verónica and Flor sought psychological and psychiatric treatment for the traumatic effects of violence in the clinical setting, underlining the convergence between antiviolence initiatives and Oaxaca's growing field of mental health services.

These narratives also reveal multiple sources of insecurity—and the "gendered effects of insecurity" (James 2008)—in Oaxacan women's lives. In Amapola's case, she was marginalized first through her status as the illegitimate child of a rape and later as an HIV-positive woman. The fact that her mother was raped and that she was infected with HIV unknowingly by her unfaithful husband speak to the not-so-invisible ways in which violence shapes Amapola's life. Like Flor, she has been subject to verbal and physical abuse from her husband (though less so since they contracted HIV; since then, he has become religious, reduced his drinking, and ceased pursuing extra-marital relationships). Like Verónica, Amapola has struggled with poverty and lack of educational opportunity. Verónica was physically and sexually abused by her father and Flor by her stepfather; in Flor's case, that earlier abuse contributed to almost total isolation once she separated from her husband and children, since she was afraid to see her stepfather and thus refused to visit her family in Puebla. Flor and Verónica both describe incapacitating sensations of fear and insecurity, and both attribute all their symptoms to the experience of violence.

Given these factors, it is clear that Amapola, Verónica, and Flor—and perhaps most other women in similar situations—have been subject to an array of violences, including structural violence. However, Verónica's and Flor's experiences complicate the cultural trope of violence that is promoted by the antiviolence campaigns and reinforced by the local clinical ethos. In line with that trope, both women were inculcated with the idea that they should endure abuse from males, and until recently neither of them had a clear means of denouncing it. The visibility of gender violence as a serious societal concern, along with the growing salience of discourse on trauma, contributes to a milieu in which it has been possible for both women to make direct links between violence and its debilitating emotional aftereffects and seek treatment for them. But while Verónica and Flor may have considered the domestic violence they suffered as "part of their life structure," as Dr. Cardozo put it, they did not express its emotional consequences as routinized or experientially mundane. Rather, both women found their symptoms—many of which were in line with the specific symptoms necessary for a diagnosis of PTSD—to be highly debilitating and disruptive. While it is important to recognize these women's agency and resilience, it can hardly be argued that they are inured to violence's effects.

Like many women at the hospital, Verónica and Flor reported great relief from antidepressants and anxiolytics and expressed profound gratitude to the psychiatrists for kind treatment and an impressive ability to treat their suffering when other professionals and healers had failed them. However, the women's stories also reveal more subtle themes of guilt, responsibility, worthlessness, and anxiety—sometimes about performing their roles as mothers and partners. Unlike the diagnosis of PTSD, which can have the effect of externalizing illness and conferring innocence on victims (Breslau 2004; French 2004), affective and personality disorder diagnoses posit illness as the internal consequence of problematic brain chemistry or unfortunate genes, potentially contributing to gendered feelings of self-blame. Experience of violence and other social factors are of course acknowledged as contributing factors to these disorders, but not in a causal sense, such that the process of diagnosis and treatment can have the effect of obscuring violence and its traumatic effects and subtly shifting responsibility for suffering to the woman.

No Oaxacan mental health practitioner would condone domestic violence or disregard its detrimental effects on mental health; however, there is little room in the context of institutional psychiatry to routinely confront domestic violence as a matter of diagnosis, treatment, and prevention.

Interestingly, observations like these have contributed to a distinct sense of antipsychiatry among many of Oaxaca's psychologists and therapists, both in institutional and private practice. These practitioners frequently critique psychiatry for pathologizing normal and adaptive emotions, for misidentifying the source of patients' problems, and for using diagnoses and medications as shortcuts when what is really needed are explicit actions to change the social situations in which Oaxacans live, like violence. The PTSD diagnosis, they say, cannot capture the essence and meaning of violence in patients' lives, or it ignores particular experiences of violence just because patients do not present with a series of specific symptoms. Although diagnoses of PTSD would not contraindicate therapy and intervention—rather, the presence of the disorder would suggest the need for such actions—psychologists consider the diagnosis a symbol of psychiatry's overmedicalization of human suffering and eschew it a priori of patient presentation. Ironically, however, the absence of PTSD as a salient means of interpreting domestic violence-related trauma results in an overreliance on other diagnoses that arguably pathologize women's distress just as much, if not more, than PTSD would.

We must also consider structural constraints on modes of expression (Jenkins 1991, 1996). In Oaxaca, as in many other places, mental health practitioners are well aware of the fear many female patients experience when faced with the option of denouncing a partner and explicitly attributing suffering to violence perpetrated by him. Especially in a region where the majority of women have not completed primary school and where a woman's place is widely considered to be the home, the costs of denunciation and full expression of emotional trauma are often considered to be quite high.[17] Second, as mentioned earlier, part of psicoeducación in Oaxaca is the incitement for Oaxacans—particularly women—to recognize and express their emotions, since it is widely thought that they do not know how to do so, and that traditional Oaxacan culture discourages such talk. Indeed, expressing feelings, especially as inner properties of individuals that merit articulation, is a very recent addition to the culture of emotional health in this region (Duncan 2012).

In this context, the particular constellation of symptoms required for a PTSD diagnosis could be quite difficult for female sufferers of domestic violence to both identify and express. On the other hand, it is also possible that local mental health practitioners themselves have internalized—and explicitly promoted—the belief that a culture of violence inures people to its traumatic effects, thus inhibiting detection of trauma-related symptoms in cases of domestic abuse. It is one thing to emphasize the extremely problematic prevalence of domestic violence in Mexico, to critique the ways in which it is symptomatic of unequal relations between the sexes, and to attempt to change those relations through state and countrywide initiatives and interventions. However, the ways in which such observations are translated to the clinical sphere can obscure the violence women are finally beginning to be able to denounce. Though it is meant to stop cultural practices from silencing distress, the cultural trope of violence may ironically silence it in other ways, by creating expectations and stereotypes, a totalizing vision of women's experience that practitioners themselves use in their own diagnostic processes.

I realize that my argument could be construed as an appeal for more diagnoses of PTSD in cases of domestic violence and abandonment of cultural explanations for violent behavior—which themselves are meant to be part of a feminist critique of machismo. However, a spike in diagnoses of PTSD in relation to domestic violence could have problematic consequences itself, particularly by silencing the important cultural critique that gender violence initiatives attempt to highlight. Although it may have unintended consequences, the heart of that critique is that only through broad cultural change and elimination of inequality can violence be addressed. If the PTSD diagnosis were widespread, it could indicate undue medicalization and problematic depoliticization of gendered violence. At the same time, more than other psychiatric diagnoses, PTSD can provide the opportunity for political and social action while also moving away from "the individual model of responsibility that pathologizes a human response to intensely frightening experiences" (Root 1996:374), which is ostensibly what the anti–gender violence initiatives—and many mental health practitioners—are working toward.

These processes draw attention to the logic and disjunctures of discourse and practice in rapidly shifting cultures of mental health. Professional practice and institutions are significant because they can act as shapers of culture: whether particular violent events are selected as potentially traumatic in the professional setting can impact local understanding of such phenomena and concepts of self and experience more generally. As such, the fact that the PTSD diagnosis is not utilized in cases of domestic violence in Oaxaca—but is growing in reference to other types of traumatic experience—acts as a weathervane for how violence, trauma, and gender are being negotiated in this setting. While expansion of Euro-American mental health practice can signify potentially homogenizing discourses, ideologies, and forms of care, it can also be generative of novel social practices and self-understandings.

Notes

1. I use the terms "domestic violence," "domestic abuse," and "gender violence" instead of "intimate partner violence" because they encompass abuse perpetrated by people beyond victims' intimate partners. Additionally, I did not hear the term "intimate partner violence" used in Oaxaca, while *violencia doméstica* (domestic violence) and *violencia de género* (gender violence) were common.

2. Metzl (2010) also uses the concept of diagnostic bracket creep as conceptualized by feminist theorist Jacquelyn Zita (1998; see also Kramer 1993) to discuss the gendered process wherein "demand, supply, and desire for [psychiatric] drugs conspire to expand diagnostic boundaries relentlessly outward, creating an ever-growing set of indications for an ever-widening set of psychiatric illnesses" (Metzl 2010:145).

3. This is despite the fact that the DSM-IV-TR and the DSM-5 specify that witnessing a traumatic event via "electronic media, television, movies, or pictures" does not qualify as a criterion for "exposure to actual or threatened death, serious injury, or sexual violence" unless exposure through those forms of media is "work-related" (American Psychiatric Association 2013).

4. Additionally, there is ongoing debate about whether the traumatic effects of domestic violence and other forms of repeated and chronic abuse may even lead to a distinct form of the disorder, known as "complex PTSD" or DESNOS (disorders of extreme stress, not otherwise specified), "an expanded set of symptoms hypothesized to better capture the phenomenology of the trauma response in highly traumatized populations" (Hinton and Lewis-Fernández 2011, see also Herman 1992).

5. All original quotations are in Spanish and translated by the author. All names have been changed to protect anonymity.

6. The UN's Millennium Development Goals, for example, explicitly target gender equality and women's empowerment as means to economic development. For discussions and critiques of female-focused development models, see Kabeer (1999) and Worthen (2012).

7. These types of violence are defined differently depending on the institution. One of the more concise definitions comes from the federal Special Prosecutor for Crimes of Violence against Women and Human Trafficking (Fiscalía Especial para los Delitos

de Violencia contra las Mujeres y Trata de Personas, known as FEVIMTRA. According to them, psychological violence exists "when someone says or does things that can
make you sad, isolate you, affect your self-esteem, make you feel fear or wish to die,
with insults, threats, or by ignoring you." Physical violence is present "when someone
uses physical force, a weapon, or any object to injure you, not only by hitting, but by
pushing you, pulling you, or pinching you, among other [aggressions]." Sexual violence
occurs when "you are degraded or when your body or sexuality is harmed; for example, being touched without your consent, forced to have sexual relations, or being subjected to offensive sexual words or signals." "Violencia patrimonial," or property
violence, occurs when a woman's belongings or those of her family are damaged or stolen. And economic violence occurs when one's income is controlled or denied or when
a woman is paid less than a man for the same type of work.

8. Wagner (2003) provides a summary of many of the domestic violence–related
initiatives, organizations, and legal reforms that have emerged over the course of the
past forty years in Mexico, beginning with Mexico City–based women's NGOs and feminist groups in the 1970s and 1980s. Programs like the Intra-Family Violence Assistance Center (CAVI) and the Grupo-Plural Pro-Víctimas in Mexico City were
established in 1990, and legal reforms have been enacted sporadically in all of Mexico's states since the 1994 Belem do Pará convention. Desjarlais et al. (1995) also note
growing institutional attention to the issue of sexual and domestic violence in Mexico
City; in the years since their volume was published, those initiatives have spread to
southern states like Oaxaca, particularly Oaxaca City but more and more to its rural
regions, as well.

9. In her piece on domestic violence, gender, and sickness in Mexico, Finkler (1997)
finds that domestic violence is disturbingly common but writes, "In Mexico, wife beating is *not* considered 'natural,' as a husband's, or mate's privilege, despite the fact that
by its prevalence a woman may have been exposed to it in her natal family, seeing her
father beat her mother: wife beating is uniformly condemned and considered evil. For
this reason, this practice in Mexico carries a moral load, resulting in anger and sickness" (Finkler 1997:1149).

10. The perception that rural indigenous cultures—particularly the Triqui and the
inhabitants of the coastal Mixteca region—are inherently violent is quite widespread
in Oaxaca. This view implies that indigenous communities commit a type of cultural
violence in which the culture itself "preaches, teaches, admonishes, eggs on, and dulls
[people] into seeing exploitation and/or repression"—of women, in this case—"as normal and natural, or not seeing them (particularly not exploitation) at all" (Galtung
1990:295). By targeting culture as culpable for these inequalities, the discourse on gender violence may reproduce historically held stereotypes of indigenous communities
as backward, uncivilized, and violent—and ignore the ways in which indigenous communities themselves have been subject to structural violence.

11. This impression stands in interesting contrast to Oscar Lewis's 1959 observation that machismo and its associated practices are "much weaker in rural areas than

in the cities and weaker among the lower classes than in the middle and upper classes"
(Lewis 1959:17).

12. The concept of a distressing event causing health-related aftereffects itself is not
new in Oaxaca: curanderos have been treating *susto* (fright sickness, also known as *espanto*) for centuries. The symptoms of susto often resemble those of depression (sadness, desperation, exhaustion, and/or insomnia), and the events leading to susto—at
least among the patients and curanderos with whom I have spoken—tend to include
things like fires, natural disasters, falling (especially near a river), being surprised by
wild animals (particularly snakes), or witnessing violence. Finkler (1997) presents a case
study of a Oaxacan woman in Mexico City who is abused by her husband and returns
to Oaxaca for treatment of espanto. In my research, however, domestic abuse was never
mentioned as a precipitating factor, even when I inquired specifically as to whether it
could cause the illness. One explanation for this is that treating susto and espanto often requires returning to the place the frightening event occurred in order to perform
a ritual. To do this in the case of domestic violence could entail identifying the perpetrator, which could invite stigma and gossip—especially in the context of a small
village.

13. Cruz del Sur is the one of the only affordable options for publicly subsidized
psychiatric care in the region. It is a Health Ministry (Servicios de Salud) facility and
offers relatively low-cost care regardless of employment. Consultations are provided at
a nominal fee; however, medications are often prohibitively expensive given patients'
incomes. The hospital is located in the Central Valley of Oaxaca, about a half hour from
Oaxaca City. Many patients travel extremely long distances from rural regions in Oaxaca and neighboring states. Initial consultations involve an hour-long medical history
and in nearly all cases result in a diagnosis (or multiple diagnoses) and medication
prescriptions. The most extreme cases result in hospitalization in the inpatient facility. Owing to the volume of patients, subsequent appointments normally consist of a
half-hour medication consultation. The hospital has on staff several outpatient psychologists, but the majority of patients either do not have the time or inclination to
participate in therapy, or are not referred to the psychologists to begin with.

14. Barricades or *barricadas* refers to the roadblocks that different neighborhoods
in Oaxaca City erected during the conflict to prevent armed forces from entering. Military forces regularly policed the streets and, reportedly, broke into people's homes to
extract those who were suspected of inciting rebellion.

15. For logistical reasons I was able administer the SPTSS to only some patients,
and even then the process had to be abbreviated. Therefore, rather than asking participants to tell me how many times they had experienced each symptom in the last
week, I asked if they frequently continued to experience them. Thus I do not have scores
for the scales I administered, but rather a general sense of posttraumatic stress symptomatology.

16. See Yarris (2009) for a discussion of "thinking too much" as related to the problem of "brainache" (*dolor de cerebro*) among marginalized Nicaraguan women. In

Flor's case, as in other Cruz del Sur hospital cases I encountered, thinking too much was presented as a symptom on its own, usually without reports of dolor de cerebro.

17. One of Oaxaca's main newspapers, *Noticias*, recently reported that 50 percent of women who begin the process of filing a domestic violence charge or complaint abandon the process (because they are not economically independent, the article argues), while 70 percent of women who experience domestic violence never report it (López 2013).

References

American Psychiatric Association
    2013 Diagnostic and Statistical Manual of Mental Disorders (5th ed.). Washington, D.C.: American Psychiatric Association.
Baker, Charlene K., Fran H. Norris, Dayna M. V. Diaz, Julia L. Perilla, Arthur D. Murphy, and Elizabeth G. Hill
    2005 Violence and PTSD in Mexico: Gender and Regional Differences. Social Psychiatry and Psychiatric Epidemiology 40:519–28.
Breslau, Joshua
    2000 Globalizing Disaster Trauma: Psychiatry, Science, and Culture After the Kobe Earthquake. Ethos 28(2):174–97.
    2004 Cultures of Trauma: Anthropology Views of Posttraumatic Stress Disorder in International Health. Culture, Medicine, and Psychiatry 28:113–26.
Brown, George W., and Tirril O. Harris
    1978 The Social Origins of Depression: A Study of Psychiatric Disorder in Women. New York: Free Press.
Carlson, Eve B.
    2001 Psychometric Study of a Brief Screen for PTSD: Assessing the Impact of Multiple Traumatic Events. Assessment 8:431–41.
Consejo Nacional de Evaluación de la Política de Desarollo Social (CONEVAL)
    2012 Informe de Pobreza en México, 2012. México: D.F. CONEVAL.
Desjarlais, Robert, Leon Eisenberg, Byron Good, and Arthur Kleinman
    1995 World Mental Health: Problems and Priorities in Low-Income Countries. New York: Oxford University Press.
Duncan, Whitney L.
    2012 The Culture of Mental Health in a Changing Oaxaca. Ph.D. diss., University of California–San Diego.
    2015 Transnational Disorders: Returned Migrants at Oaxaca's Psychiatric Hospital. Medical Anthropology Quarterly 29:24–41.
Farmer, Paul
    2003 Pathologies of Power: Health, Human Rights, and the New War on the Poor. Berkeley: University of California Press.

2004 Sidney W. Mintz Lecture for 2001: An Anthropology of Structural Violence. Current Anthropology 45:305–25.

Fassin, Didier, and Richard Rechtman
2009 The Empire of Trauma: An Inquiry into the Condition of Victimhood. Princeton, N.J.: Princeton University Press.

Finkler, Kaja
1997 Gender, Domestic Violence and Sickness in Mexico. Social Science and Medicine 45(8):1147–60.

Forché, Carolyn, ed.
1993 Against Forgetting: Twentieth Century Poetry of Witness. New York: W.W. Norton.

French, Lindsay
2004 Commentary. "Cultures of Trauma." Special issue, Culture, Medicine, and Psychiatry 28:211–20.

Friedman-Peleg, Keren, and Yehuda C. Goodman
2010 From Posttrauma Intervention to Immunization of the Social Body: Pragmatics and Politics of a Resilience Program in Israel's Periphery. Culture, Medicine, and Psychiatry 34(3):421–42.

Galtung, Johan
1969 Violence, Peace and Peace Research. Journal of Peace Research 8(2):81–117.
1990 Cultural Violence. Journal of Peace Research 27(3):291–305.

Herman, Judith Lewis
1992 Complex PTSD: A Syndrome in Survivors of Prolonged and Repeated Trauma. Journal of Traumatic Stress 5(3):377–91.
(1992) 1997 Trauma and Recovery: The Aftermath of Violence—from Domestic Abuse to Political Terror. New York: Basic Books.Hinton , Devon E., Alex L. Hinton, Vuth Pich, Reattidara J. R. Loeum, and Mark H. Pollack
2009 Nightmares Among Cambodian Refugees: The Breaching of Concentric Ontological Security. Culture, Medicine, and Psychiatry 33:219–65.

Hinton, Devon E., and Roberto Lewis-Fernández
2011 The Cross-Cultural Validity of Posttraumatic Stress Disorder: Implications for DSM-5. Depression and Anxiety 28:783–801.

Instituto Nacional de Estadística y Geografía (INEGI)
2013 Panorama de violencia contra las mujeres en Oaxaca: ENDIREH 2011. Mexico City: Instituto Nacional de Estadística y Geografía.

James, Erica Caple
2004 The Political Economy of "Trauma" in Haiti in the Democratic Era of Insecurity. Culture, Medicine, and Psychiatry 28:127–49.
2008 Haunting Ghosts: Madness, Gender, and Ensekirite in Haiti in the Democratic Era. In Postcolonial Disorders. Mary-Jo DelVecchio Good, Sandra Teresa Hyde, Sarah Pinto, and Byron J. Good, eds. Pp. 132–56. Berkeley: University of California Press.

Jenkins, Janis

1991 The State Construction of Affect: Political Ethos and Mental Health Among Salvadoran Refugees. Culture, Medicine, and Psychiatry 15:139–65.

1996 The Impress of Extremity: Women's Experience of Trauma and Political Violence. *In* Gender and Health: An International Perspective. Carolyn F. Sargent and Caroline B. Brettell, eds. Pp. 278–91. Upper Saddle River, N.J.: Prentice-Hall.

Kabeer, Naila

1999 Resources, Agency, Achievements: Reflections on the Measurement of Women's Empowerment. Development and Change 30:435–64.

Kohrt, Brandon A., and Carol Worthman

2009 Gender and Anxiety in Nepal: The Role of Social Support, Stressful Life Events, and Structural Violence. CNS Neuroscience and Therapeutics 15:237–48.

Kramer, Peter

1993 Listening to Prozac: The Landmark Book About Antidepressants and the Remaking of the Self. New York: Basic.

Lewis, Oscar

1959 Five Families: Mexican Case Studies in the Culture of Poverty. New York: Basic Books.

López, Citlalli

2013 Abandonan Proceso 50% de Mujeres con Violencia Intrafamiliar: No Cuentan con Salario, Vivienda o Seguridad Social. Noticias.Net.Mx March 14.

McNally, Richard J.

2003 Progress and Controversy in the Study of Posttraumatic Stress Disorder. Annual Review of Psychology 54:229–52.

2009 Can We Fix PTSD in DSM-V? Depression and Anxiety 26:597–600.

Metzl, Jonathan M.

2010 Gender Stereotypes in the Diagnosis of Depression: A Systematic Content Analysis of Medical Records. *In* Pharmaceutical Self: The Global Shaping of Experience in an Age of Psychopharmacology. Janis H. Jenkins, ed. Pp. 145–60. Santa Fe: School for Advanced Research Press.

Norris, Fran H., Arthur D. Murphy, Charlene K. Baker, Julia L. Perilla, Francisco Gutiérrez Rodríguez, and José de Jesús Gutiérrez Rodríguez

2003 Epidemiology of Trauma and Posttraumatic Stress Disorder in Mexico. Journal of Abnormal Psychology 112(4):646–56.

Patel, Vikram, and Arthur Kleinman

2003 Poverty and Common Mental Disorders in Developing Countries. Bulletin of the World Health Organization 81(8):609–15.

Ramirez Almanza, Patricia and Ana Laura Méndez Calderón

2007 Programa Estatal de Salud Mental 2007–2012. Servicios de Salud de Oaxaca, Dirección de Prevención y Promoción de la Salud, Subdirección de Medicina Preventiva, Departamento de Enfermedades No-Transmisibles.

Root, Maria P.

1996 Women of Color and Traumatic Stress in "Domestic Captivity": Gender and Race as Disempowering Statuses. *In* Ethnocultural Aspects of Posttraumatic Stress Disorder: Issues, Research, and Clinical Applications. Anthony J. Marsella, Matthew J. Friedman, Ellen T. Gerrity, and Raymond M. Scurfield, eds. Pp. 363–87. Washington, D.C.: American Psychological Association.

Ruiz Quiróz, R. and L. C. Vásquez

2009 Estadísticas de la población migrante oaxaqueña. Oaxaca: Instituto Oaxaqueño de Atención al Migrante.

Salis Gross, Corina

2004 Struggling with Imaginaries of Trauma and Trust: The Refugee Experience in Switzerland. Culture, Medicine and Psychiatry 28(2):151–67.

Servicios de Salud de Oaxaca (SSO)

2007 Cuenta SSO con Centros Para Atender Violencia Intrafamiliar. Comunicación Social/Comunicado de Prensa. Gobierno del Estado.

Stubbs, Paul

2005 Transforming Local and Global Discourses: Reassessing the PTSD Movement in Bosnia and Croatia. *In* Forced Migration and Mental Health: Rethinking the Care of Refugees and Displaced Persons. David Ingleby, ed. Pp. 53–66. Utrecht: Springer.

Wagner, Mary C.

2003 Comment: Belem Do Para: Moving Toward Eradicating Domestic Violence in Mexico. Penn State International Law Review 22: 349–68.

Worthen, Holly

2012 Women and Microcredit: Alternative Readings of Subjectivity, Agency, and Gender Change in Rural Mexico. Gender, Place, and Culture: A Journal of Feminist Geography 19(3):364–81.

Yarris, Kristin Elizabeth

2009 The Pain of "Thinking Too Much": *Dolor de Cerebro* and the Embodiment of Social Hardship Among Nicaraguan Women. Ethos 39(2):226–48.

Zita, Jacquelyn N.

1998 Body Talk: Philosophical Reflections on Sex and Gender. New York: Columbia University Press.

CHAPTER 7

Exploring Pathways of Distress and Mental Disorders: The Case of the Highland Quechua Populations in the Peruvian Andes

Duncan Pedersen and Hanna Kienzler

In this chapter, we aim at building a transdisciplinary framework between medicine, psychiatry, and anthropology to investigate how indigenous populations in the Peruvian Andes express their distress and suffering, and assign meaning to their experience. We further explore how troubling and traumatic experiences enter inner life processes and are expressed through narratives of distress, pain and suffering, and how these narratives are later appropriated by biomedical scientists who transform them into scientific categories, such as posttraumatic stress disorder (PTSD) and depression, classify them as diseases or disorders, and deal with them by employing some form of therapy or symptomatic treatment aimed to return to normalcy.

Our conceptual framework is based on the assumption that the mental (mind) and physical (brain and body) are linked in complex ways largely determined by social structures, modeled by culture, and mediated by social position. In attempting this mysterious leap from mind to body—as postulated by Felix Deutsch—we stay away from the linear causality model of psychosomatic medicine and adopt a more structural, and interpretative conceptual frame. Theories that consider mind and body to be distinct kinds of substances or natures are becoming increasingly contested. Instead, they give way to transdisciplinary conceptual frames that emphasize novel ways of perceiving body and mind, acknowledging the subjectivity of the illness experience and expression of distress, while recognizing that symptoms are simultaneously connected to social context and health status, and strongly modeled by culture and life experience. For instance, it is recognized that neurobiology is based on the unbreakable relationship between a person's life experience (biography) and his/her biological memory, the coding and decoding of neural networks along the history of persons, and the bio-psycho-social dynamics of higher consciousness and subjectivity (Dongier et al. 1996). Biology should not any longer be seen as a rigid, monolithic structure, but as a dynamic, interpersonal, historical, and evolutionary process (Eisenberg 1995).

Social epidemiology, which was born in the 1950s, is a continuously evolving field of enquiry. Three theoretical frameworks explaining disease distribution—psychosocial; social production of disease/political economy of health; and ecosocial and multilevel frameworks—have guided much of the discussion on the relationships between society and biology (Krieger 2001). However, little is known about the particular pathways that connect biology and inner life experiences within a context of social inequalities and violence. In the mental health field, questions remain open of how expressions of distress and symptoms are produced, constructed, and experienced by different peoples or cultures under varying social, material, political, and psychological conditions (Marmot 2005; Nichter 2010). While research on narratives of distress has emphasized the taxonomies of pain, distress, and disorder, it has not sufficiently contributed to our understanding of the interrelations between poverty and adversity as health determinants, or how history and culture mold local narratives and endow them with meaning (Bracken 2001; Almedom and Summerfield 2004).

Based on this broad conceptual frame, we focus on the following questions: How is the social world connected to psychological and biological phenomena, and, in turn, how does this translate into narratives of distress and suffering? How is this complex of interrelated phenomena perceived and reflected in the narratives of distress and suffering? How much of the idioms of distress and symptoms are due to social exclusion, persistent social and economic inequalities, and early life experiences? How are exposure to intentional violence-related stressors connected to mental health outcomes such as PTSD, depression, and anxiety? What are the processes by which poverty and trauma-related conditions relate to the soma (the body-mind) and to the expression of distress and disorder?

To provide tentative answers to these questions, we first present a focused literature review on medical, psychosocial, and anthropological approaches to the understanding of trauma exposure and mental health outcomes. We argue that while the approaches seem at first glance to be mutually exclusive, it is essential to recognize that they can influence and complement each other. Second, we show how such an integrationist approach could be achieved by revisiting our empirical data on the impact of war, trauma, and social inequality among the highland Quechua in the Peruvian Andes. We conclude by presenting an alternative framework in an attempt to show how different approaches to war- and trauma-related health problems can be brought into alignment and may provide a more holistic interpretation to better understand the complex interrelations between exposure to trauma and stressors and collective health.

Approaches to Understanding Trauma Exposure and Mental Health Outcomes

In recent years, authors have tried to identify and validate the effects of violent conflict on the mental health of those affected by focusing on concepts like war trauma, PTSD, social suffering, and idioms of distress (Bracken and Petty 1998; Fassin and Rechtman 2009; Kleinman et al. 1997; Mollica et al. 2002; Nichter 2010). While the current debate among health and social scientists seems to suggest that the various approaches to the study of trauma and mental health outcomes are mutually exclusive, we agree with Miller and Rasmussen (2010), who state that neither of them is consistent with what we are learning about the relative contribution of war exposure and long-standing stressors on mental health. In order to gain a better understanding about the multiple biological, psychological, and social pathways between the context and related expressions of distress and suffering, it is essential to adopt a more comprehensive social epidemiological framework integrating the various different approaches.

Medical Approaches

Trauma-focused approaches are most often used by health professionals, especially clinicians and psychiatrists, who tend to narrow down on the relationship between direct war exposure and PTSD as an outcome. Epidemiological research among war-affected populations has proven that war exposure, such as witnessing violent death and the killings of loved ones, separation and displacement, terrorist attacks, and bombardment and shelling, are directly linked to the development of PTSD, and that cumulative trauma is predictive of higher psychiatric symptom levels of PTSD (N. Breslau 1998; Miller and Rasmussen 2010; Mollica et al. 1998; Smith et al. 2002). This characteristic is referred to as "dose-effect relationship" and tends to assume that "each individual who has experienced or is experiencing traumatic events will develop PTSD after reaching a certain threshold of traumatic exposure" (Neuner et al. 2004:2). We may illustrate this relationship with a direct-effect conceptual model adapted from Miller and Rasmussen (2010), on which much of current trauma-focused interventions are based (Figure 7.1).

The connection between "events in the world and suffering inside individuals" (J. Breslau 2004:116) has been fairly well established through epidemiological surveys using population sampling and structured diagnostic instruments such as the Harvard Trauma Questionnaire (HTQ), the General Health Questionnaire-28 (GHQ-28), the Hopkins Symptom Check List (HSCL), and the Medical Outcomes Study-20 (MOS-20), among many others.

Studies conducted by these means have found high rates of PTSD among refugee and displaced populations affected by various forms of war trauma (Miller et al. 2006). Marshall and colleagues (2005) assessed the prevalence, comorbidity, and correlates of psychiatric disorder in the U.S. Cambodian refugee community by conducting 490 interviews on a random sample of households. The analysis revealed that all study participants had been exposed to severe trauma before immigration and, consequently, suffered from PTSD (62 percent), major depression (51 percent) , and alcohol use disorder (4 percent). PTSD and depression were comorbid findings in the population, and each showed a strong dose-response relationship with measures of traumatic exposure. Neuner and his team (2004) conducted a cross-sectional

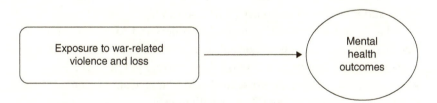

Figure 7.1. Direct effects model (adapted from Miller and Rasmussen 2010).

study among 3,339 Ugandan and Sudanese nationals and Sudanese refugees of the West Nile region. They found that 31.6 percent of the male and
40.1 percent of the female respondents fulfilled the DSM criteria for the
PTSD diagnosis. Pedersen and colleagues (2008) conducted a cross-sectional
survey among the highland Quechua indigenous peoples in the Southern
Central Andes of Peru (discussed later in this chapter), reporting relatively
high rates of mental health disorders and a 24.7 percent PTSD point prevalence rate in the adult population (N = 373). Similarly, Lopes Cardozo et al.
(2003) reported a 25 percent point prevalence of PTSD among Kosovar
Albanians; Sabin et al. (2003) found that among Mayan refugees in Mexico,
11.8 percent met PTSD symptom criteria; Dahl et al. (1998), using a self-
report measure, discerned a prevalence rate of 71 percent for current PTSD
in their sample of displaced Bosnian women in a war zone; and Sondergaard
and colleagues (2001) found a prevalence rate of 37 percent for current PTSD
in their sample of Iraqi and Kurdish refugees in Sweden using a combination of self-report measures and interview methods. Based on such and similar research, clinicians and policy makers have developed guidelines and
recommendations to determine the needs of and provide adequate treatment
to afflicted populations (Barudy 1989; Mollica and Caspi-Yavin 1991).

Psychosocial Approaches

Psychosocial approaches to war trauma argue that the diagnosis of PTSD provides a "moral paradigm" that identifies victims and perpetrators by focusing on particular traumatic events rather than on recurrent or persistent
problematic life circumstances, long-standing stressors, structural violence,
and proximal or distant social determinants of health (J. Breslau 2004; Bolton
2010). Although such stressors are difficult to assess, as they are more subjective in nature, considerable evidence exists that links social inequalities
and persistent and recurrent stressors to psychological distress, physical mor-
bidity, and mortality as outcomes (Wilkinson 1996).

It has been established that mental disorders and barriers to access to
treatment do not affect all sections of society in the same way in that at all
levels of income, health, and illness follow a social gradient: the lower the
socioeconomic position, the worse the health status (Commission on Social
Determinants of Health 2008). These health injustices are often compounded
by other social inequalities, including those emerging from gender disparities,

social discrimination, and other forms of structural violence (Bennett et al. 2008; Farmer 2004; Siegrist and Marmot 2004; Wilkinson 1994; Wilkinson and Pickett 2007). War situations generate or exacerbate stressful social and material conditions and, thus, impact negatively on the physical, social, and mental well-being of individuals and families (Miller and Rasmussen 2010). These complex interconnections may be illustrated with the partial mediation model developed by Fernando et al. (2010) and adapted by Miller and Rasmussen (2010) (Figure 7.2).

Several empirical studies are illustrative of how daily stressors mediate experiences of armed conflict: Melville and Lykes (1992) studied the psychosocial effects of civil war on displaced Guatemalan Mayan children who have witnessed the violent loss of family members and/or sudden displacement from their familial homes and communities. They found that although children and their families had suffered considerable socioemotional damage, there were several indicators of resilience: desire for freedom to express their feelings about traumatic events and desire to overcome fear, to reaffirm ethnic identity, and to prepare for future work and job opportunities. In a different context, Farhood and his team (1993) explored the stress dimensions of the Lebanese civil war and the multifaceted health effects on the Lebanese population. While the war flared up periodically, daily hassles resulting from

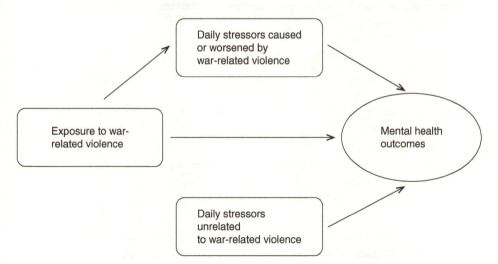

Figure 7.2. Daily stressors as partially mediating the relationship of war-related violence and loss to mental health outcomes (from Fernando et al. 2010, and adapted from Miller and Rasmussen 2010).

the breakdown in community services prevailed more uniformly and continuously. As a consequence, families reported that their mental and physical well-being was strongly impacted by the economic consequences of a process of rapid inflation, not being able to ensure the basic needs of decent living, and the reduced possibility of finding their relatives and friends. Similarly, Miller and colleagues (2008) assessed the relative contribution of daily stressors and war-related experience of violence and loss to levels of depression, PTSD, impaired functioning, and a culturally specific measure of general psychological distress among Afghanis living in Kabul. It was found that for women, daily stressors were better predictors than war experiences of all mental health outcomes except for PTSD. For men, on the other hand, daily stressors were a better predictor for depression and functional impairment, while war experiences and daily stressors were similarly predictive of general distress.

While these examples show that our bodies are "socialized bodies" that do not exist independently of the social context in which we carry out our biological functions (Horwitz 2007), the authors largely assess mental disorders according to the diagnostic criteria of the Diagnostic and Statistical Manual (DSM) classification. While the DSM is certainly not a useless tool, the following section will make apparent that its diagnostic criteria are too narrow and constrictive to capture certain expressions of distress in particular sociocultural contexts.

Anthropological Approaches

Medical anthropologists have developed discourses related to the lived experience of violence and suffering by focusing on the concept "idioms of distress." Local idioms of distress are "socially and culturally resonant means of experiencing and expressing distress in local worlds," and thus they are "evocative and index past traumatic memories as well as present stressors, such as anger, powerlessness, social marginalisation and insecurity, and possible future sources of anxiety, loss and angst" (Nichter 2010:405; see too Nichter 1981). Despite the great diversity of the cultural categories, it is assumed that such idioms share certain common features. They are believed to communicate a wide range of personal and social concerns that may or may not be related to individual distress or mental disorder (Green 2003). Consequently, such idioms are considered polysemic and idiosyncratic phenomena that bridge and, at the same time, transcend somatic, psychic, and social phenomena (Davis and Joakimsen 1997; Foss 2002). Thus, physical and psychological expressions of distress are not simple manifestations of a subjacent biological reality, but also metaphors that reflect and represent a variety of meanings that serve many social and psychological purposes (Browner and Sargent 2007; Loewenthal 2007; Pedersen et al. 2010).

For instance, Lewis-Fernández and colleagues (2010) examined the relationships in an ethnically diverse Latino psychiatric outpatient sample among interpersonal trauma, PTSD, major depressive disorder, dissociative capacity, and four cultural idioms of distress associated with the popular overall category of *nervios*. They found that the idioms of distress were largely independent from PTSD and depression, but rather were associated with trauma persistence and severity. Hinton et al. (2010), on the other hand, assessed *khyâl* (wind) attacks as traumatized Cambodian refugees experience them. They found that khyâl attacks were caused by a variety of seemingly unrelated events—such as by worry episodes, anger, trauma recall, standing up, startle, or odors—and those experiencing such attacks felt great fear that death might occur from bodily dysfunction. Their analysis makes apparent that while an idiom of distress, the symptoms of khyâl attacks are also good proxy indicators for PTSD.

The examples emphasize that it is crucial to understand not just the direct effects of war experiences on the mental health of civilian populations, but also the indirect impact of long-standing stressors that may or may not be exacerbated by war on the psychosocial well-being when designing mental health interventions in war and postwar settings. Based on this premise, we present empirical findings of the ways in which Quechua-speaking populations in the Peruvian highlands express their distress by focusing on both the direct and indirect effects of armed conflict and war, including violence in its various forms—interpersonal and collective, political and structural— which has become endemic in this region, generating and reinforcing social inequalities and health disparities.

Pathways of Distress and Disorders Among the Highland Quechua Populations

The study we are reporting here was conducted in the Huanta province (northern Ayacucho), in a picturesque highland region of the Southern Central

Peruvian Andes. Ayacucho was the epicenter of Shining Path, a radical Maoist guerrilla movement that started its operations in 1980. Over a period of a decade (1980–92), it turned into the most widespread and sustained subversive movement in the recent history of Peru (Degregori 1985; Manrique 1995; Stern 1999). With about seven thousand active combatants and many more underground partisans across the country, enrolled in the so-called Ejército Guerrillero Popular (Popular Guerrilla Army), the movement effectively controlled over half of Peru's territory. It conducted a vast operation simultaneously on various fronts—in open confrontation with military and civilian and paramilitary groups—which led to the killing and disappearing of an estimated total of 69,280 persons, the internal displacement of between 600,000 to one million people, and an undetermined amount in material and economic losses (Comisión de la Verdad y Reconciliación 2003).

According to the Peruvian Truth and Reconciliation Commission's report, three quarters of the victims were Quechua native speakers, mostly rural, poor, and illiterate. The repeated incursions of Shining Path and the Peruvian military left a trail of terror, retaliation, and revenge in the local population, where torture, murder, and other atrocities were brutally committed. The highlands of the Huanta province were among the most affected regions, and the local indigenous populations were massively exposed to a range of violence-related stressors and some of the most extreme forms of repressive violence ever experienced in the region.

In the early 1990s, Shining Path lost some of its momentum because of growing desertions and public discredit. Civil countermovements such as the Comités de Autodefensa Civil (Civil Defense Committees) and the *rondas campesinas* (local vigilantes) received tactical support from the military and police forces and, thus, confronted Shining Path and gradually improved the security at the local level (Degregori 2003; del Pino 1996, 2003). Since the apprehension and killing of Shining Path leaders in 1992, repression and political violence decreased significantly, but the context of structural violence continues to prevail.

After the cease of armed conflict between Shining Path and the military, the overall situation of the highland Quechua populations continues to be framed by poverty, social exclusion, and other forms of organized and interpersonal violence largely due to the forces of globalization and accelerated social change. A striking example is the widespread coca plantations and cocaine industry blooming along the eastern slopes of the Peruvian Andes.[1] These recent developments have given rise to a more vicious and frightening wave of organized violence, armed assaults, and crime, led by a corrupted police and criminal justice system. The area is under constant surveillance carried out by the extended presence of repressive forces, resulting in frequent clashes between the military and popular militia under the banner of Shining Path guerrillas with special drug enforcement agents and drug barons. More specifically, the number of mostly indigenous casualties or disappearances is steadily increasing, as well as the swelling numbers of women and youngsters convicted and jailed for possessing or transporting PBC (*pasta básica de cocaína*), largely due to the illegal coca production and drug trade industry. The presence of various internal battle fronts, a poorly defined and encroaching enemy territory, and above all, a context of marked social inequalities, poverty, and widespread crime and corruption configure an extremely adverse scenario where multiple sources of stress are operating in unison.

Methodology

To elicit the effects of past and present forms of structural and direct violence, this research was conducted in three subsequent phases, using a mixed qualitative and quantitative approach. The first phase, consisting of a qualitative study and a cross-sectional survey, was conducted between 2001 and 2003 and was followed by a second phase, in which a two-year intervention was implemented. A third and final phase, consisting of a longitudinal follow-up study of ninety-two cases with symptoms compatible with the diagnosis of PTSD, was conducted in 2011.[2]

The research sites included four rural villages in the highlands situated in the northern Ayacucho region and one marginal urban setting, on the outskirts of the city of Huanta, north of Ayacucho. The sample was based on an updated cartography and recent population census of the area. We visited all occupied households (N = 200) in all five settings and interviewed all adults present in the household at survey time (N = 373 adults, fifteen years old and over). Refusal rate was insignificant, as only three individuals (0.08 percent) refused to answer for illness reasons.

Our qualitative research strategy was derived from a structural-semantic approach (Corin et al. 1990), which allowed us to examine the peoples' discourse on distress and trauma-related experiences, the systems of signs and meanings associated with them, and their actions and reactions that followed.

We focused on the idioms of distress and emotions among the highland Que-chuas, expressed in their own language in connection with their past and current exposure to violence, aimed to further examine the pathways between personal narratives of distress, violence-related stressors, and the long his-tory of collective violence, repression, and cumulative adversity experienced in the region, which continues in one way or another to this date.

During the early stages of fieldwork, we collected data from secondary sources (historical sources, dictionaries, unpublished manuscripts, census registries, etc.) to build a regional and focused ethnography on the experi-ence of suffering and distress in the highlands. During the first phase of the study, we completed forty-five semistructured interviews with key in-formants, mostly carried out in Quechua, later translated into Spanish and transcribed for qualitative analysis (QSR N-Vivo). The semistructured inter-views followed a grid with themes and guiding questions regarding their sub-jective experience (idioms of distress) during the recent history of massive exposure to political violence (1980–2000). We also compiled a list of trau-matic events, which was later used in the cross-sectional survey to measure the degree of exposure to traumatic experiences. This was based on the num-ber of culture-specific traumatic events and violence-related stressors to which families were exposed, or that they witnessed and/or experienced (see Ped-ersen et al. 2008).

In 2001 we conducted the quantitative part of our study through a household cross-sectional survey consisting of three main sections. Section 1 consisted of a family questionnaire, containing sociodemographic informa-tion and two scales for assessing the degree of exposure to violence (the number of items delineating types of exposure to potentially traumatic events, drawn from the qualitative interviews) and the structure and density of so-cial support networks. Sociodemographic data were classified into categories for gender, marital status, literacy, migration status (returnee or refugee), and family gross income, if any. Age, density of social support, and degree of exposure to violence were entered as interval variables. Density of social support was established as the weighted sum of answers based on frequency of contact with family members, neighbors, and local authorities. Linear re-gression was used to model relationships between quantitative variables in the cross-sectional survey, setting the alpha level at 0.01 in order to account for multiple comparisons.

Section 2 consisted of two screening tools: the General Health Question-naire-12 (GHQ-12) and the Hopkins Symptom Check List-25 (HSCL-25).

Section 3 included the Trauma Questionnaire (TQ) that was derived from the Cambodian version of the Harvard Trauma Questionnaire (HTQ), since it was the most congruent validated version at the time and had performed well in assessing the consequences of exposure to traumatic events across different cultural settings (Mollica et al. 1992; Norris and Riad 1997). Finally, this section was different from the HTQ because symptoms and signs of distress and violence-related stress constructed on the basis of ethnographic data collected earlier in qualitative interviews, were included.

In order to address the issue of "category fallacy" raised by Kleinman (1988), all three questionnaires—GHQ-12, HSCL-25 and TQ—were subject to a semantic and cultural validation exercise (Manson 1997; van Ommeren 2003), conducted with a panel of Quechua-speaking persons. First, we conducted interviews with Quechua-Spanish speakers to elicit culturally appropriate and equivalent terms for items later included in the survey questions. Second, we tested and retested all questionnaires in focus group discussions and simulated cases until intended meanings were fully understood and cross-culturally relevant. Third, we lowered the cut-off point of the GHQ-12 to the recommended two instead of three (Goldberg 1972), which may have increased false positives and conversely, reduced false negatives. To improve the inter-rater reliability, simulated (taped) interviews were conducted with Quechua-speaking respondents. After the simulation exercises were completed, tapes were played and interviewers were requested to rate responses on the Likert scale. Interviewee response rates were then compared, and concordance among interviewers was achieved nine out of ten times. The duration of the interview was variable (between thirty to forty-five minutes), depending on the number of questionnaires administered.

The survey was carried out by six bilingual (Quechua-Spanish) trained fieldworkers, recruited among undergraduate social sciences students at University of San Cristobal de Huamanga, under close supervision of the research team (a physician, an anthropologist, and a sociologist) during a two-week survey data collection period. Finally, all quantitative data were revised and coded for electronic data processing (SPSS), which was completed in 2003.

Idioms of Distress

When mapping the experience of distress among the highland Quechua, *sassachacuy* emerges as one of the eliciting categories of the semantic network (also see Pedersen et al. 2010). Sassachacuy is equivalent to "several difficulties" and is consistently associated with experiences of violence, loss, and extreme adversity most often associated with *vida pobre* (lit. poor life or living poor). In a more strict sense, vida pobre is equivalent to impoverishment, and this is almost always presented as being at the root of all adversities. Vida pobre is the single most important cause in the chain of events leading to the appearance of other signs or symptoms of distress and suffering. When referring to the notion of "difficult times"—as the time people in Ayacucho were exposed to the atrocities of torture, war, and violence—informants used the Quechua-Hispanic two-word concept of *sassachacuy tiempu*. During the sassachacuy tiempu, people suffered displacement and were forced to migrate (*forzado a migrar*), searching for temporary refuge in nearby towns and cities, though this pattern of flight would often last for longer periods. Families were dislocated with men going to and from their *chacras* (small farms), while women stayed behind to care for children and animals and other belongings. This flight pattern is an effective adaptation response and a survival strategy to cope with the many adversities and multiple stressors. At the same time, the forced dislocation always disturbed traditional patterns of seasonal migration, impairing production and imposing a great deal of strain on the *comuneros* (natural members of a rural community) with accompanying disruption of their daily work and often devastating economic consequences, inexorably leading to vida pobre.

Traumatic Events and Violence-Related Stressors

The narratives of suffering during the sassachacuy tiempu evoked, as the worst "traumatic" event witnessed or experienced, the *muerte violenta* (violent death) of family members, friends, or close neighbors. Muerte violenta also demarcates the beginning of the sassachacuy tiempu, when people were tortured and killed at random by the military. There was consensus among the informants of the various kinds of muerte violenta: *molidos con piedra* (crushed with stone), *muerte con desmembramiento* (death by dismemberment), *muerte a bala* (death by bullet), *muerte trágica* (tragic death), and so on. Most deaths that occurred during the sassachacuy tiempu were considered muerte violenta and therefore "bad" deaths, where opportunities for proper bereavement and an adequate preparation of the body and burial—as prescribed by Quechua traditions—could not be respected.

The second single most frequently mentioned "traumatic" or extremely painful event was the experience of *huir a los cerros* (to escape to higher elevations, to the hills), a fairly common survival strategy used to avoid the incursions of Shining Path guerrillas or military patrols in more isolated communities. Material losses, such as fire and destruction of homes, burning of crops, theft or slaying of cattle or other animals, represented the third most reported violence-related stressor. Next, in order of frequency were lived or witnessed traumatic experiences such as being tortured, being threatened with dying, seriously wounded or being left for dead, being physically or sexually abused, and being forcefully enlisted in the army or as a *vigilante* (watchman).

Pinsamientuwan and Lukuyasqa

Most of the persons interviewed reiterated that during the sassachacuy tiempu people lived with *miedo* (fear) and *pena* (sorrow), and above all, with *pinsamientuwan* (worrying thoughts, worries). Pinsamientuwan is described as an internal condition, closer to an inner feeling of increasing and persistent worries, and the embodied experience of "worrying thoughts throbbing inside your head," which most often signals the imminent arrival of *pena* or *llaki* (sorrow, sadness), an idiom of distress described in more detail below.

In the semantic map, pinsamientuwan occupies a central position within a range that goes from *tutal pinsamientuwan* (full of worrying thoughts and memories), often linked to severe and lasting experiences of distress and loss, in one extreme, to *manan pinsamientuwan* (unable to think, total absence or lack of thoughts or common sense), on the opposite extreme of the range. In such way, pinsamientuwan emerges as a distinctive key category used to describe a mental state of worrying thoughts, which in turn may evolve into either two distinctive opposite conditions situated at the extremes of the range characterized by *manan* (emptiness) and *tutal* (excess of thoughts). Both conditions are considered serious and often untreatable. When we prompted our informants to explain this assertion they said cases of tutal pinsamientuwan (full of worrying thoughts and memories) are equivalent to being lukuyasqa (to be crazy, out of your mind).

> Q: You said that people with tutal pinsamientuwan are very sick, with much pena [sorrow]. How do this people behave? What do they do?

A: This people behave as in a dreamlike.

Q: Why?

A: Because they are lukuyasqa, *mamita.*

Q: What does it mean to be lukuyasqa.

A: . . . It means to be crazy, means to startle, going around making
no sense . . . singing . . . or calling names, throwing stones . . .
or "*todas las hierbitas cogiendo o lo que sea vean sus ojos, por
puro gusto*" [go picking herbs or collecting whatever he/she
sees, for no reason] . . . pinching away anything of [little] value
like a spoon, or a plate in the *comedor* [eatery] at the market, or
taking away a piece of cloth, and not paying for it . . . or [doing]
more serious things like threatening to beat or to kill your
husband. (Anita, fifty-eight years old, Catholic)

Lukuyasqa (being crazy) is often explained as an untreatable condition.
Among the comuneros, lukuyasqa is explained with behavioural descriptors
such as: *andar en vano* (aimless walking); *hablar sin sentido* (babble speech);
tirando piedras contra la gente (throwing stones against others); *botando
comida de la olla* (spilling food out of the pot); or bizarre behaviors such as
ir al mercado sin sombrero (go hatless to the market), which is often seen as
a transgression to the social norms, especially for women. *Luku* or *atacado*
often present themselves as *desgreñados* (dishevelled), dirty, and unkempt and
don't seem to care if they are wearing a hat on their heads when they congre-
gate in public places. Crazy people show distress or *tienen sobresaltos* (being
startled) or behave as *asustados* (frightened) for no reason. Extreme cases are
considered *tutal quemadu* (totally burnt out), *como el fondo de una olla* (as
the burned bottom of the pot).

Our informants also mentioned *waqay* (weeping) as an emotional state
associated with pain and distressful memories, as well as mourning and loss.
Waqay is not necessarily considered as an abnormal reaction, and as a sign
of distress may happen spontaneously, in private and/or most often in company with others. Ceremonial events involving public weeping and *qarawi*
(singing)[3] are considered a clear expression of grief and affliction, as happen
in funerals or important Catholic religious festivities such as Semana Santa
(Holy Week) in Ayacucho.[4]

We further tried eliciting emotions and similar experiences of distress
and suffering with terms and expressions of common usage among us, such

as "stressful," "being anxious," "being under pressure," or "being tense like the cords of the violin." However, our informants did not recognize stressful, anxious, or being tense as existing conditions among them; neither do they have equivalent words in Quechua language. They preferred to use instead their own metaphor of "being like *palo seco*," alluding to the fragile state of a dry wooden stick, fracturing easily under the slightest pressure (Pedersen et al. 2008).

Another metaphor used when describing those who were affected by the extreme adversities during the sassachacuy tiempu is the feeling of "being like *un pedazo de tela vieja o gastada* [an old piece of cloth, frail and eroded by use], which is beyond repair and disappears as powder in between your fingers." Connected to this metaphor, our informants used the Quechua term of *ijuyachqan* to describe the frail mental status of individuals undergoing severe distress and intense suffering, as homologous to an old and frail piece of worn cloth. According to them, people with ijuyachqan, are extremely fragile and have no cure or repair possible.

Finally, the elicitation of emotions during the sassachacuy tiempu failed at times to recall the painful memories of past experiences, and our informants either gave elusive or ambiguous responses, or in some cases, adopted a defensive silence, as they seemed more eager to forget than to remember violent or distressful events of the past. Some authors have already described this strategy of avoidance as discursive practices aimed to preserve community cohesion and solidarity by avoiding recollections of the past and safeguard the anonymity of the families of the victims and the identity of the perpetrators.

Ñakary and Llaki

In addition to feelings of fear and pinsamientuwan, almost all our informants reported that comuneros in general, but women in particular, lived with llaki (sorrow, sadness) and experienced ñakary (suffering).[5] In its widest sense, llaki is often, but not exclusively, linked to the sassachacuy tiempu and is framed by a life of worries and solitude, in which material deprivations and insecurity prevail. In addition, llaki is linked to the notion of vida pobre (impoverished life), which is equivalent to "a life without family, roof or shelter, and with no clothing and food." Single mothers and particularly widows blame their vida pobre on the sassachacuy tiempu, since after the loss of their husbands they are dependent solely on their own meager resources, as they are unable to work in the chacra or to exchange work in reciprocity with others. In these cases, women are not only confronting material insecurity but also are socially excluded and discriminated against by the comuneros and their extended family.

There seems to be a continuum between llaki following exposure to violent events, and llaki as an experience associated with poverty and daily life adversities.[6] The distinction speaks to the continuity existing between normal reactions and abnormal responses, which in the case of llaki seems to be a matter of degree: llaki (sadness) can be seen as an emotional reaction to being poor and facing adversity. Yet, this condition could drift toward a more serious form called *llumpay llaki* (sadness in excess), leading in turn to tutal pinsamientuwan, or to what some informants addressed as lukuyasqa, an equivalent of manan pinsamientuwan (unable to think, lack of thoughts or common sense), already described above.

Most narratives of llaki and ñakary contain afflictions expressed as *nanay* (pain) in various forms. A great variety of somatic pains are reported, usually referred to three different locations: *umananay* (headache), *istumaguyki pawaspan* (stomach pain), and *wirpuypi malukuna* (body pains) are the most frequent complaints. "It's *ñakaryniku* [suffering], when my body feels like this, you see? . . . Umananay [my head hurts], istumaguyki pawaspan [my stomach hurts], and my bones hurt up to the *chinila* [marrow] with the cold, wirpuypi malukuna [it hurts inside the bones all over my body] to the point I can't take it any more . . . *ñakaryniku nanaywan* we go on suffering with pain" (Teresa, sixty years old, Catholic).

Though both idioms ñakary and llaki are often found in the same narrative, we learned important differences in their respective meanings and attributions. On the one hand, ñakary, is described as a collective affliction, induced by unfortunate events (mostly external), some of them beyond control, such as heavy rains or *sequía* (drought), or natural disasters, and the like. Llaki, on the other hand, is an individual affliction, which cannot be experienced by the collective. Sorrow and sadness are feelings emerging from the inside, thought they may well be induced from the outside life events, like poverty, daily life adversities, or violent events. Another distinction must be made between the two idioms: llaki, as an individual affliction, is strongly associated with pinsamientuwan (worrying thoughts), and its occurrence implies the recollection of unpleasant or painful events not completely forgotten from the memory. Ñakary as a collective affliction is not necessarily associated with pinsamientuwan and usually subsides when the external cause is eliminated.

The Magnitude of the Problem

Turning to the quantitative results of the cross-sectional survey, the surveyed population (N = 373) consisted of adults (fifteen years old and over), two-thirds of whom were women, mostly married, with little or no schooling. About half of the population was illiterate, Catholic or evangelist, mostly working independently in farming and related agricultural activities (Table 7.1).

The results from the cross-sectional survey confirmed the high rates of mental complaints and the persistence of culture-specific symptoms among the highland Quechua populations exposed to violence-related stressors. The point prevalence of (potential and real) mental health problems detected by the GHQ-12 was elevated: 73 percent (N = 270) of the surveyed adult population (N = 373). This figure should be interpreted with caution, as it may reflect the lowering of the GHQ-12 cut-off point to two, instead of the recommended three (Goldberg 1972), which may result in an increase of the number of false positives and therefore an overestimation of mental health problems as reported among the surveyed population.

All GHQ-12 positive cases were subsequently administered the HSCL-25, and more than half of these respondents (N = 144) scored positively for anxiety and/or depression. Next, we applied the trauma questionnaire (TQ) to the population reporting anxiety and/or depression. The number of positive cases reporting symptoms within the last month compatible with a PTSD diagnosis using the DSM-III-R diagnostic categories (items 1–16) represents a point prevalence of 24.7 percent (N = 92) (Figure 7.3). The number of subjects reporting culture-specific symptoms or signs of distress, which we categorized as "local idioms of distress" (items 17–32), such as llaki (sorrow, grief), susto (fright), pinsamientuwan (worrying memories), or tutal pinsamientuwan (excess of worrying memories), represents a point prevalence of 22.5 percent (N = 84). There is an important degree of overlap between these two groups of respondents since seventy-one of the ninety-two

Table 7.1. Sociodemographic Characteristics of the Surveyed Population (n = 373)

	n	%		n	%
Age group			*Read and write*		
14–19 years	40	11.0	Yes	168	45.0
20–29 years	88	24.0	No	204	54.7
30–49 years	160	43.0	Doesn't answer	1	0.3
50 and over	85	23.0	*Religion*		
Sex			Catholic	170	46.0
Men	147	40.0	Evangelist	203	54.0
Women	226	61.0	(various categ.)		
Civil status			*Working status*		
Married	284	76.0	Independent	163	44.0
Single	47	13.0	Salaried	27	7.0
Single mother/	25	7.0	Homemaker	168	45.0
separated			(unsalaried)		
Widow	17	5.0	Other (students/	13	3.5
Schooling			pensioners)		
None	173	45.0	Doesn't answer	2	0.5
Primary incomplete	152	41.0	*Occupation*		
Primary complete	27	7.0	Shepherd/weaver/	134	36.0
Secondary incomplete	14	4.0	horticulture		
Secondary complete	5	1.0	Farmer	126	34.0
Doesn't answer	2	0.4	Housewife	48	13.0
			Crafts	11	3.0
			Merchant	19	5.0
			Shepherd only	10	3.0
			Clerk	4	1.0
			Student	14	4.0
			Maid/domestic	2	0.5
			servant		
			None declared	5	1.0

subjects scoring positive for PTSD also reported complaints and symptoms under the category of local idioms of distress. This finding implies an important commonality in reporting the experience of trauma and in the culturally bound discourse of trauma-related disorders, which should be further investigated.

Using linear regression, we found a significant association between the degree of exposure to violence—as measured by culturally significant

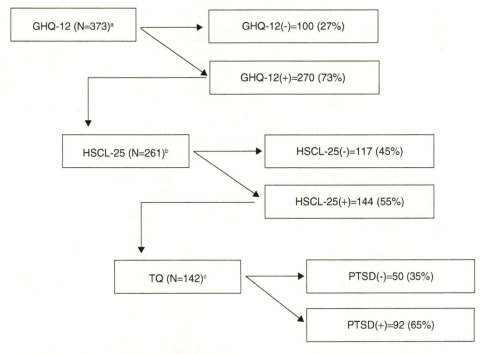

Figure 7.3. Number of respondents with positive and negative scores, by question-naire: GHQ-12, HSCL-25 and TQ modified (N=373) (from Pedersen et al. 2008).

traumatic events families were exposed to (see above)—with reported symp-toms of distress indicating the likelihood of mental illness (GHQ-12), includ-ing depression and/or anxiety (HSCL-25), as depicted in Tables 7.2 and 7.3. Another important finding was the negative association between the degree of social support and literacy, with reported mental health outcomes, as measured by the GHQ-12 (Table 7.2). Finally, being female was significantly associated with reporting symptoms of anxiety and/or depression as mea-sured by the HSCL-25 (Table 7.3).

The survey results discussed above are convergent with and supported by the focused ethnography and descriptive analyses presented elsewhere (Pedersen et al. 2003). In particular, the results confirmed that mental ill-ness, including anxiety and depression, is not randomly distributed. The most affected people were older adults (over the age of fifty), separated or widowed women (for the most part), illiterate people, those with weak or in-existent social support, and those with a higher degree of exposure to violence.

Table 7.2. General Linear Regression of GHQ-12: Total Score on Degree of Exposure to Violence, Age, Degree of Social Support, and Literacy (n = 368)

Variables	Std. Beta	t value	p value
Degree of exposure to violence	0.39	8.58	0.00
Age (in years)	0.16	3.304	0.001
Degree of social support	−0.21	−4.51	0.000
Literacy	−0.16	−3.19	0.002

Table 7.3. General Linear Regression of HSCL-25: Total Score on Age, Degree of Exposure to Violence, Gender, and Civil Status (N = 258)

Variables	Std. Beta	t value	p value
Age (in years)	0.39	6.93	0.000
Degree of exposure to violence	0.23	4.07	0.000
Gender (female)	0.17	2.93	0.004
Civil status (widowed, divorced, not married)	0.14	2.45	0.015

Second, the different types of displacement and resettlement patterns (returnees, inserted or displaced, or established populations, also called resistant) reported different degrees of exposure to violence and dissimilar mental health outcomes (Pedersen et al. 2003), although the differences turned out to be significant only for anxiety and/or depression among returnees in the linear regression analysis (Std. Beta = 0.238, t = 4.390 and p < 0.001). Finally, third, as discussed above, the results of the qualitative segment of the study support the notion that trauma-related disorders and local idioms of distress among the highland Quechua share specific meanings associated with the exposure to violence-related stressors, and the overlap of seventy-one out of ninety-two positive cases for PTSD reported above seems to confirm this assertion.

Exploring Pathways to Mental Health Outcomes in Conflict and Postconflict Settings

We began our chapter with a literature review of medical, psychosocial, and anthropological approaches to determine and interpret trauma-related mental health outcomes in conflict and postconflict settings. It became apparent that it is difficult to bring these often divergent approaches into alignment as they represent not merely different disciplines located on different poles of a continuum, but rather separate entities operating at different levels of intelligibility, that tackle similar issues from different perspectives, with different epistemologies, methodologies, and goals in mind (Kienzler 2008). Yet, this does not mean disciplines cannot influence each other. On the contrary, interdisciplinary research would lead to more holistic approaches to health and health care departing from different disciplinary perspectives and taking both professional and lay understandings of health and illness and ways of healing into consideration.

Our study among highland Quechua populations in the Peruvian Andes is a case in point as an interdisciplinary perspective combining historical, anthropological, epidemiological, and clinical approaches leading to a better understanding of how political violence and traumatic experiences inflicted by Shining Path and the military during the 1980s and 1990s have resulted in poor health outcomes, including those that are referred to as "poor mental health outcomes." While we focussed on the recent history of extreme violence and its aftermath, we can neither ignore the long history of structural violence experienced by previous generations of the highland Quechua, nor the pervasive context of poverty, discrimination, and social exclusion that followed, now aggravated by the coca and cocaine trade and its social, cultural, and ecological consequences, which in turn generate and reinforce existing social inequalities and health disparities.

We discerned several pathways operating both at micro-, meso-, and macro-level environments as well as through societal transitions that suggest that mental health outcomes, identified as idioms of distress and/or PTSD among the highland Quechua, reflect the amalgamation of distant past adversities, the exposure to multiple stressors during the last two decades of war and extreme violence, and the pervasive adversities of the current context. More specifically, our findings related to idioms of distress make apparent that the reported bodily feelings, symptoms, reactions, and emotional states are not necessarily psychopathological conditions but rather illustrate aspects of normal cognitive functioning and fall within the range of ordinary or "normal" responses to exposure to extreme violence and social adversity. However, this does not mean that the experience of such idioms of distress is not painful. On the contrary, the pains and suffering related to idioms like ñakary, llaki, pinsamientuwan, and nanay are to be taken serious by (mental) health professionals as they point to interpersonal, societal, and environmental ills that have detrimental effects on individuals' and communities' well-being (Pedersen et al. 2010).

In the context of Quechua-speaking populations, idioms of distress have distinctive features that often reveal more than one meaning. Yet, they also share a number of common traits: such idioms tend to be applied to a sense of profound malaise or illness of long duration and evolve as chronic conditions over time. This evolution does not take place at random, but roughly follows three sequential phases of construction. The first phase consists of labeling (analogical or phonemic) distressing experiences, which is followed by ascribing primary attributions of causality. Throughout the second phase, idioms are categorized, assigned meaning, and positioned within a given sequence defined by other expressions of distress. In the final phase, idioms of distress are linked with each other and, thus, arranged in discontinuous lines, loosely connected chains, loops and closed circles. In this arrangement, each element interacts dynamically with others and, thereby, establishes additional linkages, imagined or real, between them. As the scheme in Figure 7.4 illustrates, the individual idioms are interconnected into sequences and complicated webs of meanings. Interestingly, these compositions display a certain pattern in which idioms are arranged on a range with two extremes, categorized as terminal conditions, which may or may not be reversible by therapy or treatment.

From our survey data we may conclude that among the highland Quechua and after more than a decade of being exposed to political violence, one in four adults (24.7 percent) reported symptoms compatible with the diagnosis of PTSD. Both qualitative and quantitative data suggest that exposure to political violence created most of its ill effects in specific vulnerable groups, such as those unable to earn a living (unpaid domestic workers, aged, illiterate), lacking sources of emotional or material support (weak social networks), or unable to reciprocate economically (as in the case of widows). The latter strongly endorse claims made by Brewin et al. (2000) and restated by Shalev (2007), in that a combination of biological *and* biographical factors (i.e., low SES, lack of education, lack of social support, daily life stressors) increase individual vulnerability to PTSD. Most importantly, the fact that not all of those exposed to extreme traumatic experiences developed PTSD suggests that traumatic events are a *necessary* but not *sufficient* cause to explain the presence of PTSD symptoms.

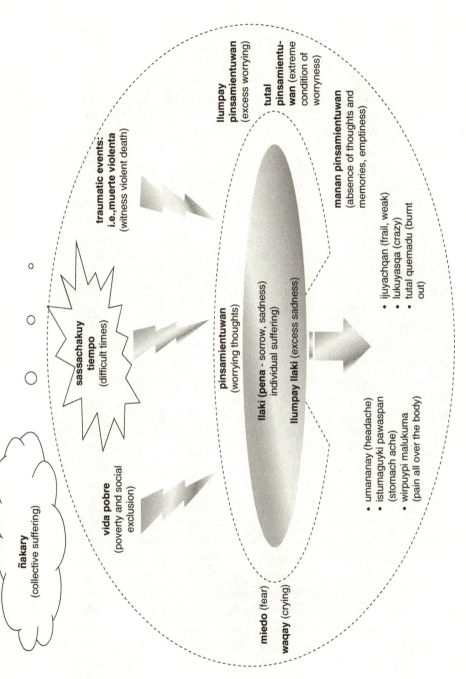

Figure 7.4. Semantic map displaying the relative position of local idioms of distress, at origin (upper portion of the map), main flows, and terminal conditions (lower portion of the map).

Moreover, it has to be kept in mind that mental disorders such as PTSD are not monolithic biomedical categories, but entities that are subject to interpretation in that they are differently understood across diverse cultural and social settings. Mental disorders may be seen as only one facet of suffering and do not account for other forms of distress that are related to a combination of traumatic events and stressful life experiences. Local idioms of distress attest to that and the ways individuals, families, and entire communities explain adversity and develop coping strategies and ways of healing. Consequently, we argue that the search for discrete disorders decontextualizes and essentializes human problems (Kienzler 2008; Lemelson et al. 2007) and that we need to be more cautious about making false attributions and drawing erroneous conclusions while ignoring the presence of confounding variables in the chain of events leading to distress, mental illness, or emotional states accompanied by painful memories of the past (Kleinman and Sung 1979).

Based on this understanding, we argue that there are multiple pathways through which social inequalities, discrimination, and violence can translate into mental health disparities (Aneshensel 1999; Dohrenwend 2000; Forget and Lebel 2001; Pearlin 1989; Schwartz and Meyer 2010). While psychosocial pathways seem to be most important, there is growing evidence of the physiological channels though which stressful negative social and environmental changes can affect endocrine and immunological processes (Cassel 1976; Dressler et al. 2005; Wilkinson 1996). This makes apparent that it is important to investigate more closely the possible overlaps between PTSD, depression, and other modes of expressing distress in order to be able to provide adequate treatment to individuals and populations living in contexts characterized by political and structural violence. In addition, it is crucial to integrate psychosocial and behavioral genetic approaches in order to better understand the causality of the pathways (Bolton 2010; Dohrenwend 2000), that is, the complex relations and interdependencies, and the various ways in which these interactions influence the distress and disease occurrence, illness experience, and well-being of individuals, families, and communities (Buitrago and Cuéllar 2004; Martin-Baro 1994).

We developed a structural interpretative framework to present in an upstream-downstream simplified metaphor these complex interrelations and interdependencies between various domains including the biomedical and biographical, the social and the cultural, and to illustrate the causes and pathways by which these interactions influence mental health outcomes of

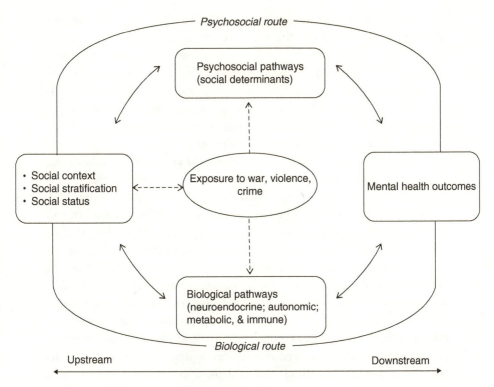

Figure 7.5. Structural interpretative framework.

individuals, families and communities (Braveman 2006; Guruge and Nazilla 2004; Lebel 2003; Waller 2001).

Looking at the structural interpretative framework (Figure 7.5), it becomes evident that there exist inextricable links between humans and their biophysical, social, political, and economic environments resulting in both individual and population health outcomes, as well as configuring their overall health status (Lebel 2003). In constructing the framework we have adopted a perspective inspired by the social determinants of health approach that is used to understand the relationships between modern conditions of life, contemporary family patterns and social organization, new cultural values, and prevalent disease categories as defined by researchers and currently used by health professionals. In addition, we used an ethnographic lens to describe and analyze the local ways through which distress, mental illness, and suffering are expressed, interpreted, reacted to, and managed on a daily basis by individuals, families, and communities. Finally, we reinforce biological pathways leading from the exposure to traumatic events and other stressful life experiences to cellular dysfunction (neuroendocrine, autonomic, metabolic, and immune) and mental health outcomes as they are outlined in DSM and similar manuals. Thus, promoting health and well-being in conflict and postconflict settings has to take into account not only a more equitable distribution of psychosocial support and medical care resources to those in need, but also address the moral dimension of the issues at stake. Above all we need to clarify the *causal* pathways among the various bio-psycho-social components, since facts and correlations per se are neither sufficient evidence to guide policy nor enough to make ethical judgements (Deaton 2011).

We conclude that it is through the development of frames, models, and practices commonly used in medicine, psychiatry, and anthropology that we will eventually better understand how distress, mental illness, and social suffering are transformed into nosographic categories and eventually absorbed in the realm of the psychiatric domain. We also acknowledge how the medicopsychiatric science and medical technologies are used both in the medicalization of the "problem" and as a form of social control, often replacing the use of local, endogenous resources. One may easily find multiple examples in industrial nations as well as in the developing world, of medical technologies aimed at controlling what is defined as deviant behaviors (i.e., hyperactivity in children, drug addictions), as well as plagues, diseases, and even natural life-cycle events (i.e., childbirth, menopause).

In our view, it remains essential to promote innovation and a greater heterogeneity of models, theories, and concepts as a counterweight to the increasing homogenization of medical and psychiatric scientific knowledge and practice. The critical perspectives we have been using in examining distress and social suffering, trauma and PTSD, may also be of relevance to a broad range of disease conditions, thus cutting across all areas pertaining to the health and well-being of populations.

Notes

We would like to express our gratitude to the Douglas Hospital Research Centre–McGill University for hosting the Trauma and Global Health (www.mcgill.ca/trauma-globalhealth) program during 2007–12 and the funding agencies, the Teasdale-Corti Grant Program and the Global Health Research Initiative (Canada), for the support received in the preparation of this manuscript. Our special thanks to Jeffrey Gamarra, a Peruvian anthropologist involved in the ethnographic work, data collection and logistical support, and to Consuelo Errazuriz, who assisted us in the survey, data collection and analysis of the field study and for her overall support in the revision and preparation of this chapter.

1. In spite of the concerted efforts of both the Peruvian and the U.S. governments to eradicate coca and replace it with alternative crops (coffee, cacao, palm oil, and rubber), the coca and cocaine trade industry has been growing steadily to the point that an estimated 15 percent of the Peruvian labor force is currently engaged in the coca industry (DEVIDA 2007).

2. In this chapter we will be reporting the results of the first phase only.

3. In Quechua, *aya-qarawi* is a mourning lament, a mix between howling and singing in a high pitch, usually performed by Quechua-speaking women attending funerals.

4. Weeping in public was explicitly forbidden by Shining Path's local *comisarios*, because crying was considered a sign of weakness and servitude, inappropriate to the "revolutionary" moral fabric.

5. In exploring the etymologies of llaki and ñakary, we consulted the following dictionaries published by Catholic priests and missionaries in the 1600s: the *Vocabulario de la lengua Quechua*, written by Fray Diego González Holguín, published in 1608; the *Vocabulario de la lengua Aymara*, written by the priest Ludovico Bertonio (circa 1612); and the Quechua-Spanish dictionary written by Fray Domingo de Santo Tomás in the 1600s (for more information see Pedersen et al. 2010).

6. An important distinction emerges between these two extremes, which is critical in differentiating between persistent symptoms and disorders, from transient emotions of lesser clinical significance.

References

Almedom, Astier M., and Derek Summerfield
    2004 Mental Well-Being in Settings of Complex Emergencies: An Overview. Journal of Biosocial Science 36(4):381–88.
Aneshensel, Carol S.
    1999 Outcomes of the Stress Process. *In* A Handbook for the Study of Mental Health, Social Contexts, Theories, and Systems. Allan V. Horowitz and Teresa Scheid, eds. Pp. 211–27. Cambridge: Cambridge University Press.
Barudy, Jorge
    1989 A Programme of Mental Health for Political Refugees: Dealing with the Invisible Pain of Political Exile. Social Science and Medicine 28(7):715–27.
Bennett, Sara, Taghreed Adam, Christina Zarowsky, Viroj Tangcharoensathien, Kent Ranson, Tim Evans, Anne Mills, and Alliance STAC

2008 From Mexico to Mali: Progress in Health Policy and Systems Research. Lancet 372(9649):1571–78.

Bolton, Derek
2010 Social, Biological and Personal Constructions of Mental Illness. *In* Principles of Social Psychiatry. Craig Morgan and Dinesh Bhugra, eds. Pp. 39–50. Hoboken: John Wiley and Sons.

Bracken, Patrick J.
2001 Post-Modernity and Post-Traumatic Stress Disorder. Social Science and Medicine 53(6):733–43.

Bracken, Patrick J., and Celia Petty, eds.
1998 Rethinking the Trauma of War. New York: Free Association Books.

Braveman, Paula
2006 Health Disparities and Health Equity: Concepts and Measurement. Annual Review of Public Health 27(1):167–94.

Breslau, Joshua
2004 Cultures of Trauma: Anthropological Views of Posttraumatic Stress Disorder in International Health. Culture, Medicine and Psychiatry 28(2):113–26.

Breslau, Naomi
1998 Epidemiology of Trauma and Posttraumatic Stress Disorder. *In* Psychological Trauma. Rachel Yehuda, ed. Pp. 1–30. Washington, D.C.: American Psychiatric Press.

Brewin, Chris R., Bernice Andrews, and John D. Valentine
2000 Meta-Analysis of Risk Factors for Posttraumatic Stress Disorder in Trauma Exposed Adults. Journal of Consulting and Clinical Psychology 68(5):748–66.

Browner, Carol H., and Carolyn F. Sargent
2007 Gender: Engendering Medical Anthropology. *In* Medical Anthropology: Regional Perspective and Shared Concerns. Francine Saillant and Serge Genest, eds. Pp. 233–51. Malden, Mass.: Blackwell.

Buitrago, Jorge, and Enrique Cuéllar
2004 Internationally Displaced Colombians: The Recovery of Victims of Violence Within a Psychosocial Framework. *In* The Mental Health of Refugees: Ecological Approaches to Healing and Adaptation. Kenneth E. Miller and Lisa M. Rasco, eds. Pp. 229–62. Mahwah, N.J.: Lawrence Erlbaum Associates.

Cassel, John
1976 The Contribution of the Social Environment to Host Resistance. American Journal of Epidemiology 104:107–23.

Comisión de la Verdad y Reconciliación
2003 General Conclusions. Final Report, vol. 8. Lima: CVR.

Commission on Social Determinants of Health
2008 Closing the Gap in a Generation: Health Equity Through Action on the Social Determinants of Health: Final Report of the Commission on Social Determinants of Health. Geneva: World Health Organization.

Corin, Ellen, Gilles Bibeau, Jean Claude Martin, and Robert Laplante
1990 Comprendre pour Soigner Autrement. Montreal: Presses de l'Université de Montréal.

Dahl, Solveig, Atifa Mutapcic, and Berit Schei
1998 Traumatic Events and Predictive Factors for Posttraumatic Symptoms in Displaced Bosnian Women in a War Zone. Journal of Traumatic Stress 11(1):137–45.

Davis, Donna Lee, and Lisa Moe Joakimsen
1997 Nerves as Status and Nerves as Stigma: Idioms of Distress and Social Action in Newfoundland and Northern Norway. Qualitative Health Research 7(3):370–90.

Deaton, Angus
2011 What Does the Empirical Evidence Tell Us About the Injustice of Health Inequalities? Unpublished MS, Center for Health and Wellbeing, Princeton University.

Degregori, Carlos Iván
1985 Sendero Luminoso Parte I. Los Hondos y Mortales Desencuentros, y Parte II. Lucha Armada y Utopía Autoritaria. Documentos de Trabajo #4 y #6. Lima: Instituto de Estudios Peruanos.
2003 Jamás tan Cerca Arremetió lo Lejos: Memoria y Violencia Política en el Perú. Lima: Instituto de Estudios Peruanos.

del Pino, Ponciano, ed.
1996 Tiempos de Guerra y de Dioses: Ronderos, Evangélicos y Senderistas. *In* Las Rondas Campesinas y la Derrota de Sendero Luminoso. Carlos Iván Degregori, José Coronel, Ponciano del Pino and Orin Starn, eds. Pp. 117–88. Lima: Instituto de Estudios Peruanos.
2003 Uchuraccay: Memoria y Representación de la Violencia Política en los Andes. *In* Jamás tan cerca Arremetió lo Lejos. Carlos Ivan Degregori, ed. Pp. 49–94. Lima: Instituto de Estudios Peruanos.

Deutsch, F. (ed.)
1959 On the Mysterious Leap from the Mind to the Body: A Workshop Study on the Theory of Conversion. New York: International Universities Press.

DEVIDA [Comisión Nacional para el Desarrollo y Vida sin Drogas]
2007 Estudio de Profundidad sobre Narcotráfico, Consumo de Drogas y Desarrollo Alternativo en las Cuencas Cocaleras. Lima: DEVIDA.

Dohrenwend, Bruce
2000 The Role of Adversity and Stress in Psychopathology, Some Evidence and Its Implications for Theory and Research. Journal of Health and Social Behavior 41:1–19.

Dongier, Maurice, William Engels, and R. Ramsay
1996 Les embuches de la psychiatrie de liaison—Consultation-liaison psychiatry. Revue médicale de Liège 51(9):590–98.

Dressler, William, Kathryn Oths, and Clarence Gravlee
2005 Race and Ethnicity in Public Health Research Models to Explain Health Disparities. Annual Review of Anthropology 34:231–52.

Eisenberg, Leon
    1995 The Social Construction of the Human Brain. American Journal of Psychiatry, 152(11):1563–75.
Farhood, Laila, Huda Zurayk, Monique Chaya, Fadia Saadeh, Garbis Meshefedjian, and Thuraya Sidani
    1993 The Impact of War on the Physical and Mental Health of the Family: The Lebanese Experience. Social Science and Medicine 36(12):1555–67.
Farmer, Paul
    2004 An Anthropology of Structural Violence. Current Anthropology 45(3): 305–25.
Fassin, Didier, and Richard Rechtman
    2009 The Empire of Trauma: An Enquiry into the Condition of Victimhood. Princeton, N.J.: Princeton University Press.
Fernando, Gaithri A., Kenneth E. Miller, and Dale E. Berger
    2010 Growing Pains: The Impact of Disaster-Related and Daily Stressors on the Psychological and Psychosocial Functioning of Youth in Sri Lanka. Child Development 81 (4):1192–210.
Forget, Gilles, and Jean Lebel
    2001 An Ecosystem Approach to Human Health. International Journal of Occupational and Environmental Health 7(Suppl 2):S3–S36.
Foss, Nina
    2002 Nerves in Northern Norway: The Communication of Emotions, Illness Experiences, and Health-Seeking Behaviors. Qualitative Health Research 12(2):194–207.
Goldberg, David P.
    1972 The Detection of Psychiatric Illness by Questionnaire. London: Oxford University Press.
Green, Bonnie L.
    2003 Traumatic Stress and Its Consequences. In Trauma Interventions in War and Peace: Prevention, Practice and Policy. Bonnie L. Green, Mathew Friedman, Joop T. V. M. de Jong, Susan Solomon, Terence Keane, John Fairbank, Brigid Donelan, Ellen Frey-Wouters, and Yael Danieli, eds. Pp. 17–32. New York: Kluwer Academic/Plenum.
Guruge, Sepali, and Khanlou Nazilla
    2004 Intersectionalities of Influence: Researching the Health of Immigrant and Refugee Women. Canadian Journal of Nursing Research 36:32–47.
Hinton, Devon, Vuth Pich, Luana Marques, Angela Nickerson, and Mark H. Pollack
    2010 Khyâl Attacks: A Key Idiom of Distress Among Traumatized Cambodia Refugees. Culture, Medicine, and Psychiatry 34(2):244–78.
Horwitz, Allan V.
    2007 Distinguishing Distress from Disorder as Psychological Outcomes of Stressful Social Arrangements. Health 11(3):273–89.

Kienzler, Hanna
  2008 Debating War-Trauma and Post-Traumatic Stress Disorder (PTSD) in an
    Interdisciplinary Arena. Social Science and Medicine 67(2):218–27.
Kleinman, Arthur
  1988 Rethinking Psychiatry. New York: Free Press.
Kleinman, Arthur, Veena Das, and Margaret Lock, eds.
  1997 Social Suffering. Berkeley: University of California Press.
Kleinman, Arthur, and Lilias H. Sung
  1979 Why Do Indigenous Practitioners Successfully Heal? Social Science and Med-
    icine. Part B: Medical Anthropology 13(1):7–26.
Krieger, Nancy
  2001 Theories for Social Epidemiology in the 21st Century: An Ecosocial Perspec-
    tive. International Journal of Epidemiology 30:668–77.
Lebel, Jean
  2003 Health: An Ecosystem Approach. Ottawa: International Development Research
    Centre.
Lemelson, Robert, Laurence Kirmayer, and Mark Barad
  2007 Trauma in Context: Integrating Cultural, Clinical and Biological Perspec-
    tives. In Understanding Trauma: Integrating Biological, Clinical, and Cultural
    Perspectives. Laurence Kirmayer, Robert Lemelson, and Mark Barad, eds. Pp. 451–74.
    Cambridge: Cambridge University Press.
Lewis-Fernández, Roberto, Magdaliz Gorritz, Greer A. Raggio, Clara Peláez, Henian
    Chen, and Peter Guarnaccia
  2010 Association of Trauma-Related Disorders and Dissociation with Four Idioms
    of Distress Among Latino Psychiatric Outpatients. Culture, Medicine, and Psy-
    chiatry 34(2):219–43.
Loewenthal, Kate
  2007 Religion, Culture and Mental Health. Cambridge: Cambridge University Press.
Lopes Cardozo, Barbara, Reinhard Kaiser, Carol A. Gotway, and Ferid Agani
  2003 Mental Health, Social Functioning, and Feelings of Hatred and Revenge
    of Kosovar Albanians One Year After the War in Kosovo. Journal of Traumatic
    Stress 16(4):351–60.
Manrique, Nelson
  1995 Political Violence, Ethnicity and Racism in Peru in the Time of War. Journal
    of Latin American Studies 4 (1):5–18.
Manson, Spiro M.
  1997 Cross-Cultural and Multiethnic Assessment of Trauma. In Assessing Psycho-
    logical Trauma and PTSD: A Handbook for Practitioners. John Preston Wilson
    and Terence Martin Keane, eds. Pp. 239–66. New York: Guilford.
Marmot, Michael
  2005 Social Determinants of Health Inequalities. Lancet 365(9464):1099–104.

Marshall, Grant N., Terry L. Schell, Marc N. Elliott, S. Megan Berthold, and Chi-Ah Chun
  2005 Mental Health of Cambodian Refugees Two Decades After Resettlement in the United States. Journal of the American Medical Association 294(5):571–79.
Martin-Baro, Ignacio
  1994 War and Mental Health. Anne Wallace, trans. In Writings for a Liberation Psychology. Adrianne Aron and Shawn Corne, eds. Pp.108–21. Cambridge, Mass.: Harvard University Press.
Melville, Margarita B., and M. Brinton Lykes
  1992 Guatemalan Indian Children and the Sociocultural Effects of Government-Sponsored Terrorisms. Social Science and Medicine 34(5):533–48.
Miller, Kenneth E., Madhur Kulkarni, and Hallie Kushner
  2006 Beyond Trauma-Focused Psychiatric Epidemiology: Bridging Research and Practice with War-Affected Populations. American Journal of Orthopsychiatry 76(4):409–22.
Miller, Kenneth E., Patricia Omidian, Andrew Rasmussen, Aziz Yaqubi, and Haqmal Daudzai
  2008 Daily Stressors, War Experiences, and Mental Health in Afghanistan. Transcultural Psychiatry 45(4):611–38.
Miller, Kenneth E., and Andrew Rasmussen
  2010 War Exposure, Daily Stressors, and Mental Health in Conflict and Post-Conflict Settings: Bridging the Divide Between Trauma-Focused and Psychosocial Frameworks. Social Science and Medicine 70(1):7–16.
Mollica, Richard F., and Yael Caspi-Yavin
  1991 Measuring Torture and Torture-Related Symptoms. Psychological Assessment 3(4):581–87.
Mollica, Richard F., Yael Caspi-Yavin, Paola Bollini, Toang Truong, Svang Tor, and James Lavelle
  1992 The Harvard Trauma Questionnaire: Validating a Cross-Cultural Instrument for Measuring Torture, Trauma, and Posttraumatic Stress Disorder in Indochinese Refugees. Journal of Nervous and Mental Disease 180(2):111–16.
Mollica, Richard F., Keith McInnes, Thang Pham, Mary Catherine Fawzi Smith, Elizabeth Murphy, and Lien Lin
  1998 The Dose-Effect Relationships Between Torture and Psychiatric Symptoms in Vietnamese Ex–Political Detainees and a Comparison Group. Journal of Nervous and Mental Disease 186(9):543–53.
Mollica, Richard F., Xing Jia Cui, Keith McInnes, and Michael Massagli P.
  2002 Science-Based Policy for Psychosocial Interventions in Refugee Camps: A Cambodian Example. Journal of Nervous and Mental Disease 190(3):158–66.
Neuner, Frank, Maggie Schauer, Unni Karunakara, Christine Klaschik, Christina Robert, and Thomas Elbert

2004 Psychological Trauma and Evidence for Enhanced Vulnerability for Posttraumatic Stress Disorder Through Previous Trauma Among West Nile Refugees. BMC Psychiatry 4(1):34.

Nichter, Mark
1981 Idioms of Distress: Alternatives in the Expression of Psychosocial Distress: A Case Study from South India. Culture, Medicine, and Psychiatry 5(4):379–408.
2010 Idioms of Distress Revisited. Culture, Medicine and Psychiatry 34(2):401–16.

Norris, Fran H., and Jasmin K. Riad
1997 Standardized Self-Report Measures of Civilian Trauma and Posttraumatic Stress Disorder. In Assessing Psychological Trauma and PTSD: A Handbook for Practitioners. John P. Wilson and Terence M. Keane, eds. Pp. 32–54. New York: Guilford.

Pearlin, Leonard
1989 The Sociological Study of Stress. Journal of Health and Social Behavior 30 (3):241–56.

Pedersen, Duncan, Jefrey Gamarra, Maria Elena Planas, and Consuelo Errázuriz
2003 Violencia Política y Salud Mental en las Comunidades Alto-andinas de Ayacucho, Perú. In La Salud Como Derecho Ciudadano: Perspectivas y Propuestas desde América Latina. Carlos Cáceres, Marcos Cueto, Miguel Ramos, and Sandra Vallenas, eds. Pp. 289–307. Lima: Universidad Peruana Cayetano Heredia.

Pedersen, Duncan, Jacques Tremblay, Consuelo Errázuriz, and Jefrey Gamarra
2008 The Sequelae of Political Violence: Assessing Trauma, Suffering and Dislocation in the Peruvian Highlands. Social Science and Medicine 67(2):205–17.

Pedersen, Duncan, Hanna Kienzler, and Jefrey Gamarra
2010 Llaki and Ñakary: Idioms of Distress and Suffering Among the Highland Quechua in the Peruvian Andes. Culture, Medicine, and Psychiatry 34(2):279–300.

Sabin, Miriam, Barbara Lopes Cardozo, Larry Nackerud, Reinhard Kaiser, and Luis Varese
2003 Factors Associated with Poor Mental Health Among Guatemalan Refugees Living in Mexico 20 Years After Civil Conflict. Journal of the American Medical Association 290(5):635–42.

Schwartz, Sharon with Ilan H. Meyer
2010 Mental Health Disparities Research. The Impact of Within and Between Group Analyses on Tests of Social Stress Hypotheses. Social Science and Medicine 70(8):111–18

Shalev, Arieh Y.
2007 PTSD: A Disorder of Recovery? In Understanding Trauma: Integrating Biological, Clinical and Cultural Perspectives. Laurence J. Kirmayer, Robert Lemelson, and Mark Barad, eds. Pp. 207–23. Cambridge: Cambridge University Press.

Siegrist, Johannes, and Michael Marmot
2004 Health Inequalities and the Psychosocial Environment—Two Scientific Challenges. Social Science and Medicine 58(8):1463–73.

Smith, Patrick, Sean Perrin, William Yule, Berima Hacam, and Rune Stuvland
  2002 War Exposure Among Children from Bosnia-Hercegovina: Psychological Adjustment in a Community Sample. Journal of Traumatic Stress 15(2):147–56.
Sondergaard, Hans Peter, Solvig Ekblad, and Tores Theorell
  2001 Self-Reported Life Event Patterns and Their Relation to Health Among Recently Resettled Iraqi and Kurdish Refugees in Sweden. Journal of Nervous and Mental Disease 189(12):838–45.
Stern, Steve. J., ed.
  1999 Los Senderos Insólitos del Perú: Guerra y Sociedad, 1980–1995. Lima: IEP/UNSCH.
Tremblay, Jacques, Duncan Pedersen, and Consuelo Errazuriz
  2009 Assessing Mental Health Outcomes of Political Violence and Civil Unrest in Peru. International Journal of Social Psychiatry 55(5):449–63.
van Ommeren, Mark
  2003 Validity Issues in Transcultural Epidemiology. British Journal of Psychiatry 182(5):376–78.
Waller, Margaret A.
  2001 Resilience in Ecosystemic Context: Evolution of the Concept. American Journal of Orthopsychiatry 71(3):290–97.
Wilkinson, Richard G.
  1994 The Epidemiological Transition: From Material Scarcity to Social Disadvantage? Daedalus 123(4):61–77.
  1996 Unhealthy Societies: The Afflictions of Inequality. London: Routledge.
Wilkinson, Richard G., and Kate E. Pickett
  2007 The Problems of Relative Deprivation: Why Some Societies Do Better Than Others. Social Science and Medicine 65(9):1965–78.

CHAPTER 8

Latinas' and Latinos' Risk for PTSD After Trauma Exposure: A Review of Sociocultural Explanations

Carmela Alcántara and Roberto Lewis-Fernández

According to national epidemiological studies conducted in the United States, the lifetime prevalence of posttraumatic stress disorder (PTSD) differs slightly between Latina/os (4.4–7.0 percent), non-Latina/o whites (6.5–7.4 percent), and African Americans (8.6–8.7 percent) (Alegría et al. 2008; Asnaani et al. 2010; Roberts et al. 2010). However, these numerical differences are not always observed and usually not statistically significant (Breslau et al. 1998; Kessler et al. 1995).

A different picture emerges when focusing on the *conditional risk of PTSD*, defined as the risk of developing a PTSD diagnosis or PTSD symptoms, of endorsing more severe PTSD symptoms, or of experiencing more persistent PTSD over time, once exposed to one or more traumatic event(s). Methodologically, conditional risk is ascertained by estimating these PTSD outcomes after controlling statistically for the effect of traumatic exposure. Sociodemographic factors, such as education and income, are often included as covariates in modeling conditional risk, in order to isolate factors associated with higher risk that are related specifically to racial/ethnic origin.

In both retrospective and prospective epidemiological studies conducted in the United States, the conditional risk of PTSD is higher among Latina/os than among non-Latina/o whites or African Americans. This is true whether the research focuses on incidence (i.e., new onset of PTSD during a determined period after a traumatic event or events) or persistence of PTSD over time, two aspects of PTSD course that affect estimates of prevalence (Dohrenwend et al. 2008; Tsuang et al. 1995). In models adjusting for differential trauma exposure, higher prevalence of PTSD among Latina/os has been found among Vietnam veterans (Kulka et al. 1990; Ortega and Rosenheck 2000; Schnurr et al. 2004), survivors of mass trauma (Galea et al. 2002, 2004, 2008; North et al. 2012; Perilla et al. 2002; Pietrzak et al. 2013), survivors of physical trauma (Marshall et al. 2009), those with histories of intimate partner violence (Stampfel et al. 2010), and urban police officers (Pole et al. 2001).

The validity of these findings of higher conditional risk among Latina/os has been questioned, however, because of methodological limitations of some studies and inconsistent findings when the issue of conditional risk has been specifically examined (Dohrenwend et al. 2008; Frueh et al. 1998; Lewis-Fernández et al. 2008; Ruef et al. 2000). In at least one study, higher persistence of PTSD among Latino veterans disappeared once the effect of sociodemographic, trauma-related, and military factors was accounted for more fully (Dohrenwend et al. 2008). Hence, whether there are *true* racial/ethnic differences in the risk of developing and/or maintaining PTSD after adjusting for differential rates of trauma exposure remains uncertain. Moreover, even if group-level differences in conditional risk are valid, much less is known about the underlying mechanisms that may contribute to higher conditional risk of PTSD among Latina/os (for brief reviews, see Hinton and Lewis-Fernández 2011; Pole et al. 2008).

In this chapter, we review the extant literature on conditional risk of PTSD among Latina/o relative to non-Latina/o white adults in the U.S. exposed to trauma. We focus our review on the differences between Latina/os and non-Latina/o whites because most of the literature provides comparisons between these racial/ethnic groups; however, we include comparisons between Latina/os and African Americans whenever these data are available. Our review distinguishes between studies that focus on overall prevalence of PTSD, versus those that distinguish between onset and/or persistence of PTSD. Studies on overall PTSD prevalence typically are not able to assess whether the PTSD began after exposure to the trauma, whereas studies that focus on PTSD onset or persistence are able to establish a temporal link between exposure to a particular trauma and the ensuing presence of PTSD. We limit our review to research that accounts for or adjusts for the effect of trauma exposure, and thereby enables exploration specifically of the conditional risk of PTSD, not only of unadjusted estimates of differential prevalence or incidence of PTSD across racial/ethnic categories. Next, we discuss potential mechanisms that may contribute to differential risk of PTSD once a person is exposed to trauma, with attention to sociocultural explanations. Lastly, we conclude with a discussion on future directions for research on conditional risk of PTSD among Latina/os. For a more comprehensive review of racial/ethnic differences in conditional risk of PTSD (prevalence, onset, persistence, and severity), as well as a discussion of the methodological characteristics of included studies and their limitations, we refer readers to our systematic review on this topic (Alcántara et al. 2013).

Conditional Risk of PTSD Among Latina/os

The literature on racial/ethnic differences in conditional risk of PTSD can be categorized into research that focuses on overall prevalence of PTSD versus that which focuses separately on onset and/or persistence of PTSD. Most of the research is on PTSD prevalence, which subsequently cannot be disaggregated into onset and persistence; furthermore, few studies assess both onset *and* persistence simultaneously.

Prevalence of PTSD

Early reports of a higher prevalence of PTSD among Latina/os relative to whites were based on data obtained from the National Vietnam Veterans Readjustment Study (NVVRS (Kulka et al. 1990). The NVVRS was conducted from 1987 to 1988 and drew from a national probability sample of veterans and civilians who participated in lay-administered and clinical interviews. Most of the published research on the NVVRS uses a definition of PTSD that is based on self-report scales that were calibrated in a diagnostic algorithm against clinician-administered Structured Clinical Interview for DSM Disorders (SCID) interviews on a subsample of veterans (Kulka et al. 1990; Lewis-Fernández et al. 2008); we refer to these estimated rates as "probable PTSD." Of note, the NVVRS occurred during a historical context when rigorous empirical research on racial/ethnic differences in PTSD among Vietnam combat veterans was sparse, despite the clinical folklore of the time that spoke of purported racial/ethnic differences in PTSD (Frueh et al. 1998). Kulka and colleagues' (1990) early report showed that Latino veterans had a higher point prevalence of probable PTSD than whites more than a decade after the end of the war, even after adjusting for war-zone stress and individual-level predisposing factors. Other reports soon followed, corroborating the results of Kulka et al. (Ortega and Rosenheck 2000; Schlenger et al. 1992). For example, Ortega and Rosenheck (2000) found that Mexican American and Puerto Rican male Vietnam veterans had increased risk and severity of probable PTSD relative to non-Latino African American and white veterans, even when controlling for both premilitary and postmilitary factors, including combat exposure.

The NVVRS results were the first to strongly raise questions about differences in conditional risk of PTSD between Latina/os and non-Latina/o whites, yet their results did not provide definitive answers to these questions. Kulka et al.'s (1990) results have been challenged mainly because of possible threats to internal and external validity in the NVVRS (e.g., representativeness of the sample, translation and measurement concerns, lack of adjustment for comorbidity of substance use disorders [Lewis-Fernández et al. 2008; Ruef et al. 2000; Schnurr et al. 2004]). For example, Lewis-Fernández and colleagues (2008) found that the effect of Latina/o ethnicity on persistence of PTSD in the SCID subsample of the NVVRS was attenuated when symptoms were assessed by clinicians using diagnostic interviews rather than by self-report measures. This raises the possibility that at least some of the observed racial/ethnic differences were due to the self-report methodology instead of true differences in PTSD prevalence (Ortega and Rosenheck 2000). In addition, Dohrenwend et al. (2008) found that differences in prevalence of PTSD between Latino and non-Latino white veterans disappear after adjusting for age, education, trauma exposure, and army qualification test scores. To our knowledge, this was the first empirical paper to explicitly challenge the notion of conditional risk differences between Latina/o and non-Latina/o white veterans using a clinician-diagnosed sample.

The second body of evidence supporting heightened conditional risk of PTSD among Latina/os—now in terms of PTSD symptom counts after trauma exposure—comes from research with trauma-specific samples such as urban police officers, war veterans, and survivors of intimate partner violence and childhood abuse. Pole and colleagues (2001) showed that Latina/o urban police officers endorsed elevated PTSD symptoms relative to non-Latina/o white and African American officers after adjusting for the effect of their most disturbing police-related critical incident, social desirability, and peritraumatic dissociation. Of note, in this sample there were no significant differences by ethnicity in exposure to duty-related critical incidents. However, the authors

did not account for differences in any non-duty/police-related trauma exposures, including childhood trauma, which may have contributed to ethnic differences in PTSD symptoms. Further evidence of higher PTSD prevalence
after exposure comes from data on Latina women relative to African American and multiracial women, in models controlling for history of intimate
partner violence (IPV) (Stampfel et al. 2010). However, these models did not
account for differential exposure to non-IPV trauma-related events. In models that adjusted for trauma exposure, higher PTSD symptom severity was
observed among Latina/os relative to non-Latina/o whites in samples of Vietnam veteran inpatients (Koopman et al. 2001) and lesbian, gay, or bisexual
adults exposed to childhood abuse (Balsam et al. 2010).

    While there are many studies indicating heightened risk of PTSD among
Latina/os relative to non-Latina/os, there are several studies that document
null results. For example, no significant racial/ethnic differences in PTSD
prevalence and PTSD severity were found in samples of residents of New York
City after 9/11 (Adams and Boscarino 2005) and inpatients suffering from
physical injuries (Zatzick et al. 2007).

    In sum, the data on the prevalence of PTSD support a higher conditional
risk of PTSD among Latina/os compared to whites, but methodological limitations, particularly with respect to the comprehensiveness of the assessments of trauma exposure, render this conclusion tentative.

Onset Versus Persistence of PTSD

Few studies analyze separately the extent to which higher conditional risk of
PTSD prevalence among Latina/os relative to non-Latina/o whites is due to
differential risk in PTSD onset versus persistence of PTSD over time. The majority of *longitudinal* data on racial/ethnic differences in conditional risk of
PTSD comes from studies on the long-standing posttraumatic effects of natural disasters (e.g., hurricanes), the 9/11 terrorist attacks, participation in
combat, or surviving physical injury. For example, in one study (n = 811) that
aggregated data from ten different disasters (e.g., natural disasters, mass
shootings, plane crash) Latina/o ethnicity was a consistent predictor of
disaster-related PTSD onset in models that adjusted for trauma exposure,
predisaster mental disorders, and standard covariates (North et al. 2012). In
this study, trauma exposure was measured as injury sustained during the
disaster, seeing someone hurt or killed, having family and/or friends hurt or

killed, or being exposed to the disaster aftermath. However, the subsample of Latina/o participants in this study was very small (<2 percent), raising questions about the stability of the model (North et al. 2012). A related study found greater risk of hurricane-related PTSD onset and PTSD severity among Mexican residents in Mexico relative to non-Latino African American and white residents in the United States who were exposed to mass trauma as a result of Hurricanes Paulina and Andrew (Norris et al. 2001a).

Moreover, a study on PTSD onset conducted six months after Hurricane Andrew devastated southern Florida in 1992 found that Latina/os who preferred to speak Spanish showed the highest rates of hurricane-related PTSD onset (35–38 percent), followed by African Americans (23–29 percent), English-preferring Latina/os (16–19 percent), and non-Latina/o whites (15–16 percent; Perilla et al. 2002). This trend persisted even after adjusting for personal trauma exposure and neighborhood trauma. We note that higher conditional risk of PTSD for Latina/os relative to African Americans and non-Latina/o whites was observed only in structural equation models among those for whom personal trauma and neighborhood trauma were high. In particular, higher rates of incident PTSD among Latina/os relative to non-Latina/o whites was found among those who perceived a high degree of personal life threat or injury and those who lived in a neighborhood with a high proportion of reported personal trauma as a result of the hurricane. This is suggestive of an interaction between social disadvantage and Latina/o ethnicity that is particularly influential on estimates of PTSD risk among vulnerable communities.

Furthermore, regional community-based epidemiological studies subsequent to the September 11 terrorist attacks in New York City (NYC) suggest increased risk of both incident PTSD and persistence of PTSD in Latina/os. Higher incidence of PTSD was documented among Latina/o adults in comparison to non-Latina/o whites, African Americans, and Asian Americans living south of 110th Street in Manhattan at five to eight weeks following the attacks (Galea et al. 2002), at six months post-9/11 among a representative sample of NYC residents (Galea et al. 2004), at thirty months post-9/11 in a large population-based cohort of NYC residents (Galea et al. 2008), and at two to three years post-9/11 among a sample of Manhattan residents living south of Canal Street (Adams and Boscarino 2006; Farfel et al. 2008). The elevated PTSD risk persisted even when controlling for trauma exposure, which was measured as, for example, sustained injuries during the attack, lost possessions or property, friend/relative killed in the attack, involved in rescue effort, lost job as a result of the attack, lived below Fourteenth Street, or evacuated the workplace.

We note that results from Galea et al. (2003) suggest no conditional risk differences in PTSD onset between Latina/o and non-Latina/o whites at six months post-9/11 attack, which counters the results presented in Galea et al. (2004). The diverging results, however, may be due to differences in sample composition and sample size. For example, Galea et al. (2003) drew from a smaller total sample (n = 1,570) and used an aggregated Latina/o sample, whereas Galea et al. (2004) drew from a larger total sample size (n = 2,616) and disaggregated the Latina/o group into Dominicans, Puerto Ricans, and other Hispanics to make comparisons to non-Latina/o groups. Thus, Galea et al. (2003) may have had limited power to detect statistically significant differences in PTSD risk.

Higher rates of PTSD over a period of two to three years after 9/11 was especially profound among Latina/os living south of Canal Street relative to white residents after adjusting for trauma exposure (DiGrande et al. 2008). Trauma exposure was assessed as a dichotomous variable (e.g., caught in dust cloud, injured on 9/11, witnessed horror on 9/11, being in other destroyed/ damaged buildings on 9/11). Similarly elevated onset rates of probable PTSD based on the PTSD Checklist—Civilian Version (PCL-17; a PTSD symptom checklist survey) cutoff scores have been observed in Latino male police first responders relative to white police responders over a two-to-three year period after 9/11 in models adjusting for trauma exposure (e.g., inside a Twin Tower or adjacent building at time of attack, and sustained injury on 9/11 (Bowler et al. 2010). This same pattern holds true among a sample of adult civilian survivors of 9/11 and persons who were in the World Trade Center (WTC) Towers at the time of the attack. Latina/o survivors had higher PTSD rates relative to non-Latina/o whites over the two-to-three year period after 9/11 in models adjusting for exposure severity. One limitation of the research on 9/11, however, is that some studies inferred but did not clarify whether PTSD began after exposure to the events of 9/11 and was directly related to it (e.g., in the character of the intrusive and avoidant symptoms), raising the question whether the findings truly represent PTSD incidence as opposed to prevalence.

Additional evidence of higher onset of PTSD comes from studies with adult survivors of physical trauma. Latina/o adult survivors living in Los Angeles County showed higher odds of a probable PTSD diagnosis based on PCL-17 scores at six to twelve months after traumatic physical injury relative to their white counterparts (Shih et al. 2010); however, these investigators did not adjust for the effect of more specific differential trauma exposure characteristics both before and after physical injury.

The relationship between ethnicity and persistence of PTSD over time appears to suggest a similar trend to what we observe when we focus on PTSD onset. For example, in a population-based prospective study after 9/11 of a representative sample of 2,752 NYC residents, Latina/o ethnicity was persistently associated with PTSD at each of three time points over a two-year period in analyses (Galea et al. 2008). Galea and colleagues adjusted for the effect of respondents' peri-event emotional reaction (i.e., endorsement of panic symptoms hours following WTC attacks), and whether respondents were directly affected by 9/11 (e.g., injured during attacks, lost possession or property, friend/relative killed, involved in rescue effort, or lost job as a result of attack). The effect of Latina/o ethnicity was also observed by Marshall et al. (2009) in a sample of Latina/o (mostly Mexican) survivors of physical injury when assessed prospectively for posttraumatic symptoms within days, six months, and twelve months after the trauma. The elevated PTSD risk among Latina/os persisted across time, even when the ethnic groups were matched by type and severity of trauma using propensity weights. In yet another prospective study, Latino ethnicity was a significant predictor of chronic and severe PTSD among police and nontraditional WTC responders who were followed for eight years after the WTC attack (Pietrzak et al. 2013). In contrast, Schnurr and colleagues (2004) found that Latino ethnicity among male veterans was associated only with increased risk of PTSD onset but not with persistence of PTSD.

In sum, the emerging trend documented across these studies is that Latina/os relative to non-Latina/o whites exhibit an increased risk of developing a diagnosis of PTSD or PTSD symptoms after exposure to a traumatic event, even when adjusting for differential exposure and sociodemographic factors. Furthermore, conditional risk differences in PTSD appear to persist over time. In other words, once Latina/o individuals develop PTSD at higher rates, the rates of PTSD are likely to remain high over time relative to non-Latina/o whites. Thus, Latinos are more likely than non-Latino whites to exhibit more chronic and severe PTSD symptom trajectories. We note that although adjusting for trauma exposure is the norm, most of the adjustments use proxy measures of trauma exposure. Further, most of the epidemiological research uses PTSD symptom checklists to derive estimations of PTSD risk and infer a *probable* PTSD diagnosis. A probable PTSD diagnosis refers to instances when prevalence of PTSD is estimated based on whether a respondent meets symptom scale cutoff criteria for PTSD, rather than estimations based on the use of a diagnostic instrument. In addition, studies typically do not track PTSD persistence at the individual level; instead, aggregate PTSD rates are presented for the full sample at each time point, obscuring the exact relationship between new onset and persistence of PTSD for each individual. Thus, although there is strong evidence to support conditional risk differences in PTSD between Latina/os and non-Latina/o whites, the limitations inherent in the measurement of PTSD caution us to interpret these findings judiciously, especially in the absence of a discussion on the potential reasons for these differences. The section that follows focuses on various sociocultural explanations that have been offered to understand the observed differences in conditional risk related to PTSD onset and persistence.

Sociocultural Explanations of Differences in Conditional Risk for PTSD

In order to meet criteria for a PTSD diagnosis in the fifth edition of the *Diagnostic and Statistical Manual of Mental Disorders* (DSM-5), an individual must be exposed to actual or threatened death, serious injury, or sexual violence; develop a set number of symptoms from the intrusion, avoidance, mood/cognition, and hyperarousal clusters; and meet duration and distress criteria (American Psychiatric Association 2013). Specifically, exposure to the traumatic event must occur through one of four means: direct experience of the traumatic event, witnessing (in person) the traumatic event as experienced by others, learning that the traumatic event occurred to a close family member or close friend, or experiencing repeated exposure to aversive details of the traumatic event (American Psychiatric Association 2013). Unadjusted racial/ethnic differences in PTSD prevalence therefore may result from the following: (a) differential distribution of exposure to certain types of traumatic events (Roberts et al. 2010); (b) differential vulnerability to onset and/or persistence of PTSD (Perilla et al. 2002); or (c) differential expression of PTSD symptoms, which complicates assessment (Hinton and Lewis-Fernández 2011). Many of the aforementioned studies document elevated prevalence, incidence, and/or persistence of PTSD among Latina/os relative to non-Latina/o whites that persist even when accounting for differential levels and characteristics of trauma exposure (Galea et al. 2002; North et al.

2012; Pole et al. 2001; Roberts et al. 2010; Shih et al. 2010). Differential exposure then does not fully explain the observed differences, although we
note the need for additional research using more thorough and direct assessments of trauma exposure characteristics in order to fully endorse this
conclusion.

The remainder of this chapter reviews five sociocultural explanations that
may help clarify the reasons for the apparently higher conditional risk of
onset and persistence of PTSD among Latina/os relative to non-Latina/o
whites. These include: cross-cultural variation of PTSD symptom structure,
relationship between peritraumatic responses and cultural syndromes
(e.g., *ataque de nervios*), expressive style, variations in acculturation and adherence to cultural interpretations, and uneven distribution of social disadvantage. The five explanations are reviewed in detail below.

Structure of PTSD

While research on the cross-cultural validity of PTSD as defined in the
DSM-5 is at the moment nonexistent, prior research on the cross-cultural
equivalence of the PTSD diagnosis as defined in the DSM-IV-TR (American
Psychiatric Association 2000) supports the validity of PTSD across cultures
(Hinton and Lewis-Fernández 2011; Karam et al. 2014). For example, several
studies have examined the factor structure of the DSM-IV-TR PTSD symptoms across cultural settings, and most of the findings differ little from what
is found in Western samples, although the prevalence might differ slightly
across countries (Fawzi et al. 1997; Karam et al. 2014; Lim et al. 2009; Norris
et al. 2001b; Palmieri et al. 2007; Sack et al. 1997; Yufik and Simms 2010).
However, the relative salience of symptom clusters may show greater variation
across cultural groups. For example, the symptom clusters of reexperiencing and possibly avoidance as defined in the DSM-IV-TR are more commonly endorsed by U.S. Latina/os in comparison to non-Latina/o white
Americans across a range of trauma-exposed samples (Marshall et al. 2009;
Norris et al. 2001b; Ortega and Rosenheck 2000; Perilla et al. 2002; Pole et al.
2005). In addition, the degree to which specific symptom clusters are endorsed
may vary by Latina/o ethnic subgroup. For example, Ortega and Rosenheck
(2000) found unequal endorsement rates of reexperiencing, avoidance, and
hyperarousal symptoms in Puerto Rican and Mexican American Vietnam

veterans relative to non-Latina/o whites. Specifically, Puerto Rican veterans more frequently endorsed symptoms of reexperiencing, hyperarousal, guilt, and avoidance compared to non-Latina/o whites, whereas Mexican Americans more frequently endorsed symptoms of hyperarousal relative to white veterans. Furthermore, Marshall and colleagues (2009) found that Latina/o survivors of physical injury reported more positive symptoms of PTSD than whites, including hypervigilance, flashbacks, and intrusive thoughts.

These unique symptom patterns raise the possibility that the salience of particular constellations of PTSD symptoms, and therefore the structure of PTSD, may vary across Latina/o subgroups as a function of culture-of-origin characteristics, and that unidimensional models of PTSD may mask these differences (see Norris et al. 2001b). We note that most of the epidemiological studies on differences in conditional PTSD risk across racial/ethnic groups make inferences about the likelihood of a DSM-IV-TR PTSD diagnosis and severity based on PTSD symptom checklists (e.g., PTSD Checklist—Civilian Version, Mississippi Scale for Combat-Related PTSD, National Women's Study posttraumatic stress module) rather than clinician-administered diagnostic interviews. Seven of the seventeen PTSD symptoms in these checklists refer explicitly to reexperiencing or avoidance of stimuli. Thus, in cases where a *probable* PTSD diagnosis is derived from symptom checklists that rely on cutoff scores, it is possible that the experiential salience of avoidance and reexperiencing/intrusion symptoms among Latina/os may result in a greater likelihood of endorsing more PTSD symptoms, and therefore a greater likelihood of meeting symptom cutoff scores, and subsequently a probable PTSD diagnosis. It remains an open question whether these higher rates of PTSD diagnoses would also be observed with clinician-rated diagnostic instruments, such as the SCID. In fact, our systematic review indicates that these racial/ethnic differences are attenuated when diagnoses are made by clinicians, suggesting that clinicians may adjust for differential symptom expression in their diagnostic interviews (Alcántara et al. 2013). Cross-cultural variation in trauma subtypes and corresponding symptoms, in coping responses (e.g., avoidance, numbing), in comorbidity profiles (e.g., depression and PTSD, panic attacks and PTSD) and their interplay with cultural syndromes, and in the meaning of symptoms and symptom clusters: all these are potential explanations for the variation in the relative salience of PTSD clusters across cultures (Hinton and Lewis-Fernández 2011). We also lack data on potential racial/ethnic variations in the endorsement of the negative alterations in cognition and mood symptom cluster as described in the recently published DSM-5 (American Psychiatric Association 2013).

Peritraumatic Responses and *Ataque de Nervios*

Peritraumatic responses refer to the reactions that occur during or immediately after the traumatic event, such as peritraumatic dissociation and peri-event panic attack symptoms. Endorsement of peritraumatic responses has been linked to a higher likelihood of developing PTSD across racial/ethnic groups (Ozer et al. 2003). For example, peritraumatic dissociation may account for a twelve- to eighteen-fold increased odds of subsequent PTSD among an ethnically diverse sample of Vietnam veterans (Schnurr et al. 2004). The relationship between peritraumatic dissociation and PTSD has not been consistently replicated, however, and in some cases is attenuated when other variables are considered (Breh and Seidler 2007; Briere et al. 2005; van der Hart et al. 2008).

Latina/os are found to endorse more peritraumatic dissociation (e.g., depersonalization, derealization) and peri-event panic attack symptoms relative to non-Latina/o whites (Galea et al. 2008; Pole et al. 2001; Santos et al. 2008). Greater peritraumatic dissociation accounted for a large proportion of the racial/ethnic variance in PTSD symptom severity among police officers (Pole et al. 2005). For example, in the study conducted by Pole and colleagues (2005), 21 percent of the variance between Latina/os and African Americans and 20 percent of the variance between Latina/os and non-Latina/o whites was due to peritraumatic dissociation. The next factor, wishful-thinking/self-blame coping, explained only 12 percent and 0 percent of the variance in symptom severity between Latina/o and non-Latina/o white officers and Latina/o and African American officers, respectively (Pole et al. 2005). Similarly, peritraumatic dissociation was associated with increased PTSD symptom severity in a sample of Latina/os exposed to community violence after adjusting for trauma characteristics (e.g., injury severity, length of hospitalization, method of injury [e.g., gunshot]; see Denson et al. 2007). Of note, the effect of peritraumatic dissociation largely disappeared when a measure of five-day PTSD symptom severity was included in the model. This implies that the severity of PTSD symptoms in the days following exposure to a traumatic event may mediate the relationship between PTSD and peritraumatic dissociation occurring during or within moments of the trauma.

In regard to peri-event panic, endorsement of panic symptoms immediately following the trauma was a robust predictor of risk of PTSD among a sample of New York City residents at six months after the September 11 terrorist attacks (Galea et al. 2004), and also over time, at two and three years post attack (Galea et al. 2008).

The elevated rates of peritraumatic dissociation and peri-event panic among Latinos have been linked to the cultural predisposition to experiencing an *ataque de nervios* [attack of nerves] in response to acute stress (Lewis-Fernández et al. 2002; Ruef et al. 2000). Ataque de nervios is a cultural concept of distress that often involves typical and atypical panic and dissociation symptoms, such as intense anxiety, loss of control, rage, aggressiveness, amnesia, depersonalization, and derealization (American Psychiatric Association 2013). Ataques de nervios are popularly endorsed among Latina/os from Caribbean countries such as Puerto Rico and the Dominican Republic and are also linked to interpersonal conflict, loss, psychiatric vulnerability, and social adversity (Alcántara et al. 2012; Guarnaccia et al. 1989, 2003, 2010). Prevalence of ataques is associated with prevalence of panic disorder, PTSD, depressive disorders, anxiety sensitivity, childhood trauma, dissociative symptoms, dissociative predisposition, and noncriterion PTSD symptoms (Cintrón et al. 2005; Guarnaccia et al. 1996, 2010; Hinton et al. 2008; Lewis-Fernández et al. 2002, 2010; Norris et al. 2001c; Schechter et al. 2000). These associations make it plausible that once exposed to a traumatic event Latina/os may experience a peritraumatic or peri-event emotional response in the form of an ataque de nervios, and this in turn may lead to increased odds of PTSD onset or persistence.

The predisposition to experience ataques de nervios in the context of trauma and other adverse experiences may result from the presence of cultural scripts that sanction communication of overwhelming distress (e.g., anger, anxiety) and/or strategic resolution of interpersonal conflict through an ataque (Guarnaccia et al. 2003; Hinton et al. 2009; Lewis-Fernández 1998). Ataques may also stem in part from fear of negative emotional states (e.g., anxiety, anger), fear of psychological and physiological arousal symptoms, and/or fear of interpersonal consequences (Hinton et al. 2009). These negative emotions and physiological states may activate trauma memories, catastrophic cognitions, and/or metaphoric networks related to life stressors that may heighten fear and arousal and thereby increase the likelihood of an ataque (Hinton et al. 2009). A positive feedback loop may thereby be created that engenders the occurrence and likelihood of the cultural syndrome, similarly to what has been proposed for Cambodian *khyâl* attacks (Hinton and Otto 2006). Thus, it is possible that ataques de nervios may operate on fear-based, anger-based, or communication/resolution-based pathways, resulting in different types of ataques that may be differentially associated to psychiatric categories such as PTSD. Any of these mechanisms may engender ataque experiences in the context of peritraumatic distress. In fact, whether there are different pathways to ataques and their relationship to PTSD remains an empirical question. It is also plausible that an ataque de nervios is an epiphenomenon of peritraumatic distress with a particular cultural phenomenology, much like Fikretoglu and colleagues (2006) suggest that peritraumatic dissociation is an epiphenomenon of peritraumatic distress (Fikretoglu et al. 2006). Interestingly, in one of the only studies examining the relationship between lifetime ataque de nervios and current PTSD among a diverse sample of Latina/os, a statistically significant relationship was not documented (Lewis-Fernández et al. 2010). Instead, a relationship was found with *padecer de los nervios ahora* (currently ill with nerves), an idiom of distress strongly related to ataque. This may indicate a lack of relationship specifically between ataque and PTSD or, given the substantial lag between the traumatic events and the assessment of PTSD, a limited relationship between ataque and PTSD persistence over time. "Currently ill with nerves" may thus be a marker of more persistent posttraumatic symptoms, possibly due to the disproportionately low rates of mental health service utilization relative to the high percentage of lifetime traumas and political violence reported by Latina/o immigrants (Fortuna et al. 2008). It is also possible that some Latina/o ethnic groups and not others may be particularly at risk to experience an ataque de nervios peritraumatic response. For example, in the first epidemiological study of ataque de nervios in the United States, lifetime history of ataques was endorsed most frequently by Puerto Ricans (15 percent), followed by Mexicans (9.6 percent), Cubans (9 percent), and other Latinos (7 percent) (Guarnaccia et al. 2010). Similarly, Dominicans and Puerto Ricans were more likely than other Latinos to experience a peri-event panic attack six months after the September 11 attack. Peri-event panic emerged as a particularly important predictor of PTSD for Dominicans (Galea et al. 2004).

There is evidence to suggest that variation in peritraumatic responses (both peritraumatic dissociation and peri-event panic) accounts for a substantial percentage of the variance in the conditional risk of PTSD onset between Latina/os and non-Latina/o whites. Given the relationships between dissociative capacity, panic attack, and ataque de nervios, it is possible that this cultural syndrome facilitates and channels the expression of peritraumatic dissociation and peri-event panic in at least some Latina/o subgroups and thereby increases the risk of PTSD onset after trauma. However, no study has examined the concurrent relationship between trauma exposure, peritraumatic dissociation, peri-event panic, ataque de nervios, and PTSD onset. Lewis-Fernández et al. (2010) found a relationship between related constructs (twelve-month PTSD prevalence, lifetime trauma exposure, general dissociative capacity, and being currently ill with nerves), but a more rigorous study of these constructs at the time of trauma exposure remains to be done. Furthermore, specific Latina/o subethnicity (e.g., Dominican and Puerto Rican origin) may moderate the relationship between ataque de nervios or another peritraumatic response and PTSD risk, yet this hypothesis remains largely untested.

Expressive Style

The notion that Latina/os overendorse or overreport PTSD symptoms as a function of a "culturally-based expressive style" (Ortega and Rosenheck 2000: 619; see also Ruef et al. 2000) has been suggested as one explanation for higher conditional risk of PTSD among Latina/os relative to non-Latina/o whites. Overendorsement or overreporting may result from either a cultural predisposition to amplify symptom experience during the experience itself, a tendency to report more symptoms subsequent to the experience despite the same level of resulting clinical severity, or to both kinds of expressiveness. The expressive style hypothesis was initially based on NVVRS data (Ortega and Rosenheck, 2000), which showed that Puerto Rican and Mexican American veterans endorsed more PTSD symptoms than non-Latina/o white veterans after adjusting for premilitary (e.g., educational attainment, childhood poverty) and military factors (e.g., degree of war-zone experience), but without showing the higher functional impairment that would be expected with greater symptomatology. However, recent research provides mixed support for the expressive style hypothesis. Pole et al. (2005) did not find an overreporting bias, finding evidence instead for a pattern of distress underreporting. When Lewis-Fernández and colleagues (2008) tested the expressive-style hypothesis with the NVVRS subsample that was also interviewed by clinicians using the SCID—rather than the full sample assessed only with self-report PTSD symptom scales—they found evidence of heightened expressive style among Hispanic male Vietnam veterans only when PTSD was assessed via self-report. Moreover, Puerto Rican male veterans showed a more profound pattern of self-reported symptom overendorsement than Mexican Americans. In this SCID subsample, however, there was no evidence of higher PTSD symptom reporting in clinician-administered diagnostic interviews or a consistent trend of reduced functional impairment among Hispanics compared to African Americans and non-Hispanic whites. Thus, it appears that cultural patterns of expressive style may contribute only a partial explanation for variation in conditional risk between Latina/os and whites, especially when diagnostic inferences are made by clinicians (for a more detailed discussion see Alcántara et al. 2013).

Fatalism, Familism, and Acculturation

Variations in adherence to the cultural values of fatalism and familism, which are common among Latina/os, and in acculturation to U.S. society have also been suggested as potential mediators in the relationship between Latina/o ethnicity and PTSD owing to their influence on posttrauma coping strategies. Fatalism refers to the deterministic notion that the causal influence of external forces is greater than the causal influence of individual/internal forces (Perilla et al. 2002). Familism is a cultural value that prizes interconnectedness among members of the family unit, including the extended family and godparents, and privileges family priorities above individual priorities (Laria and Lewis-Fernández 2006; Sabogal et al. 1987). In one of the few studies to examine a mediation model, Perilla et al. (2002) found that cultural values such as fatalism and familism did mediate the relationship between certain PTSD symptom clusters (e.g., reexperiencing) and Latina/o ethnicity (e.g., versus African American ethnicity), as well as between the symptom clusters and minority (versus majority) ethnicity. Fatalism and familism were conceptualized as proxies of the values dimension of the acculturation process. These investigators measured familism as the extent to which respondents positively endorsed the view that aging parents should live at home and that children should live at home until marriage. Fatalism was measured by the extent to which respondents endorsed coping strategies based on an external versus internal locus of control. The mediational role of fatalism in the onset of PTSD may be due to the postulated relationship between this cultural value and the use of passive rather than active

coping strategies (Neff and Hoppe 1993), which may lead to higher vulnerability to PTSD. This hypothesis is supported by the finding that Latina/o
police officers use self-blaming and wishful-thinking coping strategies more
often than white officers, and that use of these coping strategies has a partial
effect on PTSD severity (Pole et al. 2005). However, an equally plausible
competing theory stipulates that endorsement of fatalistic values could result in more adaptive functioning owing to use of mindfulness acceptance,
which may lead to decreased anxiety and greater sense of self-efficacy (Markowitz et al. 2009), and possibly lower risk of PTSD. To date, these alternative hypotheses have not been tested.

Perilla et al. (2002) hypothesized that familism would mediate the relationship between Latina/o ethnicity and PTSD because of the decreased likelihood to seek medical care stemming from a strong reliance on kin networks
for social support as well as the increased likelihood of interpersonal distress in the face of familial obligations. These kin social support networks may
be compromised, and family-related interpersonal distress may be increased
in the context of a natural disaster if relatives are among those affected. Perilla and colleagues (2002) found that familism mediated the relationship
between PTSD intrusion symptoms and Latina/o ethnicity in the expected
direction. On the other hand, lower levels of familism were associated
with greater levels of hyperarousal in one of the initial mediation models,
suggesting that familism could confer at least a partially protective effect
on PTSD onset and PTSD symptom clusters. However these effects did not
hold in the full mediation model, suggesting that other pathways beyond
familism are more central to the development of PTSD symptomatology.

Studies examining the extent to which differential levels of acculturation
explain higher conditional risk of PTSD among Latina/os relative to non-
Latina/o whites have been inconclusive. For example, among Mexican
American women, those who were born in the United States had higher PTSD
symptom scores than Mexico-born women from a range of age-at-migration
cohorts (e.g., those who immigrated in childhood, adolescence, or adulthood).
These differences held in models that adjusted for number of lifetime traumatic experiences (Heilemann et al. 2005). However, Perilla et al. (2002) found
the opposite effect of acculturation on PTSD when acculturation was measured by language preference. In cases where personal trauma and neighborhood trauma exposure were high, Spanish-speaking Latina/os showed the
highest rates of PTSD, followed by African Americans, Latina/os who prefer
English, and non-Latina/o whites. Similarly, Marshall and colleagues (2002)

found an association between lower levels of acculturation to U.S. society (as measured by language preference) and increased dissociative symptoms even when controlling for assault characteristics (e.g., injury severity, duration of attack, gunshot wound or other mechanism) and lifetime exposure to community violence among a sample of physical injury survivors (Marshall et al. 2002). It is possible that Spanish-speaking respondents or those with low acculturation to U.S. American society exhibit a greater predisposition toward peritraumatic dissociation, which results in higher rates of PTSD in this group on account of the association between peritraumatic dissociation and PTSD (Ozer et al. 2003). Other studies do not find a statistically significant bivariate effect of acculturation (measured as language of survey administration, country of origin, or language preference as child/adult) on PTSD symptoms or peritraumatic responses (Galea et al. 2004; Ortega and Rosenheck 2000).

In sum, research is sparse on the extent to which cultural values such as fatalism and familism, as well as levels of acculturation, mediate the relationship between conditional risk of PTSD and Latina/o ethnicity. In cases where these cultural mediators are included, often studies are conducted with proxy measures of acculturation (e.g., language preference/proficiency in lieu of multidimensional scales of acculturation) and of cultural values (e.g., locus of control in lieu of fatalism). Thus, the lack of an association in some studies may be due to measurement limitations.

Social Disadvantage

Repeated exposure to sociocontextual risk factors, such as discrimination and poverty, may place individuals in disadvantaged social positions that predispose them to develop and maintain PTSD. This possibility is supported by research indicating that limited socioeconomic resources at baseline and over the life course are linked to PTSD symptoms among NYC residents following 9/11, even after adjusting for the effect of lifetime trauma history (i.e., number of lifetime traumatic experiences), trauma characteristics (i.e., caught in dust cloud, suffered injury on 9/11, lost possessions, witnessed horror on 9/11, friend or relative killed in attack), posttrauma consequences (i.e., involved in rescue and recovery effort, evacuation from residence, lost employment due to attack), and demographic variables (DiGrande et al. 2008; Galea et al. 2008). In particular, socioeconomic position accounted for approximately 14–17 percent of the observed variance in onset of probable

PTSD among Dominicans and Puerto Ricans in models adjusting for differential trauma exposure (Galea et al. 2004). In addition, lower prewar educational attainment (in addition to younger age and lower Armed Forces Qualification Test scores) accounted for elevated rates of PTSD incidence among a SCID-diagnosed subsample of the NVVRS after adjusting for severity of exposure to war-zone stressors (Dohrenwend et al. 2008). College education was also associated with lower disaster-related PTSD onset after adjusting for demographics, ethnicity, history of mental disorder, and trauma exposure in a large population-based sample (n = 811) (North et al. 2012). Other studies have shown that perceived discrimination mediates the relationship between Latina/o ethnicity and PTSD prevalence in a representative sample of Vietnam veterans (Ruef et al. 2000) and urban police officers (Pole et al. 2005) in models adjusting for either war-zone trauma exposure or peritraumatic dissociation.

The possibility that social disadvantage, such as low socioeconomic position, poverty, and discrimination, could mediate the relationship between ethnicity and poor mental health status or fundamentally cause poor mental health outcomes (Cook et al. 2009) fits well within a *vulnerable populations* framework. Frohlich and Potvin (2008:218) define a vulnerable population as a "subgroup or subpopulation who, because of shared social characteristics, is at higher risk of risks." If we accept that Latina/os are a vulnerable U.S. subpopulation because of their disadvantaged socioeconomic position (U.S. Census Bureau 2002; DeNavas-Walt et al. 2011), the higher conditional risk of PTSD may be understood as the consequence of an accumulation of risk factors that in turn generate greater exposure to risks. In relation to trauma-specific risks, Latina/os have been shown to report disproportionately higher exposure to political violence (Eisenman et al. 2003), higher rates of positive lifetime histories of intimate partner violence (Fedovskiy et al. 2008; Rodriguez et al. 2008), lower social support (Galea et al. 2004), and higher exposure to childhood maltreatment (Roberts et al. 2010) relative to U.S. whites and Americans of Asian, Hawaiian, or Pacific Island descent. All of these risk factors have been linked to posttraumatic stress outcomes. Furthermore, among those experiencing posttraumatic stress, Latina/os are less likely to use mental health services (Brinker et al. 2007; Fortuna et al. 2008; Roberts et al. 2010). Therefore, uneven distribution of social disadvantage—including disparities in access and use of treatment for Latina/os exhibiting posttraumatic stress symptoms as well as increased likelihood of being at "risk of risks" (i.e., multiple traumas, socioeconomic disadvantage, poor physical health)—over the lifespan may contribute to a higher conditional risk of PTSD for Latina/os relative to non-Latina/o whites.

Social disadvantage may account for higher conditional risk of onset and persistence of PTSD in two ways. First, the lived experience of a life at risk of risks and of social vulnerability may not be well captured in models that adjust for trauma exposure with dichotomous or ordinal measures. Similarly, individual-level assessments of socioeconomic position may not adequately capture lifetime exposure to social vulnerability (Williams et al. 2010). Second, treatment disparities and exposure to social disadvantage may place Latina/os relative to whites on life trajectories where they are more likely to remain symptomatic over extended periods of time, and thereby to exhibit a pattern of high conditional risk of PTSD that persists over time.

Future Directions

Research on racial/ethnic differences in PTSD prevalence and conditional risk of PTSD has grown exponentially since the early work of Penk and colleagues (Penk et al. 1989) and the call from Frueh, Brady, and de Arellano (1998) for rigorous empirical research on this topic. Nonetheless, much remains unknown about the mechanisms responsible for racial/ethnic differences in conditional risk of PTSD. Based on our review, we propose five areas for further study to help address the limitations of available research and clarify the reasons behind differential conditional risk of PTSD between Latina/os and non-Latina/o whites. These research areas focus on: (a) assessment of PTSD diagnosis and PTSD symptoms, (b) mechanisms involved in onset versus persistence of PTSD, (c) Latina/o subgroup-level analyses, (d) objective and subjective measures of trauma exposure and severity, and (e) interaction between gender, ethnicity, culture, and socioeconomic position.

First, future research would benefit from the use of multimethod assessments of PTSD symptoms and diagnoses. As mentioned previously, many of the epidemiological studies reviewed were based on lay-administered structured diagnostic interviews or self-report symptom checklists and cutoff scores. Studies that rely strictly on symptom cutoff scores to infer a probable PTSD diagnosis may be problematic given the preliminary evidence of cross-cultural variation in PTSD symptom constellations. For example, the apparently higher endorsement of avoidance and reexperiencing/intrusion symptoms among Latina/os relative to non-Latina/o whites may result in a higher false-positive rate of PTSD diagnoses. Use of lay-administered diagnostic instruments, while preferable to scale-based assessments, are less desirable than clinician-administered semistructured diagnostic interviews, in light of the low concordance between these two methods when applied to PTSD (Alegria et al. 2009; Lewis-Fernández et al. 2008). We also encourage reliance on prospective rather than retrospective assessments of PTSD, and evaluations that combine diagnostic interviews with assessments of functional impairment, in order to ascertain the impairment criterion for the diagnosis (Lewis-Fernández et al. 2008). These multimethod assessments could provide needed data for sensitivity analyses that permit estimation of the magnitude and reliability of the effects observed.

Second, more in-depth research is needed on the moderators and mediators of the relationship between Latina/o ethnicity and higher conditional risk of PTSD, particularly as these affect onset versus persistence of PTSD. It is actually likely that different mediators may be involved at each of these two stages of the condition. Future research should explore biological, psychological, and social mechanisms that may be more closely linked to onset (e.g., physiological reactivity) and persistence of psychopathology (e.g., emotion regulation skills). Third, future studies should examine subgroup-level racial and ethnic differences in the conditional risk of PTSD symptoms and diagnoses (Triffleman and Pole 2010). Many researchers aggregate Latino subgroups as a single undifferentiated category, despite findings of subgroup differences in conditional risk of PTSD (Galea et al. 2004; Ortega and Rosenheck 2000), as well as in differential psychiatric risk profiles more generally (Alegría et al. 2008). We recommend further research on the variation of cultural and psychosocial characteristics by Latina/o subgroup and their relative influence on PTSD risk.

Fourth, this review focused on conditional risk of PTSD among Latina/os relative to non-Latina/o whites, that is, on studies that adjusted for the effect of trauma exposure. We note that the quality and scope of the adjustments made for trauma exposure (and in some cases severity) were not uniform across studies. Moreover, many studies used objective measures of direct exposure (e.g., number of days hospitalized, distance from epicenter of disaster, injuries incurred) and tended not to include subjective measures of trauma exposure, severity, and subsequent distress (as discussed in Alcántara et al. 2013). Yet participants' subjective perceptions of the severity of their traumas provide additional information beyond that obtained from objective indicators (Fikretoglu et al. 2006), which may help explain the findings of differential conditional risk. In addition, these objective indicators of trauma exposure seldom accounted for other lifetime traumatic events. Even when such assessments were conducted, the methods used for adjustment may not have fully captured the impact of accumulated vulnerability, or the extent of a life at risk of risks (Frohlich and Potvin 2008). It is possible that individuals at risk of risks have different thresholds for peritraumatic responses and PTSD. We recommend that future research more closely address differential pathways to PTSD.

Fifth, a next wave of studies should more closely examine gender and, in particular, the intersection between gender, ethnicity, culture, and socioeconomic position on PTSD risk. Most studies on differential racial/ethnic PTSD risk have been conducted with predominantly male samples, or in male-dominated work contexts, such as the military or police work. Very few studies have examined gender differences in the conditional risk of PTSD. This is surprising, given the extensive body of research demonstrating gender differences in trauma exposure and PTSD prevalence (Olff et al. 2007; Tolin and Foa 2006). In addition, there is preliminary evidence that Latina women are at increased odds of receiving a PTSD diagnosis or exhibiting higher symptom severity than their counterparts, even when controlling for socioeconomic status and adversity (Galea et al. 2008; Montoya et al. 2003). Female gender has also been associated with increased peritraumatic responses, such as peritraumatic dissociation and endorsement of ataque de nervios among Latina/os (Guarnaccia et al. 2010; Lewis-Fernández et al. 2010), which in turn may place Latina women at higher risk of developing PTSD. Future research must examine the interplay between gender, race/ethnicity, culture, and socioeconomic position on differential risk and mediators of PTSD.

Conclusion

Various regional epidemiological studies conducted in the United States suggest that the conditional risk for PTSD (prevalence, and in some cases onset and persistence separately) once exposed to one or more traumatic events is higher among Latina/os than non-Latina/o whites. In this chapter we reviewed several sociocultural explanations that may account for the observed ethnic differences in conditional risk of PTSD. These included cross-cultural variation in the structure of PTSD; the relationship between peritraumatic responses and ataque de nervios, and expressive style; and variation in adherence to cultural values (e.g., familism, fatalism), level of acculturation, and distribution of social disadvantage. Based on the limitations of the available studies, we recommend that researchers in future studies (a) use multimethod assessments of PTSD diagnosis and PTSD symptoms, (b) separately examine mechanisms involved in onset versus persistence of PTSD, (c) assess Latina/o subgroup differences, (d) include adjustment for both objective and subjective measures of trauma exposure and severity, and (e) examine the interaction between gender, ethnicity, culture, and socioeconomic position on PTSD risk.

Acknowledgments

Portions of this chapter appeared previously in Carmela Alcántara, Melynda D. Casement, and Roberto Lewis-Fernández 2013 (Conditional Risk for PTSD Among Latinos: A Systematic Review of Racial/Ethnic Differences and Sociocultural Explanations, in *Clinical Psychology Review* 33[1]:107–19).

References

Adams, Richard E., and Joseph A. Boscarino
  2005 Differences in Mental Health Outcomes Among Whites, African Americans, and Hispanics Following a Community Disaster. Psychiatry: Interpersonal and Biological Processes 68(3):250–65.
  2006 Predictors of PTSD and Delayed PTSD After Disaster: The Impact of Exposure and Psychosocial Resources. Journal of Nervous and Mental Disease 194(7):485–93.
Alcántara, Carmela, James L. Abelson, and Joseph P. Gone
  2012 Beyond Anxious Predisposition: Do Padecer de Nervios and Ataque de Nervios Add Incremental Validity to Predictions of Current Distress Among Mexican Mothers? Depression and Anxiety 29(1):23–31.
Alcántara, Carmela, Melynda D. Casement, and Roberto Lewis-Fernández
  2013 Conditional Risk for PTSD Among Latinos: A Systematic Review of Racial/Ethnic Differences and Sociocultural Explanations. Clinical Psychology Review 33(1):107–19.

Alegría, Margarita, Glorisa Canino, Patrick E. Shrout, Meghan Woo, Naihua Duan, Doryliz Vila, Maria Torres, Chih-nan Chen, and Xiao-Li Meng
   2008 Prevalence of Mental Illness in Immigrant and Non-Immigrant U.S. Latino Groups. American Journal of Psychiatry 165(3):359–69.
Alegria, Margarita, Patrick E. Shrout, Maria Torres, Roberto Lewis-Fernández, Jamie M. Abelson, Meris Powell, Alejandro Interian, Julia Lin, Mara Laderman, and Glorisa Canino
   2009 Lessons Learned from the Clinical Reappraisal Study of the Composite International Diagnostic Interview with Latinos. International Journal of Methods in Psychiatric Research 18(2):84–95.
American Psychiatric Association
   2000 Diagnostic and Statistical Manual of Mental Disorder. 4th edition. Text revision. Washington, D.C.: American Psychiatric Association.
   2013 Diagnostic and Statistical Manual of Mental Disorder. 5th edition. Text revision. Washington, D.C.: American Psychiatric Association.
Asnaani, Anu, Anthony J. Richey, Ruta Dimaite, Devon E. Hinton, and Stefan G. Hofmann
   2010 A Cross-Ethnic Comparison of Lifetime Prevalence Rates of Anxiety Disorders. Journal of Nervous and Mental Disease 198(8):551–55.
Balsam, Kimberly F., Keren Lehavot, Blair Beadnell, and Elizabeth Circo
   2010 Childhood Abuse and Mental Health Indicators Among Ethnically Diverse Lesbian, Gay, and Bisexual Adults. Journal of Consulting and Clinical Psychology 78(4):459–68.
Bowler, Rosemari M., Hui Han, Vihra Gocheva, Sanae Nakagawa, Howard Alper, Laura DiGrande, and James E. Cone
   2010 Gender Differences in Probable Posttraumatic Stress Disorder Among Police Responders to the 2001 World Trade Center Terrorist Attack. American Journal of Industrial Medicine 53(12):1186–96.
Breh, Doris C., and Günter H. Seidler
   2007 Is Peritraumatic Dissociation a Risk Factor for PTSD? Journal of Trauma and Dissociation 8(1):53–69.
Breslau, Naomi, Ronald C. Kessler, Howard D. Chilcoat, Lonni R. Schultz, Glenn C. Davis, and Patricia Andreski
   1998 Trauma and Posttraumatic Stress Disorder in the Community: The 1996 Detroit Area Survey of Trauma. Archives of General Psychiatry 55(7):626–32.
Briere, John, Catherine Scott, and Frank Weathers
   2005 Peritraumatic and Persistent Dissociation in the Presumed Etiology of PTSD. American Journal of Psychiatry 162(12):2295–301.
Brinker, Michael, Joseph Westermyer, Paul Thuras, and Jose Canive
   2007 Severity of Combat-Related Posttraumatic Stress Disorder Versus Noncombat-Related Posttraumatic Stress Disorder: A Community-Based Study in American

Indian and Hispanic Veterans. Journal of Nervous and Mental Disease 195(8): 655–61.

Cintrón, Jennifer A., Michele M. Carter, and Tracy Sbrocco
2005 Ataques de Nervios in Relation to Anxiety Sensitivity Among Island Puerto Ricans. Culture, Medicine and Psychiatry 29(4):415–31.

Cook, Benjamin, Margarita Alegría, Julia Y. Lin, and Jing Guo
2009 Pathways and Correlates Connecting Latinos' Mental Health with Exposure to the United States. American Journal of Public Health 99(12):2247–54.

DeNavas-Walt, Carmen, Bernadette D. Proctor, and Jessica C. Smith
2011 U.S. Census Bureau, Current Population Reports, P60–239, Income, Poverty, and Health Insurance Coverage in the United States: 2010. Washington, D.C.: U.S. Census Bureau.

Denson, Thomas F., Grant N. Marshall, Terry L Schell, and Lisa H. Jaycox
2007 Predictors of Posttraumatic Distress 1 Year After Exposure to Community Violence: The Importance of Acute Symptom Severity. Journal of Consulting and Clinical Psychology 75(5):683–92.

DiGrande, Laura, Megan A. Perrin, Lorna E. Thorpe, Lisa Thalji, Joseph Murphy, David Wu, Mark Farfel, and Robert M. Brackbill
2008 Posttraumatic Stress Symptoms, PTSD, and Risk Factors Among Lower Manhattan Residents 2–3 years After the September 11, 2001 Terrorist Attacks. Journal of Traumatic Stress 21(3):264–73.

Dohrenwend, Bruce P., J. Blake Turner, Nicholas A. Turse, Roberto Lewis-Fernández, and Thomas J. Yager
2008 War-Related Posttraumatic Stress Disorder in Black, Hispanic, and Majority White Vietnam Veterans: The Roles of Exposure and Vulnerability. Journal of Traumatic Stress 21(2):133–41.

Eisenman, David P., Lillian Gelberg, Honghu Liu, and Martin F. Shapiro
2003 Mental Health and Health-Related Quality of Life Among Adult Latino Primary Care Patients Living in the United States with Previous Exposure to Political Violence. Journal of the Amercian Medical Association 290(5): 627–34.

Farfel, Mark, Laura DiGrande, Robert Brackbill, Angela Prann, James Cone, Stephen Friedman, Deborah J. Walker, Grant Pezeshki, Pauline Thomas, Sandro Galea, David Williamson, Thomas R. Frieden, and Lorna Thorpe
2008 An Overview of 9/11 Experiences and Respiratory and Mental Health Conditions Among World Trade Center Health Registry Enrollees. Journal of Urban Health 85(6):880–909.

Fawzi, Mary Catherine Smith, Thang Pham, Lien Lin, Tho Viet Nguyen, Dung Ngo, Elizabeth Murphy, and Richard F. Mollica
1997 The Validity of Posttraumatic Stress Disorder Among Vietnamese Refugees. Journal of Traumatic Stress 10(1):101–8.

Fedovskiy, Kaney, Stacy M. Higgins, and Anuradha Paranjape
    2008 Intimate Partner Violence: How Does it Impact Major Depressive Disorder and Post Traumatic Stress Disorder Among Immigrant Latinas? Journal of Immigrigant and Minority Health 10(1):45–51.
Fikretoglu, Deniz, Alain Brunet, Suzanne Best, Thomas Metzler, Kevin Delucchi, Daniel Weiss, Jeffrey Fagan, and CharlesMarmar
    2006 The Relationship Between Peritraumatic Distress and Peritraumatic Dissociation: An Examination of Two Competing Models. Journal of Nervous and Mental Disease 194(11):853–58.
Fortuna, Lisa R., Michelle V. Porche, and M. Alegria
    2008 Political Violence, Psychosocial Trauma, and the Context of Mental Health Services Use Among Immigrant Latinos in the United States. Ethnicity and Health 13(5):435–63.
Frohlich, Katherine L., and Louise Potvin
    2008 Transcending the Known in Public Health Practice: The Inequality Paradox: The Population Approach and Vulnerable Populations. American Journal of Public Health 98(2):216–21.
Frueh, B. Christopher, Kristine L. Brady, and Michael A. de Arellano
    1998 Racial Differences in Combat-Related PTSD: Empirical Findings and Conceptual Issues. Clinical Psychology Review 18(3):287–305.
Galea, Sandro, Jennifer Ahern, Heidi Resnick, Dean Kilpatrick, Michael Bucuvalas, Joel Gold, and David Vlahov
    2002 Psychological Sequelae of the September 11 Terrorist Attacks in New York City. New England Journal of Medicine 346(13):982–87.
    2004 Hispanic Ethnicity and Post-Traumatic Stress Disorder After a Disaster: Evidence from a General Population Survey After September 11, 2001. Annals of Epidemiology 14(8):520–31.
Galea, Sandro, Jennifer Ahern, Melissa Tracy, Alan Hubbard, Magdalena Certa, Emily Goldmann, and David Vlahov
    2008 Longitudinal Determinants of Posttraumatic Stress in a Population-Based Cohort Study. Epidemiology 19(1):47–54.
Galea, Sandro, David Vlahov, Heidi Resnick, Jennifer Ahern, Ezra Susser, Joel Gold, Michael Bucuvalas, and Dean Kilpatrick
    2003 Trends of Probable Post-Traumatic Stress Disorder in New York City After the September 11 Terrorist Attacks. American Journal of Epidemiology 158(6):514–24.
Guarnaccia, Peter J., Victor DeLaCancela, and Emilio Carrillo
    1989 The Multiple Meanings of Ataques de Nervios in the Latino Community. Medical Anthropology 11(1):47–62.
Guarnaccia, Peter J., Roberto Lewis-Fernández, and Melissa Rivera Marano
    2003 Toward a Puerto Rican Popular Nosology: Nervios and Ataque de Nervios. Culture, Medicine and Psychiatry 27(3):339–66.

Guarnaccia, Peter J., Roberto Lewis-Fernández, Igda Martinez Pincay, Patrick Shrout, Jing Guo, Maria Torres, Glorisa Canino, and Margarita Alegria
    2010 Ataque de Nervios as a Marker of Social and Psychiatric Vulnerability: Results from the NLAAS. International Journal of Social Psychiatry 56(3):298–309.
Guarnaccia, Peter J., Melissa Rivera, Felipe Franco, and Charlie Neighbors
    1996 The Experiences of Ataques de Nervios: Towards an Anthropology of Emotions in Puerto Rico. Culture, Medicine and Psychiatry 20(3):343–67.
Heilemann, Marysue V., Felix S. Kury, and Katheryn A. Lee
    2005 Trauma and Posttraumatic Stress Disorder Symptoms Among Low Income Women of Mexican Descent in the United States. Journal of Nervous and Mental Disease 193(10):665–72.
Hinton, Devon E., Roberto Chong, Mark H. Pollack, David H. Barlow, and Richard J. McNally
    2008 Ataque de Nervios: Relationship to Anxiety Sensitivity and Dissociation Predisposition. Depression and Anxiety 25(6):489–95.
Hinton, Devon E., and Roberto Lewis-Fernández
    2011 The Cross-Cultural Validity of Posttraumatic Stress Disorder: Implications for DSM-5. Depression and Anxiety 28(9):783–801.
Hinton, Devon E., Roberto Lewis-Fernández, and Mark H. Pollack
    2009 A Model of the Generation of Ataque de Nervios: The Role of Fear of Negative Affect and Fear of Arousal Symptoms. CNS Neuroscience and Therapeutics 15(3):264–75.
Hinton, Devon E., and Michael W. Otto
    2006 Symptom Presentation and Symptom Meaning Among Traumatized Cambodian Refugees: Relevance to a Somatically Focused Cognitive-Behavior Therapy. Cognitive and Behavioral Practice 13(4):249–60.
Karam, E. G., Matthew J. Friedman, Eric D. Hill, Ronald C. Kessler, Katie A. McLaughlin, Maria Petukhova, Laura Sampson, Victoria Shahly, Matthias C. Angermeyer, Evelyn J. Bromet, Giovanni de Girolamo, Ron de Graaf, Koen Demyttenaere, Finola Ferry, Silvia E. Florescu, Josep Maria Haro, Yanling He, Aimee N. Karam, Norito Kawakami, Viviane Kovess-Masfety, María Elena Medina-Mora, Mark A. Oakley Browne, José A. Posada-Villa, Arieh Y. Shalev, Dan J. Stein, Maria Carmen Viana, Zahari Zarkov, and Karestan C. Koenen
    2014 Cumulative Traumas and Risk Thresholds: 12-Month PTSD in the World Mental Health (WMH) Surveys. Depression and Anxiety 31(2):130–42.
Kessler, Ronald C., Amanda Sonnega, Evelyn Bromet, Michael Hughes, Christopher B. Nelson
    1995 Posttraumatic Stress Disorder in the National Comorbidity Survey. Archives of General Psychiatry 52(12):1048–60.
Koopman, Cheryl, Kent Drescher, Stephen Bowles, Fred Gusman, Dudley Blake, Harvey Dondershine, Vickie Chang, Lisa D. Butler, and David Spiegel

2001 Acute Dissociative Reactions in Veterans with PTSD. Journal of Trauma and Dissociation 2(1):91–111.

Kulka, Richard A., William E. Schlenger, John A. Fairbanks, Richard L. Hough, B. Kathleen Jordan, Charles R. Marmar, Daniel S. Weiss, David A. Grady, and Senator Alan Cranston

1990 Trauma and the Vietnam War Generation: Report of Findings from the National Vietnam Veterans Readjustment Study. Philadelphia: Brunner/Mazel.

Laria, Amaro J., and Roberto Lewis-Fernández

2006 Latino Patients. *In* Clinical Manual of Cultural Psychiatry. R. F. Lim, ed. Pp. 119–73. Arlington, Va.: American Psychiatric Publishing.

Lewis-Fernández, Roberto

1998 "Eso No Estaba en Mí . . . No Pude Controlarme": El Control, la Identidad y Las Emociones en Comunidades Puertorriqueñas ["That Was Not in Me . . . I Could Not Control Myself": Control, Identity, and Emotion in Puerto Rican Communities]. Revista de Ciencias Sociales (4):268–99.

Lewis-Fernández, Roberto, Magdaliz Gorritz, Greer A. Raggio, Clara Peláez, Henian Chen, and Peter J. Guarnaccia

2010 Association of Trauma-Related Disorders and Dissociation with Four Idioms of Distress Among Latino Psychiatric Outpatients. Culture, Medicine and Psychiatry 34(2):219–43.

Lewis-Fernández, Roberto, Magdaliz Gorritz, Greer A. Raggio, Clara Peláez, Henian Chen, and Peter J. Guarnaccia

2002 Comparative Phenomenology of Ataques de Nervios, Panic Attacks, and Panic Disorder. Culture, Medicine and Psychiatry 26(2):199–223.

Lewis-Fernández, Roberto, J. Blake Turner, Randall Marshall, Nicholas Turse, Yuval Neria, and Bruce P. Dohrenwend

2008 Elevated Rates of Current PTSD Among Hispanic Veterans in the NVVRS: True Prevalence or Methodological Artifact? Journal of Traumatic Stress 21(2):123–32.

Lim, Hyun-Kook, Jong-Min Woo, Tae-Suk Kim, Tae-Hyung Kim, Kyeong-Sook Choi, Sang-Keun Chung, Ik-Seoung Cheef, Kyoung-Uk Lee, Ki Chung Paik, Ho-Jun Seo, Won Kim, Bora Jin, and Jeong-Ho Chae

2009 Reliability and Validity of the Korean Version of the Impact of Event Scale-Revised. Comprehensive Psychiatry 50(4):385–90.

Markowitz, John C., Sapana R. Patel, Ivan C. Balan, Michelle A. Bell, Carlos Blanco, Maria Yellow Horse Brave Heart, Stephanie Buttacavoli Sosa, and Roberto Lewis-Fernández

2009 Toward an Adaptation of Interpersonal Psychotherapy for Hispanic Patients with DSM-IV Major Depressive Disorder. Journal of Clinical Psychiatry 70(2): 214–22.

Marshall, Grant N., and Maria Orlando

2002 Acculturation and Peritraumatic Dissociation in Young Adult Latino Survivors of Community Violence. Journal of Abnormal Psychology 111(1):166–74.

Marshall, Grant N., Terry L. Schell, and Jeremy N. V. Miles
  2009 Ethnic Differences in Posttraumatic Distress: Hispanics' Symptoms Differ
  in Kind and Degree. Journal of Consulting and Clinical Psychology 77(6):
  1169–78.
Montoya, Isaac D., Laura D Covarrubias, Janeene Patek, and Jason A. Graves
  2003 Posttraumatic Stress Disorder Among Hispanic and African-American Drug
  Users. American Journal of Drug and Alcohol Abuse 29(4):729–41.
Neff, James A., and Sue K. Hoppe
  1993 Race/Ethnicity, Acculturation, and Psychological Distress: Fatalism and
  Religiosity as Cultural Resources. Journal of Community Psychology 21(1):
  3–20.
Norris, Fran H., Julia L. Perilla, Gladys E. Ibanez,and Arthur D. Murphy
  2001a Sex Differences in Symptoms of Posttraumatic Stress: Does Culture Play a
  Role? Journal of Traumatic Stress 14(1):7–28.
  2001b Postdisaster Stress in the United States and Mexico: A Cross-Cultural Test of
  the Multicriterion Conceptual Model of Posttraumatic Stress Disorder. Journal
  of Abnormal Psychology 110(4):553–63.
Norris, Fran H.,Deborah L. Weisshaar, M. Lori Conrad, Eolia M. Diaz, Arthur D.
  Murphy, and Gladys E. Ibañez
  2001c A Qualitative Analysis of Posttraumatic Stress Among Mexican Victims of
  Disaster. Journal of Traumatic Stress 14(4):741–56.
North, Carol S., Julianne Oliver, and Anand Pandya
  2012 Examining a Comprehensive Model of Disaster-Related Posttraumatic Stress
  Disorder in Systematically Studied Survivors of 10 Disasters. American Journal
  of Public Health 102(10):e40–e48.
Olff, Miranda, Willie Langeland, Nel Draijer, and Berthold P. R. Gersons
  2007 Gender Differences in Posttraumatic Stress Disorder. Psychological Bulletin
  133(2):183–204.
Ortega, Alexander N., and Robert Rosenheck
  2000 Posttraumatic Stress Disorder Among Hispanic Vietnam Veterans. American
  Journal of Psychiatry 157(4):615–19.
Ozer, Emily J., Suzanne R. Best, Tami L. Lipsey, and Daniel S. Weiss
  2003 Predictors of Posttraumatic Stress Disorder and Symptoms in Adults: A Meta-
  Analysis. Psychological Bulletin 129(1):52–73.
Palmieri, Patrick A., Grant N. Marshall, and Terry L. Schell
  2007 Confirmatory Factor Analysis of Posttraumatic Stress Symptoms in Cambo-
  dian Refugees. Journal of Traumatic Stress 20(2):207–16.
Penk, Walter E., Ralph Robinowitz, John Black, Michael Dolan, William Bell, Dovalee
  Dorsett, Michael Ames, and Lori Noriega
  1989 Ethnicity: Post-Traumatic Stress Disorder (PTSD) Differences Among Black,
  White, and Hispanic Veterans Who Differ in Degrees of Exposure to Combat in
  Vietnam. Journal of Clinical Psychology 45(5, Mono Suppl):729–35.

Perilla, Julia L., Fran H. Norris, and Evelyn A. Lavizzo
    2002 Ethnicity, Culture, and Disaster Response: Identifying and Explaining Ethnic
    Differences in PTSD Six Months After Hurricane Andrew. Journal of Social and
    Clinical Psychology 21(1):20–45.
Pietrzak, Robert H., Adriana Feder, Ritika Singh, Clyde B. Schechter, Evelyn J.
    Bromet, Craig L. Katz, Dori B. Reissman, Fatih Ozbay, Vansh Sharma, Michael
    Crane, Denise Harrison, Robin Herbert, Stephen M. Levin, Benjamin J. Luft,
    Jacqueline M. Moline, Jeanne M. Stellman, Iris G. Udasin, Philip J. Landrigan,
    and Steven M. Southwick
    2013 Trajectories of PTSD Risk and Resilience in World Trade Center Responders:
    An 8-Year Prospective Cohort Study. Psychological Medicine 44(1):205–19.
Pole, Nnamdi, Suzanne R.Best, Thomas Metzler, and Charles R. Marmar
    2005 Why Are Hispanics at Greater Risk for PTSD? Cultural Diversity and Ethnic
    Minority Psychology 11(2):144–61.
Pole, Nnamdi, Suzanne R. Best, Daniel S. Weiss, Thomas Metzler, Akiva Liberman,
    Jeffrey Fagan, and Charles R. Marmar
    2001 Effects of Gender and Ethnicity on Duty-Related Posttraumatic Stress Symp-
    toms Among Urban Police Officers. Journal of Nervous and Mental Disease
    189(7):442–48.
Pole, Nnamdi, Joseph P. Gone, and Madhur Kulkarni
    2008 Posttraumatic Stress Disorder Among Ethnoracial Minorities in the United
    States. Clinical Psychology: Science and Practice 15(1):35–61.
Roberts, Andrea L., Stephen E. Gilman, Joshua Breslau, Naomi Breslau, and Kares-
    tan C. Koenen
    2010 Race/Ethnic Differences in Exposure to Traumatic Events, Development of
    Post-Traumatic Stress Disorder, and Treatment-Seeking for Post-Traumatic Stress
    Disorder in the United States. Psychological Medicine 41(1):71–83.
Rodriguez, Michael A., MarySue V. Heilemann, Eve Fielder, Alfonso Ang, Faustina
    Nevarez, and Carol M. Mangione
    2008 Intimate Partner Violence, Depression, and PTSD Among Pregnant Latina
    Women. Annals of Family Medicine 6(1):44–52.
Ruef, Anne Marie, Brett T. Litz, and William E. Schlenger
    2000 Hispanic Ethnicity and Risk for Combat-Related Posttraumatic Stress Disor-
    der. Cultural Diversity and Ethnic Minority Psychology 6(3):235–51.
Sabogal, Fabio, Bob G. Knight, Maria Marquez-Gonzalez, Ignacio Montori, Igone
    Etxeberria, and Cecilia Penacoba
    1987 Hispanic Familism and Acculturation: What Changes and What Doesn't?
    Hispanic Journal of Behavioral Sciences 9(4):397–412.
Sack, William H., John R. Seeley, and Gregory N. Clarke
    1997 Does PTSD Transcend Cultural Barriers? A Study from the Khmer Adoles-
    cent Refugee Project. Journal of the American Academy of Child and Adolescent
    Psychiatry 36(1):49–54.

Santos, Monica R., Joan Russo, Gino Aisenberg, Edwina Uehara, Angela Ghesquiere, and Douglas F. Zatzick
2008 Ethnic/Racial Diversity and Posttraumatic Distress in the Acute Care Medical Setting. Psychiatry: Interpersonal and Biological Processes 71(3):234–45.

Schechter, Daniel S., Randall Marshall, Ester Salmán, Deborah Goetz, Sharon Davies, and Michael R. Liebowitz
2000 Ataque de Nervios and History of Childhood Trauma. Journal of Traumatic Stress 13(3):529–34.

Schlenger, William E., Richard A. Kulker, John A. Fairbank, Richard L. Hough, B. Kathleen Jordan, Charles R. Marmar, and Daniel S. Weiss
1992 The Prevalence of Post-Traumatic Stress Disorder in the Vietnam Generation: A Multimethod, Multisource Assessment of Psychiatric Disorder. Journal of Traumatic Stress 5(3):333–63.

Schnurr, Paula P., Carole A. Lunney, and Anjana Sengupta
2004 Risk Factors for the Development Versus Maintenance of Posttraumatic Stress Disorder. Journal of Traumatic Stress 17(2):85–95.

Shih, Regina A., Terry L. Schell, Katrin Hambarsoomian, Howard Belzberg, and Grant Marshall
2010 Prevalence of Posttraumatic Stress Disorder and Major Depression After Trauma Center Hospitalization. Journal of Trauma 69(6):1560–66.

Stampfel, Caroline C., Derek A. Chapman, and Andrea E. Alvarez
2010 Intimate Partner Violence and Posttraumatic Stress Disorder Among High-Risk Women: Does Pregnancy Matter? Violence Against Women 16(4):426–43.

Tolin, David F., and Edna B. Foa
2006 Sex Differences in Trauma and Posttraumatic Stress Disorder: A Quantitative Review of 25 Years of Research. Psychological Bulletin 132(6):959–92.

Triffleman, Elisa G., and Nnamdi Pole
2010 Future Directions in Studies of Trauma Among Ethnoracial and Sexual Minority Samples: Commentary. Journal of Consulting and Clinical Psychology 78(4):490–97.

Tsuang, Ming T., Mauricio Tohen, and Gwendolyn E. P. Zahner
1995 Textbook in Psychiatric Epidemiology. New York: Wiley-Liss.

U.S. Census Bureau
2002 The Hispanic Population in the United States: March 2002. Washington, D.C.: U.S. Census Bureau.

van der Hart, Onno, Jacobien M. van Ochten, Maarten J. M. van Son, Kathy Steele, and Gerty Lensvelt-Mulders
2008 Relations Among Peritraumatic Dissociation and Posttraumatic Stress: A Critical Review. Journal of Trauma and Dissociation 9(4):481–505.

Williams, David R., Selina A. Mohammed, Jacinta Leavell, and Chiquita Collins
2010 Race, Socioeconomic Status, and Health: Complexities, Ongoing Challenges, and Research Opportunities. Annals of the New York Academy of Sciences 1186:69–101.

Yufik, Tom, and Leonard J. Simms
  2010 A Meta-Analytic Investigation of the Structure of Posttraumatic Stress Disorder Symptoms. Journal of Abnormal Psychology 119(4):764–76.
Zatzick, Douglas F., Frederick P. Rivera, Avery B. Nathens, Gregory J. Jurkovich, Jin
      Wang, Ming-Yu Fan, Joan Russo, David S. Salkever, and Ellen J. Mackenzie
  2007 A Nationwide U.S. Study of Post-Traumatic Stress After Hospitalization for
  Physical Injury. Psychological Medicine: A Journal of Research in Psychiatry and
  the Allied Sciences 37(10):1469–80.

CHAPTER 9

Karma to Chromosomes: Studying the Biology of PTSD in a World of Culture

Brandon A. Kohrt, Carol M. Worthman,
and Nawaraj Upadhaya

Four hundred kilometers west of Kathmandu in a rural mountain village, Sushmita spoke to a community health worker. She explained that Maoists had taken over her home during a battle with the Nepal Army. During the firefight, Maoists brought wounded soldiers into her house to tend their injuries. Sushmita stayed locked in her bedroom with her children until Maoists forced their way into the room. The Maoists demanded she boil water for treating the injured. She heard bombs exploding as she went outside. She ran back into the house before getting the water. A Maoist girl soldier threatened to kill her if she did not bring water. Sushmita quickly returned with an overflowing bucket. She repeated this throughout the night. Before daybreak, the Maoists fled.

Four years passed between the battle and Sushmita's recounting to the health worker. Sushmita explained that whenever she sees Nepal Army soldiers, she is worried they will abduct her and beat her for helping the Maoists. "Fear consumes my heart-mind; I think I will die." She avoids going to the bazaar because the path crosses in front of the army barracks. She has difficulty falling asleep. "My heart-mind is empty except for worries. There is no room for happiness because I am filled with worry." She repeatedly has called traditional healers to her house. Their healing ceremonies help for a few weeks, then her worries and pains return.

Others in her community endured similar hardship during the war. However, most of them are not troubled with such suffering. Sushmita blames her continued distress on her bad karma. "Because my grandfather stole others' lands, I must bear this sadness." Sushmita's karma is not the only thing that separates her from other women in her village. She also has higher levels of the stress hormone cortisol when she awakes in the morning.

Sushmita's suffering raises the question of how culture and biology interact to create group differences in posttraumatic stress disorder (PTSD). The goal of this chapter is to investigate biocultural variation related to PTSD risk factors, prevalence, and symptom presentation. We propose a developmental biocultural model to explain group differences in PTSD.

Biocultural Approaches to Human Experience

Theorists create divides between biology and culture, and methods of investigation are often split between cultural and biological research techniques. However, in a holistic view, these divisions—while useful for research—ultimately do not reflect the human condition, which is the product of processes variably labeled as "cultural" and "biological" (Hruschka et al. 2005). Some psychiatrists and anthropologists have argued that culture and biology operate in interactive pathways, neither existing without the other (Kirmayer 2006; Worthman 2009; Worthman and Brown 2005; Worthman and Costello 2009). Culture is a product of human neurobiology, and human neurobiology is shaped by the experience of culture (Alarcon et al. 2002; Kirmayer 2006).

The biocultural perspective has been defined as "a critical and productive dialogue between biological and cultural theories and methods in answering key questions in anthropology" (Hruschka et al. 2005). A biocultural approach is one path toward understanding the experience of PTSD and exploring possible group differences along lines of culture, ethnicity, and other social categories.

In order to warrant a biocultural discussion of PTSD, one must begin with evidence for cultural differences in PTSD. Hinton and Lewis-Fernández (2011) have summarized such group variation. They concluded that while PTSD is generally "valid," that is, it reflects reality of human experience across populations (Kendell and Jablensky 2003), there is considerable cultural variability. Hinton and Lewis-Fernández (2011) highlight cultural differences in the meaning and interpretation of trauma symptoms, the prevalence of the diagnosis across groups, the prevalence of specific symptoms such as those related to avoidance and numbing, the likelihood that a person of one culture will develop PTSD compared to a person of another culture given the same trauma exposure, and the association with nontraumatic stressors. Below we review the existing biological models of PTSD, then we discuss a biocultural framework to explain cultural variability.

Biological Theories of PTSD

Rooted in animal models of conditioning, the heart of dysfunction in PTSD is thought to lie in the fear-learning pathway. Exemplar stimuli in animal models are predator exposure, shocks, and air puffs to the eye (Jovanovic and Ressler 2010; Quirk et al. 2007; Rau and Fanselow 2007). The amygdala is the part of the central nervous system that mediates fear conditioning (Figure 9.1). When an animal in a laboratory setting is exposed to a shock, the amygdala associates that aversive stimuli with other contextual details, such as a preceding tone or the setting (Quirk et al. 2007). The amygdala facilitates emotionally salient traumatic memories (McEwen and Sapolsky 1995). However, the amygdala has different activation based on the salience within a culture (Han and Northoff 2008). For example, there is greater amygdala activity when one sees a fearful expression on an individual within one's cultural group and less amygdala activity when witnessing fear in a person not from one's cultural group (Chiao et al. 2008).

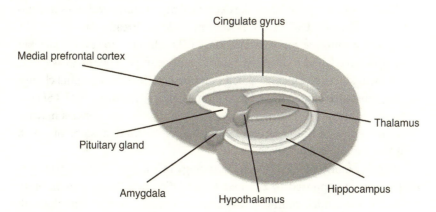

Figure 9.1. Neuroanatomical structures involved in PTSD

The reduction in fear over time—a process that goes awry in PTSD—is mediated by the planning centers of the brain in the prefrontal cortex, which has outputs to inhibit the amygdala (Jovanovic and Ressler 2010). The prefrontal cortex transforms an individual's life history into action plans for acute stressful or traumatic exposures. Based on one framework, the prefrontal cortex is underactive and/or the amygdala is overactive in persons with PTSD (Lanius et al. 2010). This is also an area for individual and cultural difference because the prefrontal cortex will be influenced by prior life experience and salience of events. East Asians and European Americans were found to perceive stimuli differently in regions of the prefrontal cortex (Gutchess et al. 2006). When these two groups viewed the same stimuli, there was differential activation of areas related to object processing, semantic memory, and abstraction. While the significance and implications are unknown, this could influence what types of exposures would be more or less salient as traumatic cues. Differential object processing could influence therapeutic efficacy of PTSD treatments involving imagery and reexperiencing protocols.

In addition to associating danger cues, the amygdala has outputs to the hippocampi (the center of declarative memory consolidation) and the rest of the body via the hypothalamic-pituitary-adrenal axis (HPA), another part of the fight-or-flight response. Some researchers consider damaged hippocampi a key to PTSD (Bremner 2002; Elzinga and Bremner 2002). In Bremner's model, traumatic events trigger the HPA axis, which elevates cortisol levels and causes hippocampal damage. The reduced volume of the hippocampus then theoretically impairs contextual processing and learning. Bremner (2002:61) rests his argument on the decreased hippocampal volumes in combat veterans with PTSD and survivors of child maltreatment with PTSD, when both groups are compared to non-PTSD subjects. However, a number of studies have failed to identify reduced hippocampal volume (Vasterling and Brewin 2005). The inconsistencies may be explained by a gradual change in size, substance abuse, or reduced volume being a risk factor for PTSD but not a result of trauma (Teicher et al. 2003). Or, the inconsistencies may reflect differences in the experience and response to trauma, some of which could vary along cultural lines.

Another model of PTSD locates pathology in low cortisol profiles (hypocortisolism) as opposed to elevated cortisol (Yehuda 2002; Yehuda et al. 1993). In this model, traumatic experiences evoke fear reactions through activation of the amygdala and sympathetic nervous system. Among normal individuals (i.e., those who do not develop PTSD) the HPA axis curbs excess sympathetic activation (Davis and Whalen 2001). For normal subjects, although the memories are highly emotional, the severity is not in a pathological realm that would contribute to later reexperiencing, hyperarousal, and avoidance/numbing—the three clusters of PTSD—because cortisol levels are high enough to moderate the intensity of amygdala activity and memory formation.

Individuals with hypocortisolism are hypothesized to be unable to inhibit this sympathetic activity (Yehuda 2002), thus memories remain vivid and distressing when triggered. The individual suffers overwhelming recollections (flashbacks) and extreme emotional distress comparable to the original experience. Hypocortisolism has been observed among some PTSD populations as well as increased sympathetic activity, suggesting lack of cortisol feedback (Yehuda 2002). However, many studies have failed to replicate findings of low cortisol levels in PTSD patients (van der Kolk 2003; Yehuda 2002). Two large community epidemiological studies find elevated cortisol only among persons with both PTSD and depression (E. Young and Breslau 2004; E. Young et al. 2004). In a meta-analysis, low cortisol was associated with PTSD only among women and those experiencing sexual and/or physical abuse (Meewisse et al. 2007).

Based on our research in Nepal, we were unable to identify any difference in daily salivary cortisol concentration across the day when comparing persons with PTSD against those without the disorder (Figure 9.2, part a). In addition, trauma burden was not associated with any differences in diurnal cortisol (Figure 9.2, part b). However, when the reexperiencing symptoms of cluster B of PTSD are evaluated separately, we see that individuals with intrusive memories and flashbacks had higher levels of cortisol when waking (Figure 9.2 parts c and e). Sushmita, whose case was presented at the beginning of this chapter, was one of the individuals in Nepal who displayed higher levels of cortisol when waking.

In a recent review, Rachel Yehuda (2009) depicts a field plagued with contrasting conclusions about PTSD. She noted that PTSD was associated with lower ambient cortisol levels in thirteen studies and normal or variable levels of cortisol in eight studies. She reported elevated cortisol levels in five studies among persons with PTSD, as we observed in our Nepal sample. Yehuda suggests differing HPA axis functioning may pre-date traumatic exposure rather than be an outcome of it. It may reflect genetic or developmental differences rather than traumatic sequelae.

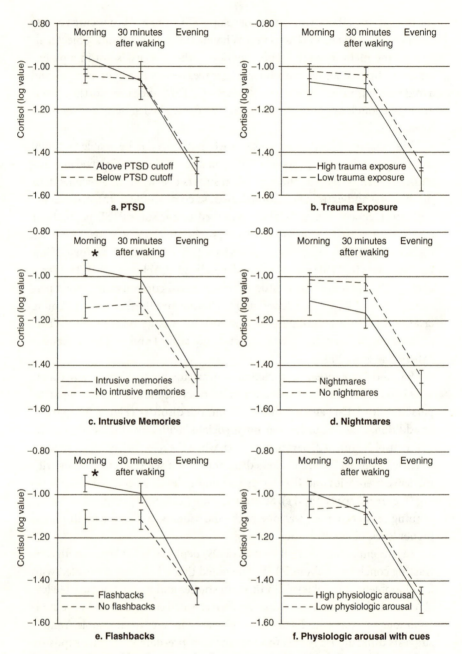

Figure 9.2. Cortisol levels across the day among 119 Nepali adults. Total cortisol samples=1,071. Asterisks denote statistically significant differences in cortisol levels between groups.

Gene-by-environment (GxE) studies are an area of inquiry to explain individual differences in mental health outcomes. Genetic differences (polymorphisms) in a serotonin gene (the serotonin transporter [5-HTT] gene-linked polymorphic region, 5-HTTLPR) confer variable risk to depression and suicide based on high versus low stress and trauma exposure (Caspi et al. 2003). Based on these studies, individuals who carry two copies of the short allele of 5-HTTLPR are at greater risk of depression at higher levels of stress and trauma exposure when compared with person carrying one or two copies of the long allele. The short allele also is associated with greater amygdala activity, which is associated with PTSD (Munafo et al. 2008). The 5-HTTLPR short allele polymorphism also is associated with greater cortisol release to social stressors that include negative appraisals (Way and Taylor 2010). There are genetic differences in other components of the hypothalamic pituitary adrenal axis and cortisol pathway that also appear to confer psychological risk versus resilience in the face of trauma (Binder et al. 2008).

In a review by Caspi and colleagues (2010), forty-four studies of GxE interaction for 5-HTTLRP were identified; nine of these studies examined the childhood maltreatment as the environment stressor. Of the forty-four studies in the review, 89 percent had been in conducted in high-income countries in Europe or English-speaking high-income countries such as United States, Australia, and New Zealand. The only other countries including populations not of European descent were Japan (one study), Korea (two studies), China (one study), and Taiwan (one study). However, none of the studies of child maltreatment as the environmental stressor were conducted with populations of non-European descent. Of note, while the Asian studies in Caspi and colleagues review (2010) represented only 11 percent of studies reviewed, they represented 33 percent of associations in the opposite direction of commonly reported pattern in the literature; that is, the long allele posed greater risk than the short allele (Zhang et al. 2009). Among the 5-HTTLRP studies, the Taiwanese sample was shown to have a greater frequency of the short-short allele combination compared with European groups; they also carry an extra-long variant (XL), which is rare in European groups (Goldman et al. 2010). This raises questions about whether risk and resilience alleles may operate differently across cultural settings. Ultimately, one must be cautious in making any causative claims about ethnic differences in genetic polymorphisms, as there is more variation within ethnic and racial groups than between groups (Brown and Armelagos 2001).

Rather than focusing on static group differences, a life history approach will likely be the key to unlocking group and individual differences in PTSD. Yehuda (2009) concludes her review of PTSD and cortisol biology by calling for more attention to "developmental issues, the longitudinal course of the disorder, and individual differences that affect these processes" (p. 63). The diversity of findings point toward multiple possible pathways to PTSD and a need for better evaluation of personal, contextual, and cultural differences that may be reflected in biological differences.

Biocultural Approaches to PTSD Diversity Across the Life Course

The cultural diversity and biological variability suggest there may be an interaction of cultural processes and biological mechanisms to create the heterogeneity subsumed under the label of PTSD. Rather than group differences explained by genetic polymorphisms, we would argue that the key is cultural context, which shapes the biological response into psychopathology. Unfortunately, to our knowledge, there has been an absence of studies exploring biological differences associated with cultural variation in PTSD. Therefore, our goal is to present a life course model that highlights areas for further research.

Figure 9.3 is a schematic of interacting cultural and biological processes at four time periods: child development, pretrauma, trauma exposure, and posttrauma. Cultural variation in social structures, political policies, conceptions of the body, and social stigma toward trauma survivors influence and are influenced by biological processes to create variation in the individual experience of trauma.

Development

Early child development, including prenatal development, may set the stage for whether or not an adult develops PTSD after exposure to a traumatic event. The prenatal environment influences chronic disease and similarly may confer psychological vulnerability (Worthman and Kuzara 2005). Childhood PTSD influences adult health (Baker et al. 2009), and, child physical health

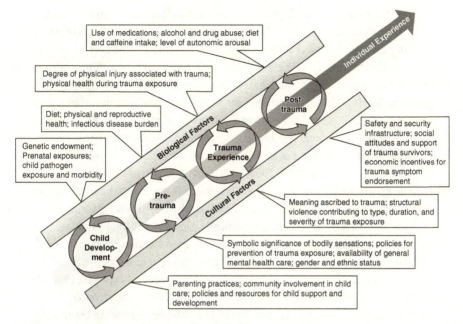

Figure 9.3. Life course biocultural model of trauma experience.

may also influence PTSD vulnerability. Cultural context will influence what impact these biological factors may have. Early childhood stress and trauma increase the risk of PTSD in adults (Binder et al. 2008; Brewin et al. 2000; Friedman et al. 2007; Tolin and Foa 2006), and genetic risk factors appear to be most salient when there is a history of child abuse (Binder et al. 2008).

Anthropologists are interested in how cultural attitudes shape rearing environments, such as cultural beliefs that exacerbate or mitigate child maltreatment. Punjabi families in rural India that regard female children as an unproductive burden direct more violence toward daughters than sons (Pettigrew 1986). Among indigenous Hawaiians, hitting a child is thought to anger ancestral spirits and cause illness in the abuser, and in Papua New Guinea, violence toward children tarnishes a woman's status within the community and is stigmatized (Korbin 2002). Community involvement in child care also improves child mental and physical health outcomes (Earls and Carlson 2001; Earls et al. 2008). Policies that support child development programs such as Head Start and Women, Infants, and Children (WIC) also improve well-being in later life (Beeber et al. 2007; Currie 2009).

The putative PTSD biological marker cortisol may have childhood antecedents of abnormal rhythms. Flinn (2006) found that cortisol levels briefly
rose in response to social stresses and physical illness. However, there was
not a stable and predictable elevation or decline in cortisol among children
exposed to greater psychosocial stressors (Flinn 2009). In Mongolia, caregivers endorsing physical punishment were more likely to have boys with
lower basal cortisol levels (Kohrt et al. 2005a; Kohrt et al. 2014). In Nepal,
homeless street children resembled school children in their cortisol levels,
whereas squatter children and village children displayed hypocortisolism
(Worthman and Panter-Brick 2008). It is unclear which of these profiles confers the greatest PTSD risk. This raises questions about what constitutes an
adverse environment and what is considered a healthy HPA pattern.

Neuroendocrine differences, specifically glucocorticoid physiology, may
be a pretrauma predisposition to PTSD rather than a consequence of it. Children of Holocaust survivors with PTSD and children of women with PTSD
following 9/11 both have hypocortisolism without personal exposure (Yehuda
2009). "The role of glucocorticoid alterations in PTSD pathophysiology may
be more as precipitants or facilitators of the disorder following trauma exposure that as consequences of exposure *per se*" (Yehuda 2009, p. 59).

Developmental psychologists propose that early childhood experience influenced by culture and biology sets the stage for variation in adult behavior
and mental health, and this is mediated through HPA functioning (Bagot
et al. 2007; Ellis et al. 2005; McGowan et al. 2009; Pluess and Belsky 2010).
Neurobiological changes reflect alternate developmental trajectories that
favor survival in conditions of deprivation and violence (Teicher et al. 2003).
Children with difficult temperaments are not inherently on a trajectory to
poor adult well-being. Rather, difficult temperaments in the presence of high
quality parenting result in improved social and academic outcomes over children with easy temperaments (Belsky et al. 2009; Belsky and Pluess 2009;
Pluess and Belsky 2010). However, children with difficult temperaments in
the presence of poor parenting develop negative social, behavioral, and emotional outcomes.

Adaptations in childhood to adversity, which varies across cultures, may
set the stage for vulnerability to psychopathology as adults. Early behavioral
adaptations may manifest later as socioemotional mismatch of person and
environment in adulthood (Pluess and Belsky 2010). For example, increased
environmental sensitivity in early childhood may favor social competence
in high adversity environments (Ellis et al. 2005), but this may lead to

oversensitivity to traumatic events and predisposition to PTSD in adults (Jovanovic and Ressler 2010).

Pretrauma Context

Pretrauma factors are those biocultural factors that place one at risk of trauma exposure and developing PTSD. The symbolic significance and interpretation of bodily sensations may create feedback loops that accentuate distress. For example, in western Nepal, the experience of parasthesia (numbness and tingling) in one's hands, feet, or head can be interpreted as spirit possession (Kohrt et al. 2005b). If an individual has a traumatic experience that is associated with parasthesia (which can easily arise from hyperventilation), this can be a cue that something is spiritually and physically wrong, thus leading to distress-related cognitions.

Hinton and colleagues (2010) describe this process among Cambodian refugees in relation to orthostasis and associated symptoms (lightheadedness and dizziness seemingly resulting in part from a drop in blood pressure). The cultural significance of orthostasis leads to dizziness upon standing resulting in catastrophic cognitions about having a serious disorder of bodily physiology. In an orthostatic challenge, Hinton and colleagues (2010) demonstrated that the severity of drop in systolic blood pressure was associated with greater catastrophic cognitions, flashbacks, and panic symptoms; this process is referred to as biolooping, in which biology and catastrophic cognitions interact to create vicious cycles of worsening. This concept could be further extended as biocultural looping, whereby early disadvantage leads to physical vulnerability to trauma—as well as differential exposure to trauma, resulting in PTSD and poor context for coping posttrauma, which diminishes functioning, and thus heightens vulnerability.

Social, economic, environmental, and occupational policies and legislation play an important role in the exposure to traumatic events. For example, vehicle safety policies minimize automobile collisions. Gun control laws limit exposure to domestic and criminal violence (Killias 1993). Twelve-month prevalence rates of PTSD in the United States are 3.5 percent compared with 0.9 percent in Europe, 0.4 percent in Japan, and 0.7 percent in South Korea (Hinton and Lewis-Fernández 2011); in these latter countries, there is significantly less gun ownership (Krug et al. 1998). The U.S. PTSD prevalence rate is more than threefold greater than other high-income countries, and the U.S. firearm mortality rate is eight times greater than other high-income countries (Krug et al. 1998). Gun ownership rates are correlated with homicide rates internationally (Killias 1993). In Brazil, firearm-related mortality was reduced with the increase in gun control legislation (Marinho de Souza et al. 2007). Drug enforcement and rehabilitation policies also play a role in differential exposure to violence, as has been observed in both the United States and Latin America (Briceno-Leon et al. 2008; Miron 2001). Therefore, cultural differences in social and criminal policies may influence differences in exposure to traumatic events, thus contributing to international variability in PTSD prevalence.

Gender and ethnic status within a culture influence PTSD risk. For example, chronic exposure to nontraumatic stressors such as poverty and discrimination may increase the likelihood of developing PTSD after trauma exposure (Hinton and Lewis-Fernández 2011), as well as the likelihood of being exposed to trauma (Pedersen 2002). In cultures where there is little economic and legal recourse for survivors of domestic violence, women may be at greater risk for PTSD. In the United States there are high rates of PTSD among African Americans in urban centers (Schwartz et al. 2005), which may be associated with the syndemic of poverty, lack of access to mental health care, and racial discrimination.

Biological pretrauma risk factors include diet, physical and reproductive health, and infectious disease burden. These physical stressors may lead to somatic and neurobiologic vulnerability to the somatic sequelae of trauma. The experience of social stressors also may contribute to biological vulnerability through changes in gene transcription (Cole et al. 2007). Social stress contributes to higher rates of infectious disease, higher cortisol levels, and more chronic diseases such as diabetes and heart disease (Lupien et al. 2000; Sapolsky et al. 2000). Social support is associated with lower cortisol levels and better health outcomes (Cacioppo et al. 2002).

Traumatic Experiences

Cultural differences are also related to biological and cultural differences in the trauma experiences. In a cultural group, the type, duration, and severity of a trauma will vary based on social, political, economic, and health structures. In Nepal, obstetric trauma is prevalent because of the lack of salaried trained health workers in many rural areas (Maes et al. 2010). In the United

States an individual is likely to experience gun violence or an automobile accident. In Liberia, domestic violence and other gender-based violence was widespread during the war owing to the collapse of infrastructure to prevent perpetration (K. Johnson et al. 2008). Thus, cultural context influences the trauma landscape.

Taking the type of traumatic event and posttraumatic context into account, it is not surprising that the symptom profile across cultures may be very different, even when using the same instrument that has been validated cross-culturally. We found that when using the Child PTSD Symptom Scale (CPSS) to assess trauma-affected children, the PTSD symptoms associated with impairment vary significantly across cultural and traumatic context. PTSD symptom discriminant validity varied significantly between children exposed to civil war in Nepal (Kohrt et al. 2011) and children exposed to an earthquake in the United States (Foa et al. 2001). In the original U.S. sample, the six items with lowest discriminant validity included traumatic amnesia and foreshortened future—items that showed the strongest validity in the Nepali children. Moreover, the three items that showed the strongest validity in the American youth sample performed poorly in the Nepali sample: distress with reminders, less interest in activities, and overly careful.

It is unclear whether this is due to the nature of trauma studied—a single earthquake in California versus a decade of war in Nepal—or other cultural differences. In Nepal, avoidance of sites of political violence is likely a behavior of both healthy and impaired children. In our focus groups in Nepal, children described how all children engaged in avoidance behaviors regardless of mental health issues. This is supported by ethnographic accounts of children in Nepal during the civil war (Pettigrew 2007). Moreover, there are also cultural factors at play. In Nepal, children and adults, regardless of mental health status, told us that *bhut* (ghosts/spirits) afflicted the sites where war atrocities had occurred. Therefore, all individuals avoided those sites. This has been reported in Rwanda as well, where avoidance is common among all children because of belief systems related to genocide atrocity sites (Neugebauer et al. 2009). Ultimately, it is crucial to undertake mixed methods qualitative and quantitative PTSD assessment tool adaptation and validation to determine which symptoms discriminate between those with and without psychosocial impairment (Kohrt et al. 2011; Van Ommeren et al. 1999) (Table 9.1).

The types of trauma experienced will also have biological influences. Traumas that involve bodily harm are more likely to produce aberrations in

Table 9.1. Differences in PTSD Symptoms That Discriminate Between Children with High and Low Functional Impairment Associated with Trauma Exposure

	American children exposed to an earthquake (Foa et al. 2001)	Nepali children exposed to civil war (Kohrt et al. 2011)
Symptoms with *high* PTSD discriminant validity	• distress with reminders[a] • less interest in activities[a] • overly careful[a]	• nightmares • flashbacks • traumatic amnesia[b] • foreshortened future[b] • easily angered/ irritated
Symptoms with *low* PTSD discriminant validity	• traumatic amnesia[b] • emotionally distant • restricted affect • foreshortened future[b] • insomnia • easily startled	• intrusive thoughts • distress with reminders[a] • avoiding activities • less interest in activities[a] • overly careful[a] • easily startled

[a] Items with high PTSD discriminant validity for American children exposed to an earthquake but with low discriminant validity for Nepali children exposed to civil war.
[b] Items with high PTSD discriminant validity for Nepali children exposed to civil war but with low discriminant validity for American children exposed to an earthquake.

cortisol whereas traumas without injury are not associated with differences in cortisol secretion (Delahanty et al. 2003) based on our current limited data on nonphysical traumatic events. One's physical health during trauma exposure also plays a role. Hinton and colleagues (2010) write that Cambodian survivors of trauma were often malnourished and dehydrated related to prolonged forced labor, and that this often caused dizziness. Therefore, the experience of orthostasis, as mentioned above, reminds them of the context in which trauma occurred, and also dizziness itself serves as a trauma cue.

The cultural meaning ascribed to a traumatic event may play a significant role in the development and severity of psychological sequelae. Survivors of torture who had identified an ideological reason for their persecution reported fewer PTSD symptoms (Basoglu et al. 1996; Holtz 1998; Kanninen et al. 2002). In Nepal, voluntarily associated child soldiers had lower levels of distress after traumatic exposure than children forcibly conscripted (Kohrt et al. 2010a). Hinton and Lewis-Fernández's review (2011) summarizes studies of Tibetan refugees that suggest witnessing destruction of religious artifacts may be more traumatic than suffering personal injury (Sachs et al. 2008; Terheggen et al. 2001). The cultural differences in meaning may be mediated through different levels of physical arousal during the traumatic event. If an event, such as destruction of Buddhist artifacts, has special religious significance, it may produce a greater activation on emotional centers in the amygdala, less inhibition from the frontal cortex, and then more disruption of hippocampal activity.

Posttrauma Context

There is increasing evidence that posttrauma context is profoundly influential on the development, severity, and duration of PTSD symptoms. Survivors of trauma in settings of livelihood insecurity and political instability are at greater risk of PTSD (de Jong et al. 2001). Daily stressors mediate the impact of trauma events on current psychosocial distress (Miller and Rasmussen 2010). Social support consistently protects against PTSD in humans (Brewin et al. 2000; Ozer et al. 2003). Negative homecoming experiences among Vietnam veterans were a crucial determinant of who developed PTSD (Fontana and Rosenheck 1994; D. Johnson et al. 1997). Former child soldiers in Nepal explained that their war experiences were not traumatic for them; the return home to unwelcoming families was far more threatening (Kohrt et al. 2010b). Traumatic events in Nepal are commonly seen as the consequences of deeds in previous lives that are transmitted through karma into misfortune in the present life (Kohrt and Hruschka 2010), as described by Sushmita at the beginning of this chapter.

According to Bista (1991), karma is the unalterable consequence of one's prior misdeeds. Families may be reluctant to acknowledge or seek help for traumatized relatives because it reflects badly on the family's and ancestors' piety. The burden of blame typically falls on women, who have poorer karma by virtue of not being born as men (Bennett 1983). Families and communities often blame and ostracize widows for the deaths of their husbands (Dahal 2008). Interestingly, attributing trauma to karma predicts greater risk of PTSD among North American participants (Davidson et al. 2005). The importance of social contact in relation to development of posttraumatic behavioral and physiological changes has also been observed in animals. Social isolation after social stressors place organisms at tremendous risk of physiological changes in animal models of PTSD, while socially housed animals do not display severe physiological changes after stress exposures (Buwalda et al. 2005).

Whereas lack of social support and cultural models of blame may influence posttraumatic distress, pecuniary motives contribute to pursuit of a PTSD label. Economic changes and other forms of compensation influence endorsement of distress after a traumatic event as Allan Young (1995) has outlined describing the history of the PTSD diagnosis. The secondary gain from psychological trauma was central to theories of psychiatric complaints as an excusal from military action (McNally 2003; Summerfield 2001; A. Young 1995). Women in Sri Lanka who used posttraumatic stress labels and trauma narratives of suffering were also the people most likely to pursue monetary compensation from the government for disappeared male relatives (Argenti-Pillen 2003). In the political asylum system, PTSD is nearly requisite as evidence of torture (Bracken et al. 1995; Summerfield 1999). From automobile collisions to overhearing sexual jokes in the workplace, identifying with the discourse of psychological trauma may provide the foundation for compensation (Kontorovich 2001).

Symptoms and severity will vary based on the biological milieu. For example, use of alcohol and other drugs is likely to impair recovery from the social and biological sequelae of PTSD (Flynn and Brown 2008). Moreover, being in an environment where one is perpetually in a state of arousal will lead to prolongation of PTSD symptoms and impairment (Hinton and Lewis-Fernández 2011; Miller and Rasmussen 2010).

There can be significant meaning to continued experience of symptoms or resistance to treatment. Researchers working with veterans and refugees have reported that PTSD symptoms can be a form of bonding and social connection with others, whereas recovering may be seen as neglecting the suffering and loss of others. A Vietnam veteran explained, "I do not want to take drugs for my nightmares, because I must remain a memorial to my dead friends" (Caruth 1995:vii). Similarly, among Cambodian refugees, "remembering, despite the pain it causes, constitutes a political activity that protests injustice and inhumanity. In such circumstances, forgetting is unthinkable" (Becker et al. 2000:341). As with grief, this may represent one of many possible coping mechanisms (Bonanno 2004), which could be reflected in lower physiological distress despite participation in the narrative of suffering.

Conclusion

To best understand the suffering associated with PTSD and work toward its alleviation, it is important to understand the disorder in a biocultural framework. Treating culture and biology as separate independent processes will produce incomplete and possibly misleading interpretations. An interactive model that examines how biology and culture coproduce life experience, including PTSD, is optimal for elucidating risk and recovery factors. Given the wide range of biological findings in PTSD in relation to the HPA axis, it is improbable that there is a unitary PTSD biological profile. Instead, there are likely different pathways produced through variations in developmental environments, pretrauma context, types and meanings of traumatic experiences, and circumstances after traumatic exposures. Through better contextualization of traumatic experiences, not only will we have more accurate biocultural models, but ultimately we ideally will promote effective treatment and prevention of PTSD for children, women, and men across cultures, settings, and context.

Acknowledgments

The first author was supported by a National Institute of Mental Health National Research Service Award (F31 MH075584) and a Wenner-Gren Foundation Doctoral Dissertation Improvement Grant (GR7473). The authors gratefully acknowledge Gary Carbell for his insightful comments in the revision of this manuscript.

References

Alarcon, Renato D., Margarita Alegria, Carl C. Bell, Cheryl Boyce, Laurence J. Kirmayer, Keh-Ming Lin, Steven Lopez, Bedirhan Ustun, and Katherine L. Wisner
2002 Beyond the Funhouse Mirrors: Research Agenda on Culture and Psychiatric Diagnosis. In A Research Agenda for DSM-V. David J. Kupfer, Michael B. First, and Darrel A. Reiger, eds. Pp. 219–81. Washington, D.C.: American Psychiatric Press.

Argenti-Pillen, Alex
   2003 Masking Terror: How Women Contain Violence in Southern Sri Lanka. Phila-
      delphia: University of Pennsylvania Press.
Bagot, Rosemary, Carine Parent, Timothy W. Bredy, Tieyann Zhang, Alain Gratton,
      and Michael J. Meaney
   2007 Developmental Origins of Neurobiological Vulnerability for PTSD. *In* Under-
      standing Trauma: Integrating Biological, Clinical, and Cultural Perspectives.
      Laurence J. Kirmayer, Robert Lemelson, and Mark Barad, eds. Pp. 98–117. New
      York: Cambridge University Press.
Baker, Charlene K., Fran H. Norris, Eric C. Jones, and Arthur D. Murphy
   2009 Childhood Trauma and Adulthood Physical Health in Mexico. Journal of Be-
      havioral Medicine 32(3):255–69.
Basoglu, Metin, Erdogan Ozmen, Dogan Sahin, Murat Paker, Ozgun Tasdemir, Ayten
      Ceyhanli, Cem Incesu, and Nusin Sarimurat
   1996 Appraisal of Self, Social Environment, and State Authority as a Possible Me-
      diator of Posttraumatic Stress Disorder in Tortured Political Activists. Journal of
      Abnormal Psychology 105(2):232–36.
Becker, Gay, Yewoubdar Beyene, and Pauline Ken
   2000 Memory, Trauma, and Embodied Distress: The Management of Disruption in
      the Stories of Cambodians in Exile. Ethos 28(3):320–45.
Beeber, Linda S., Rachel Chazan-Cohen, Jane Squires, Brenda J. Harden, Neil W. Bo-
      ris, Sherryl S. Heller, and Neena M. Malik
   2007 The Early Promotion and Intervention Research Consortium (E-PIRC): Five
      Approaches to Improving Infant/Toddler Mental Health in Early Head Start. In-
      fant Mental Health Journal 28(2):130–50.
Belsky, Jay, C. Jonassaint, Michael Pluess, M. Stanton, B. Brummett, and R. Williams
   2009 Vulnerability Genes or Plasticity Genes? Molecular Psychiatry 14(8):746–54.
Belsky, Jay, and Michael Pluess
   2009 Beyond Diathesis Stress: Differential Susceptibility to Environmental Influ-
      ences. Psychological Bulletin 135(6):885–908.
Bennett, Lynn
   1983 Dangerous Wives and Sacred Sisters: Social and Symbolic Roles of High-Caste
      Women in Nepal. New York: Columbia University Press.
Binder, Elisabeth B., Rebekah G. Bradley, Wei Liu, Michael P. Epstein, Todd C. De-
      veau, Kristina B. Mercer, Yilang Tang, Charles F. Gillespie, Christine M. Heim,
      Charles B. Nemeroff, Ann C. Schwartz, Joseph F. Cubells, and Kerry J. Ressler
   2008 Association of FKBP5 Polymorphisms and Childhood Abuse with Risk of
      Posttraumatic Stress Disorder Symptoms in Adults. Journal of the American
      Medical Association 299(11):1291–305.
Bista, Dor Bahadur
   1991 Fatalism and Development. Calcutta: Orient Longman.

Bonanno, George A.

2004 Loss, Trauma, and Human Resilience: Have We Underestimated the Human Capacity to Thrive After Extremely Aversive Events? American Psychologist 59(1):20–28.

Bracken, Patrick J., Joan E. Giller, and Derek Summerfield

1995 Psychological Responses to War and Atrocity: The Limitations of Current Concepts. Social Science and Medicine 40(8):1073–82.

Bremner, J. Douglas

2002 Does Stress Damage the Brain? Understanding Trauma-Related Disorders from a Mind-Body Perspective. New York: W. W. Norton.

Brewin, Chris R., Bernice Andrews, and John D. Valentine

2000 Meta-Analysis of Risk Factors for Posttraumatic Stress Disorder in Trauma-Exposed Adults. Journal of Consulting and Clinical Psychology 68(5):748–66.

Briceno-Leon, Roberto, Andres Villaveces, and Alberto Concha-Eastman

2008 Understanding the Uneven Distribution of the Incidence of Homicide in Latin America. International Journal of Epidemiology 37(4):751–57.

Brown, Ryan A., and George J. Armelagos

2001 Apportionment of Racial Diversity: A Review. Evolutionary Anthropology 10(1):34–40.

Buwalda, Bauke, Maarten H. P. Kole, Alexa H. Veenema, Mark Huininga, Sietse F. de Boer, S. Mechiel Korte, and Jaap M. Koolhaas

2005 Long-Term Effects of Social Stress on Brain and Behavior: A Focus on Hippocampal Functioning. Neuroscience and Biobehavioral Reviews 29(1):83–97.

Cacioppo, John T., Louise C. Hawkley, L. Elizabeth Crawford, John M. Ernst, Mary H. Burleson, Ray B. Kowalewski, William B. Malarkey, Eve Van Cauter, and Gary G. Berntson

2002 Loneliness and Health: Potential Mechanisms. Psychosomatic Medicine 64(3):407–17.

Caruth, Cathy, ed.

1995 Trauma : Explorations in Memory. Baltimore: Johns Hopkins University Press.

Caspi, A., K. Sugden, T. E. Moffitt, A. Taylor, I. W. Craig, H. Harrington, J. McClay, J. Mill, J. Martin, A. Braithwaite, and R. Poulton

2003 Influence of Life Stress on Depression: Moderation by a Polymorphism in the 5-HTT Gene . Science 301(5631):386–89.

Caspi, Avshalom, Ahmad R. Hariri, Andrew Holmes, Rudolf Uher, and Terrie E. Moffitt

2010 Genetic Sensitivity to the Environment: The Case of the Serotonin Transporter Gene and Its Implications for Studying Complex Diseases and Traits. American Journal of Psychiatry 167(5):509–27.

Chiao, Joan Y., Tetsuya Iidaka, Heather L. Gordon, Junpei Nogawa, Moshe Bar, Elissa Aminoff, Norihiro Sadato, and Nalini Ambady

2008 Cultural Specificity in Amygdala Response to Fear Faces. Journal of Cognitive Neuroscience 20(12):2167–74.

Cole, Steve W., Louise C. Hawkley, Jesusa M. Arevalo, Caroline Y. Sung, Robert M. Rose, and John T. Cacioppo

2007 Social Regulation of Gene Expression in Human Leukocytes. Genome Biology 8(9):R189.

Currie, Janet

2009 Policy Interventions to Address Child Health Disparities: Moving Beyond Health Insurance. Pediatrics 124 (Suppl 3):S246–54.

Dahal, Kapil Babu

2008 Medical Anthropology in Nepal. Innovia Foundation Newsletter 6:7–9.

Davidson, Jonathan R. T., Kathryn M. Connor, and Li-Ching Lee

2005 Beliefs in Karma and Reincarnation Among Survivors of Violent Trauma—A Community Survey. Social Psychiatry and Psychiatric Epidemiology 40(2): 120–25.

Davis, Michael, and Paul J. Whalen

2001 The Amygdala: Vigilance and Emotion. Molecular Psychiatry 6(1):13–34.

de Jong, Joop T., Ivan H. Komproe, Mark Van Ommeren, Mustafa El Masri, Mesfin Araya, Noureddine Khaled, Willem van De Put, and Daya Somasundaram

2001 Lifetime Events and Posttraumatic Stress Disorder in 4 Postconflict Settings. Journal of the American Medical Association 286(5):555–62.

Delahanty, Douglas L., A. Jay Raimonde, Eileen Spoonster, and Michael Cullado

2003 Injury Severity, Prior Trauma History, Urinary Cortisol Levels, and Acute PTSD in Motor Vehicle Accident Victims. Journal of Anxiety Disorders 17(2): 149–64.

Earls, Felton, and Mary Carlson

2001 The Social-Ecology of Child Health and Wellbeing. Annual Review of Public Health 22:143–66.

Earls, Felton, Giuseppe J. Raviola, and Mary Carlson

2008 Promoting Child and Adolescent Mental Health in the Context of the HIV/ AIDS Pandemic with a Focus on Sub-Saharan Africa. Journal of Child Psychology and Psychiatry and Allied Disciplines 49(3):295–312.

Ellis, Bruce J., Marilyn J. Essex, and W. Thomas Boyce

2005 Biological Sensitivity to Context: II. Empirical Explorations of an Evolutionary-Developmental Theory. Development and Psychopathology 17(2):303–28.

Elzinga, Bernet, and J. Douglas Bremner

2002 Are the Neural Substrates of Memory the Final Common Pathway in Post-traumatic Stress Disorder (PTSD)? Journal of Affective Disorders 70(1):1–17.

Flinn, Mark V.

2006 Evolution and Ontogeny of Stress Response to Social Challenges in the Human Child. Developmental Review 26(2):138–74.

2009 Are Cortisol Profiles a Stable Trait During Child Development? American Journal of Human Biology 21(6):769–71.

Flynn, Patrick M., and Barry S. Brown
2008 Co-Occurring Disorders in Substance Abuse Treatment: Issues and Prospects. Journal of Substance Abuse Treatment 34(1):36–47.

Foa, Edna B., Kelly M. Johnson, Norah C. Feeny, and Kimberli R. Treadwell
2001 The Child PTSD Symptom Scale: A Preliminary Examination of Its Psychometric Properties. Journal of Clinical Child Psychology 30(3):376–84.

Fontana, Alan, and Robert Rosenheck
1994 Posttraumatic Stress Disorder Among Vietnam Theater Veterans. A Causal Model of Etiology in a Community Sample. Journal of Nervous and Mental Disease 182(12):677–84.

Friedman, Matthew J., John Jalowiec, Gregory McHugo, Sheila Wang, and Annmarie McDonagh
2007 Adult Sexual Abuse Is Associated with Elevated Neurohormone Levels Among Women with PTSD Due to Childhood Sexual Abuse. Journal of Traumatic Stress 20(4):611–17.

Goldman, Noreen, Dana A. Glei, Yu-Hsuan Lin, and Maxine Weinstein
2010 The Serotonin Transporter Polymorphism (5-HTTLPR): Allelic Variation and Links with Depressive Symptoms. Depression and Anxiety 27(3):260–69.

Gutchess, Angela H., Robert C. Welsh, Aysecan Boduroglu, and Denise C. Park
2006 Cultural Differences in Neural Function Associated with Object Processing. Cognitive Affective and Behavioral Neuroscience 6(2):102–9.

Han, Shihui H., and Georg Northoff
2008 Culture-Sensitive Neural Substrates of Human Cognition: A Transcultural Neuroimaging Approach. Nature Reviews Neuroscience 9(8):646–54.

Hinton, Devon E., Stefan G. Hofmann, Scott P. Orr, Roger K. Pitman, Mark H. Pollack, and Nnamdi Pole
2010 A Psychobiocultural Model of Orthostatic Panic Among Cambodian Refugees: Flashbacks, Catastrophic Cognitions, and Reduced Orthostatic Blood-Pressure Response. Psychological Trauma—Theory, Research, Practice, and Policy 2(1):63–70.

Hinton, Devon E., and Roberto Lewis-Fernández
2011 The Cross-Cultural Validity of Posttraumatic Stress Disorder: Implications for DSM-5. Depression and Anxiety 28(9):783–801

Holtz, Timothy H.
1998 Refugee Trauma Versus Torture Trauma: A Retrospective Controlled Cohort Study of Tibetan Refugees. Journal of Nervous and Mental Disease 186(1):24–34.

Hruschka, Daniel J., Daniel H. Lende, and Carol R. M. Worthman
2005 Biocultural Dialogues: Biology and Culture in Psychological Anthropology. Ethos 33(1):1–19.

Johnson, David R., Hadar Lubin, Robert Rosenheck, Alan Fontana, Steven Southwick, and Dennis Charney

1997 The Impact of the Homecoming Reception on the Development of Posttraumatic Stress Disorder: The West Haven Homecoming Stress Scale (WHHSS). Journal of Traumatic Stress 10(2):259–77.

Johnson, Kirsten, Jana Asher, Stephanie Rosborough, Amisha Raja, Rajesh Panjabi, Charles Beadling, and Lynn Lawry

2008 Association of Combatant Status and Sexual Violence with Health and Mental Health Outcomes in Postconflict Liberia. Journal of the American Medical Association 300(6):676–90.

Jovanovic, Tanja, and Kerry J. Ressler

2010 How the Neurocircuitry and Genetics of Fear Inhibition May Inform Our Understanding of PTSD. American Journal of Psychiatry 167(6):648–62.

Kanninen, Katri, Raija-Leena Punamaki, and Samir Qouta

2002 The Relation of Appraisal, Coping Efforts, and Acuteness of Trauma to PTS Symptoms Among Former Political Prisoners. Journal of Traumatic Stress 15(3):245–53.

Kendell, Robert, and Assen Jablensky

2003 Distinguishing Between the Validity and Utility of Psychiatric Diagnoses. American Journal of Psychiatry 160(1):4–12.

Killias, Martin

1993 International Correlations Between Gun Ownership and Rates of Homicide and Suicide. CMAJ: Canadian Medical Association Journal 148(10):1721–25.

Kirmayer, Laurence J.

2006 Beyond the New Cross-Cultural Psychiatry: Cultural Biology, Discursive Psychology and the Ironies of Globalization. Transcultural Psychiatry 43(1):126–44.

Kohrt, Brandon A., and Daniel J. Hruschka

2010 Nepali Concepts of Psychological Trauma: The Role of Idioms of Distress, Ethnopsychology and Ethnophysiology in Alleviating Suffering and Preventing Stigma. Culture, Medicine and Psychiatry 34(2):322–52.

Kohrt, Brandon A., Daniel J. Hruschka, Holbrook E. Kohrt, Victor G. Carrion, Irwin D. Waldman, and Carol M. Worthman

2014 Child Abuse, Disruptive Behavior Disorders, Depression, and Salivary Cortisol Levels Among Institutionalized and Community-Residing Boys in Mongolia. Asia-Pacific Psychiatry. doi. 10.1111/appy.12141

Kohrt, Brandon A., Daniel J. Hruschka, Richard D. Kunz, Holbrook E. Kohrt, Victor G. Carrion, and Carol M. Worthman

2005a Low Cortisol Levels and Disruptive Behaviors in Mongolian and Nepali boys. Foundation for Psychocultural Research, University of California, Los Angeles.

Kohrt, Brandon A., Mark J. D. Jordans, Wietse A. Tol, Nagendra P. Luitel, Sujen M. Maharjan, and Nawaraj Upadhaya

2011 Validation of Cross-Cultural Child Mental Health and Psychosocial Research Instruments: Adapting the Depression Self-Rating Scale and Child PTSD Symptom Scale in Nepal. BMC Psychiatry 11(1):e127.

Kohrt, Brandon A., Mark J. D. Jordans, Wietse A. Tol, Em Perera, Rohit Karki, Suraj Koirala, and Nawaraj Upadhaya

2010a Social Ecology of Child Soldiers: Child, Family, and Community Determinants of Mental Health, Psychosocial Well-Being, and Reintegration in Nepal. Transcultural Psychiatry 47(5):727–53.

Kohrt, Brandon A., Richard D. Kunz, Jennifer L. Baldwin, Naba R. Koirala, Vidya D. Sharma, and Mahendra K. Nepal

2005b "Somatization" and "Comorbidity": A Study of Jhum-Jhum and Depression in Rural Nepal. Ethos 33(1):125–47.

Kohrt, Brandon A., Wietse A. Tol, Judith Pettigrew, and Rohit Karki

2010b Children and Revolution: The Mental Health and Psychosocial Wellbeing of Child Soldiers in Nepal's Maoist Army. In The War Machine and Global Health. Merrill Singer and G. Derrick Hodge, eds. Pp. 89–116. Lanham, Md.: Rowan and Littlefield.

Kontorovich, Eugene

2001 The Mitigation of Emotional Distress Damages. University of Chicago Law Review 68(2):491–520.

Korbin, Jill E.

2002 Culture and Child Maltreatment: Cultural Competence and Beyond. Child Abuse and Neglect 26(6–7):637–44.

Krug, Etienne G., Kenneth E. Powell, and Linda L. Dahlberg

1998 Firearm-Related Deaths in the United States and 35 Other High- and Upper-Middle-Income Countries. International Journal of Epidemiology 27(2):214–21.

Lanius, Ruth A., Eric Vermetten, Richard J. Loewenstein, Bethany Brand, Christian Schmahl, J. Douglas Bremner, and David Spiegel

2010 Emotion Modulation in PTSD: Clinical and Neurobiological Evidence for a Dissociative Subtype. American Journal of Psychiatry 167(6):640–47.

Lupien, Sonia J., Suzanne King, Michael J. Meaney, and Bruce S. McEwen

2000 Child's Stress Hormone Levels Correlate with Mother's Socioeconomic Status and Depressive State. Biological Psychiatry 48(10):976–80.

Maes, Kenneth C., Brandon A. Kohrt, and Svea Closser

2010 Culture, Status and Context in Community Health Worker Pay: Pitfalls and Opportunities for Policy Research. A Commentary on Glenton et al. (2010). Social Science and Medicine 71(8):1375–78; discussion 1379–80.

Marinho de Souza, Maria de Fatima, James Macinko, Airlane Pereira Alencar, Deborah Carvalho Malta, and Otaliba Libanio de Morais Neto

2007 Reductions in Firearm-Related Mortality and Hospitalizations in Brazil after Gun Control. Health Affairs 26(2):575–84.

McEwen, Bruce S., and Robert M. Sapolsky
    1995 Stress and Cognitive Function. Current Opinion in Neurobiology 5(2): 205–16.
McGowan, Patrick O., Aya Sasaki, Ana C. D'Alessio, Sergiy Dymov, Benoit Labonte, Moshe Szyf, Gustavo Turecki, and Michael J. Meaney
    2009 Epigenetic Regulation of the Glucocorticoid Receptor in Human Brain Associates with Childhood Abuse Nature Neuroscience 12(3):342–48.
McNally, Richard J.
    2003 Progress and Controversy in the Study of Posttraumatic Stress Disorder. Annual Review of Psychology 54:229–52.
Meewisse, Marie-Louise, Johannes B. Reitsma, Giel-Jan de Vries, Berthold P. R. Gersons, and Miranda Olff
    2007 Cortisol and Post-Traumatic Stress Disorder in Adults: Systematic Review and Meta-Analysis. British Journal of Psychiatry 191:387–92.
Miller, Kenneth E., and Andrew Rasmussen
    2010 War Exposure, Daily Stressors, and Mental Health in Conflict and Post-Conflict Settings: Bridging the Divide Between Trauma-Focused and Psychosocial Frameworks. Social Science and Medicine 70(1):7–16.
Miron, Jeffrey A.
    2001 Violence, Guns, and Drugs: A Cross-Country Analysis. Journal of Law and Economics 44(2):615–33.
Munafo, Marcus R., Sarah M. Brown, and Ahmad R. Hariri
    2008 Serotonin Transporter (5-HTTLPR) Genotype and Amygdala Activation: A Meta-Analysis. Biological Psychiatry 63(9):852–57.
Neugebauer, Richard, Prudence W. Fisher, J. Blake Turner, Saori Yamabe, Julia A. Sarsfield, and Tasha Stehling-Ariza
    2009 Post-Traumatic Stress Reactions Among Rwandan Children and Adolescents in the Early Aftermath of Genocide. International Journal of Epidemiology 38(4):1033–45.
Ozer, Emily J., Suzanne R. Best, Tami L. Lipsey, and Daniel S. Weiss
    2003 Predictors of Posttraumatic Stress Disorder and Symptoms in Adults: A Meta-Analysis. Psychological Bulletin 129(1):52–73.
Pedersen, Duncan
    2002 Political Violence, Ethnic Conflict, and Contemporary Wars: Broad Implications for Health and Social Well-Being. Social Science and Medicine 55(2):175–90.
Pettigrew, Judith
    1986 Child Neglect in Rural Punjabi Families. Journal of Comparative Family Studies 17(1):63–85.
    2007 Learning to Be Silent: Change, Childhood and Mental Health in the Maoist Insurgency in Nepal. In Nepalis Inside and Outside Nepal: Political and Social Transformations. H. Ishi, David N. Gellner, and K. Nawa, eds. Pp. 307–84. Japanese Studies on South Asia. New Delhi: Manohar.

Pluess, Michael, and Jay Belsky
    2010 Differential Susceptibility to Parenting and Quality Child Care. Developmen-
    tal Psychology 46(2):379–90.
Quirk, Gregory J., Mohammed R. Milad, Edwin Santini, and Kelimer Lebron
    2007 Learning Not to Fear: A Neural Systems Approach. *In* Understanding
    Trauma: Integrating Biological, Clinical, and Cultural Perspectives. Laurence J.
    Kirmayer, Robert Lemelson, and Mark Barad, Eds. Pp. 60–77. New York: Cam-
    bridge University Press.
Rau, Vinuta, and Michael S. Fanselow
    2007 Neurobiological and Neuroethological Perspectives on Fear and Anxiety. *In*
    Understanding Trauma: Integrating Biological, Clinical, and Cultural Perspec-
    tives. Laurence J. Kirmayer, Robert Lemelson, and Mark Barad, eds. Pp. 27–40.
    New York: Cambridge University Press.
Sachs, Emily, Barry Rosenfeld, Dechen Lhewa, Andrew Rasmussen, and Allen Keller
    2008 Entering Exile: Trauma, Mental Health, snd Coping Among Tibetan Refugees
    Arriving in Dharamsala, India. Journal of Traumatic Stress 21(2):199–208.
Sapolsky, Robert M., L. Michael Romero, and Allan U. Munck
    2000 How Do Glucocorticoids Influence Stress Responses? Integrating Permissive,
    Suppressive, Stimulatory, and Preparative Actions. Endocrine Reviews 21(1):55–89.
Schwartz, Ann C., Rebekah L. Bradley, Melissa Sexton, Alissa Sherry, and Kerry J.
    Ressler
    2005 Posttraumatic Stress Disorder Among African Americans in an Inner City
    Mental Health Clinic. Psychiatric Services 56(2):212–15.
Summerfield, Derek A.
    1999 A Critique of Seven Assumptions Behind Psychological Trauma Programmes
    in War-Affected Areas. Social Science and Medicine 48(10):1449–62.
    2001 The Invention of Post-Traumatic Stress Disorder and the Social Usefulness of
    a Psychiatric Category. British Medical Journal 322(7278):95–98.
Teicher, Martin H., Susan L. Andersen, Ann Polcari, Carl M. Anderson, Carryl P. Na-
    valta, and Dennis M. Kim
    2003 The Neurobiological Consequences of Early Stress and Childhood Maltreat-
    ment. Neuroscience and Biobehavioral Reviews 27(1–2):33–44.
Terheggen, Maaike A., Margaret S. Stroebe, and Rolf J. Kleber
    2001 Western Conceptualizations and Eastern Experience: A Cross-Cultural Study
    of Traumatic Stress Reactions Among Tibetan Refugees in India. Journal of
    Traumatic Stress 14(2):391–403.
Tolin, David F., and Edna B. Foa
    2006 Sex Differences in Trauma and Posttraumatic Stress Disorder: A Quantitative
    Review of 25 Years of Research. Psychological Bulletin 132(6):959–92.
van der Kolk, Bessel A.
    2003 The Neurobiology of Childhood Trauma and Abuse. Child and Adolescent
    Psychiatric Clinics of North America 12(2):293–317.

Van Ommeren, Mark, Bhogendra Sharma, Suraj Thapa, Ramesh Makaju, Dinesh Pra-
    sain, Rabindra Bhattaria, and Joop T. V. M. de Jong
    1999 Preparing Instruments for Transcultural Research: Use of the Translation
    Monitoring Form with Nepali-Speaking Bhutanese. Transcultural Psychiatry
    36(3):285–301.
Vasterling, Jennifer J., and Chris Brewin
    2005 Neuropsychology of PTSD : Biological, Cognitive, and Clinical Perspectives.
    New York: Guilford Press.
Way, Baldwin M., and Shelley E. Taylor
    2010 The Serotonin Transporter Promoter Polymorphism Is Associated with Corti-
    sol Response to Psychosocial Stress. Biological Psychiatry 67(5):487–92.
Worthman, Carol M.
    2009 Habits of the Heart: Life History and the Developmental Neuroendocrinology
    of Emotion. American Journal of Human Biology 21(6):772–81.
Worthman, Carol M., and Ryan A. Brown
    2005 A Biocultural Life History Approach to the Developmental Psychobiology of
    Male Aggression. In Developmental Psychobiology of Aggression. David M. Stoff
    and Elizabeth J. Susman, eds. Pp. 187–221. New York: Cambridge University Press.
Worthman, Carol M., and E. Jane Costello
    2009 Tracking Biocultural Pathways in Population Health: The Value of Biomark-
    ers. Annals of Human Biology 36(3):281–97.
Worthman, Carol M., and Jennifer Kuzara
    2005 Life History and the Early Origins of Health Differentials. American Journal
    of Human Biology 17(1):95–112.
Worthman, Carol M., and Catherine Panter-Brick
    2008 Homeless Street Children in Nepal: Use of Allostatic Load to Assess the Bur-
    den of Childhood Adversity. Development and Psychopathology 20(1):233–55.
Yehuda, Rachel
    2002 Post-Traumatic Stress Disorder. New England Journal of Medicine 346(2):
    108–14.
    2009 Status of Glucocorticoid Alterations in Post-Traumatic Stress Disorder. An-
    nals of the New York Academy of Sciences 1179:56–69.
Yehuda, Rachel, Steven M. Southwick, John H. Krystal, Douglas Bremner, Dennis S.
    Charney, and John W. Mason
    1993 Enhanced Suppression of Cortisol Following Dexamethasone Administration
    in Posttraumatic Stress Disorder. American Journal of Psychiatry 150(1):83–86.
Young, Allan
    1995 The Harmony of Illusions: Inventing Post-Traumatic Stress Disorder. Prince-
    ton, N.J.: Princeton University Press.
Young, Elizabeth A., and Naomi Breslau
    2004 Saliva Cortisol in Posttraumatic Stress Disorder: A Community Epidemio-
    logic Study. Biological Psychiatry 56(3):205–9.

Young, Elizabeth A., Richard Tolman, Kristine Witkowski, and George Kaplan
    2004 Salivary Cortisol and Posttraumatic Stress Disorder in a Low-Income Community Sample of Women. Biological Psychiatry 55(6):621–66.
Zhang, Kerang, Qi Xu, Yong Xu, Hong Yang, Jinxiu Luo, Yan Sun, Ning Sun, Shan Wang, and Yan Shen
    2009 The Combined Effects of the 5-HTTLPR and 5-HTR1A Genes Modulates the Relationship Between Negative Life Events and Major Depressive Disorder in a Chinese Population. Journal of Affective Disorders 114(1–3):224–31.

CHAPTER 10

Square Pegs and Round Holes: Understanding Historical Trauma in Two Native American Communities

Tom Ball and Theresa D. O'Nell

> I thought she was sleeping, but she suddenly popped up her head and started talking. She was just doing like her mom and aunties; she had been deep in prayer and meditation, searching her indigenous knowledge bank for an indigenous answer to an indigenous problem. And this is what she had to say, "What you are really talking about here is healing. We have five steps in our healing process, and what you are talking about is the first step—identifying what it is that is really hurting you." It was a profound "aha" moment, and we all sat nodding our heads, knowing she had put into words what we all knew in our hearts, that historical trauma and unresolved grief are the silent killers of our first nation peoples, and that the solution must come from us.
> —Planning meeting, Healing Our Wounded Spirits II Conference, Warm Springs Indian Reservation, 2002

In many tribes, *identifying what it is that is really hurting you* is the first step in healing. In this chapter we argue that Historical Trauma (HT) identifies with better accuracy (than does posttraumatic stress disorder [PTSD] and other nomenclature of the DSM) the root causes underlying the high rates of mental and behavioral pathology in Native American communities and families. We argue further that for healing to take place, clinicians must validate the profound realities of the well-known and devastating losses that drive the symptoms. The way to do this is by calling them what they really are—historical traumas, unresolved grief, and soul wounds.

This is not an argument that pits PTSD against HT in a simple way. PTSD usually deals with a single traumatic event and always within the sufferer's lifetime. Native Americans, however, have collectively suffered from generations of repeated and prolonged trauma. While PTSD can be found in Native American populations or communities, its application remains blind to their histories of profound losses. Across Indian Country there is an increasing awareness that historical trauma is a predominant cause of the many difficulties experienced by native peoples today. Psychological and symbolic theories of healing call our attention to the need for a shared assumptive world between patient and healing practitioner.[1] In other words, they need to agree in their identification of what it is that is really hurting them. For a clinician to attempt to treat what they recognize as PTSD naively—without an awareness of the realities and vocabulary of HT—is akin to showing up at a gunfight armed only with a knife (please forgive the colloquialism). The knowledge base around PTSD does not equip the clinician with the right tools for the complex healing task at hand. Moreover a narrow diagnosis of PTSD ignores the resources, insights, and solutions that native peoples may provide in the solution of the problem. We are arguing that HT is a potentially powerful indigenous answer to an indigenous problem. In the following pages, we draw attention to important research on historical trauma and draw parallels with the experiences of Vietnam veterans and their efforts to get help during their postwar adjustment.

Historical Trauma

In a recent article about a project investigating the meaning of healing among First Nations clinicians, and after years of initial skepticism about the construct of "historical trauma," Gone (2009) changes his mind and makes two points relevant to our current discussion. First, he notes that historical trauma is an important part of the local indigenous language of pathology and healing not only in the mental health clinic where he conducted his research but across Indian Country as a whole. As a result, he argues, we cannot afford simply to ignore this crucial language of distress. Second, in discussing the relationship between historical trauma and the constructs of Euro-American psychiatric nosology, including PTSD, he points out that the two sets of constructs do not match each other in "content, form, or function" (2009:758). In particular, Gone suggests that historical trauma serves not as an attempt to reliably diagnose specific syndromes but rather to embed pathologies and disorders within a historical and political context that highlights intergenerational and community factors. He concludes, in opposition to current APA guidelines, that therapists working with Native populations must start with the indigenous ways of understanding, rather than simply bringing in established Euro-American "evidence-based treatments" and then making minor modifications. The title of our chapter gives our similarly stark conclusion: that to use Euro-American nosology, namely PTSD, with Native Americans who are suffering from the repeated assaults of historical traumas is like trying to force square pegs into round holes.

It will not be a surprise to many of our readers to learn that Gone has not been alone in his skepticism about historical trauma. The fact of the matter, though, is that widespread academic and mental health practitioner skepticism about historical trauma is being dispelled by the rich and compelling materials emerging from the work of a handful of scholars. In what is perhaps the most far-reaching statement in the field, Duran and Duran (1995) posit that most of the ills that face the Native American communities—high rates of poverty, unemployment, substance abuse, violence, and poor health and mental health indicators—are a result of historical traumas that Native Americans have endured during the various stages of their colonization at the hands of Europeans and Americans. In Duran and Duran's terms, historical traumas have resulted in soul wounds for many Native Americans. Describing what they, and others, call the American Indian Holocaust, Brave Heart and DeBruyn (1998), conceptual leaders in the field of historical trauma, concur and emphasize unresolved grief as central to the intergenerational effects of historical trauma. They argue that the tremendous losses incurred by Native Americans since the arrival of non-Indians to these lands—of loved ones, means of subsistence, lands, and language, for example—were amplified as traditional mechanisms for dealing with grief (primarily ceremonies and prayers) were outlawed and suppressed.

In addition to the works of these leading thinkers, historical trauma has also begun to appear in the articles of social workers, nurses, and others who form the front lines of health care for Native Americans (Cedar Project Partnership et al. 2008; Hazel and Mohatt 2001; Jones-Saumty 2002; Moffitt 2004; Struthers and Lowe 2003; Weaver 1998). Drawing on similar concerns with historical losses, Walters et al. (2002) call for an "indigenist" framework for understanding the rates of substance use among American Indians and Alaska Natives (see also Walters and Simoni 2002). An indigenist model, the authors argue, not only shifts the focus away from the isolated individual with symptoms to the historical individual whose problems arise out of the stresses of colonization but also to an embedding of the person within the coping resources of family, community, and spirituality. Other writers, from a variety of disciplines, are contributing to the growing area of interest (Denham 2008; Evans-Campbell 2008; Kawamoto 2001; Manson 1996; Morrissette 1994; Tafoya and DelVecchio 1996). Interestingly, some formulations of historical trauma have made it into a seminal volume on multigenerational effects of trauma (Gagne 1998; Duran et al. 1998). Yet, as Maviglia (2002) notes, despite the deep resonance within Indian Country of the notion of historical trauma, the idea has failed so far to enter fully into mainstream nosology. There are likely many reasons for this state of affairs. In part, however, the slow response to take up this powerful notion is probably traceable to the perceived lack of empirical validation.

There are, however, two important studies that have explored the prevalence of historical trauma in community settings. They are worth a closer look. In the more well known of the two studies, Whitbeck et al. (2004), in consultation with tribal elders and a tribal advisory board, developed and pilot tested with 143 midwestern tribal adults a Historical Loss Scale, consisting of twelve types of historical losses. The researchers also constructed a Historical Loss Associated Symptoms Scale that measured the frequency of different kinds of feelings respondents had when they thought about historical losses. The authors found that a majority of the adults thought at least occasionally about historical losses, and that 20–50 percent of the adults thought daily about one or more of the specific losses. Moreover, while few respondents indicated severe symptoms when thinking about historical losses (i.e., rage or loss of sleep), the majority reported sadness, anger, mistrust of whites, and alienation.

The importance of the Whitbeck et al. research cannot be overemphasized. It elegantly confirmed that historical traumas are on the minds of Native Americans in this midwestern tribal community, and that feelings of distress are often the result. This is similar to the lesson that emerged from a second, lesser-known empirical study. Using an expanded PTSD measure, Ball (1998) surveyed ninety-eight adults of one northwestern tribe to determine lifetime exposure to different kinds of traumas, including historical traumas, and evidence of PTSD symptoms and syndromes. Of particular interest in this study was the degree of association between the symptoms and syndrome of PTSD and the "termination" of the tribe by the federal government in the 1950s.[2] Strikingly, Ball found that 72 percent of a sample of the adult population (n = 98) had a diagnosis of PTSD due to the specific historical trauma of termination.

The sample was also surveyed to determine lifetime exposure to different kinds of traumas and evidence of PTSD symptoms and syndromes. Results from the tribal sample were compared to a non-Indian community sample, n = 1,002 (Stein et al. 1996). The tribal sample had significantly higher rates of exposure in all trauma categories. In the categories "threatened with a weapon," "other terrible experiences," "and beaten up or attacked," the rates for the tribal sample were over three times higher. Rates of more than two times higher were found "in death of a friend or family member due to an accident, homicide, or suicide," "witnessing severe injury or death," "being in a motor vehicle accident serious enough to cause injury to yourself or someone else," "and suffering injury or property damage due to fire." The total number of traumatic experiences was also quite different for the two samples: 78 percent of the community sample experienced at least one traumatic event versus 100 percent of the tribal sample. Only 50 percent of the community sample reported multiple traumas; 98 percent of tribal sample reported multiple traumas.

The rates of PTSD for the two samples were also significantly different. Notably, the prevalence rate for full PTSD in the tribal sample (11.2 percent) was significantly higher (p < 0.001) than in the community sample (2.0 percent). The rate for partial PTSD was also significantly higher (p < 0.001) in the tribal sample (17.2 percent) compared to (1.9 percent) in the community sample. Rates of lifetime PTSD were also significantly higher in the tribal sample. Of central concern to the present proposal, posttraumatic symptoms arising from the federal policy of termination were examined. As noted above, a total of 72 percent of the tribal sample reported symptoms of PTSD as a result of termination.

These two studies lend full support to the increasingly accepted idea that historical trauma is of tremendous importance in understanding the mental and behavioral health of Native Americans. With this chapter we hope to contribute to this growing body of work. Specifically, we detail the results of a project on historical trauma in two Northwest Native American communities and present our analysis of the materials.

Intergenerational Trauma and Unresolved Grief (ITUG 2004)

Author Tom Ball's dissertation led to a series of conferences that were held in six different Northwest reservation communities from 2000 to 2005. The Healing Our Wounded Spirits (HOWS) Conferences were funded through the Oregon Social Learning Center Prevention and Intervention Research Center Grant. These conferences introduced the theory and terminology of historical trauma and unresolved grief. These conferences included both research studies, and traditional Native beliefs and practices. The Intergenerational Trauma and Unresolved Grief (ITUG 2004) project came about after Ball read about the use of family genograms as a counseling tool, and the often asked question at the HOWS conferences, of what is the next step. Author Theresa O'Nell and Ball came up with the idea of creating tribal-specific historical trauma genograms that could be used as counseling tools by tribal mental health and alcohol and drug counselors. The authors selected the Umatilla Tribe because of the extensive contacts Dr. Ball had with the tribe, and the working relationship they both had with the local HOWS committee. We added the Klamath Tribes to give a comparative dimension. We were interested in similarities and differences in tribal trauma histories and were also interested in whether this was a process that could be replicated. Using Tribal Participatory Research (TPR) methodology, the research aim was presented to the respective tribal governments for their approval.[3] The tribes supplied us with the names of tribal elders. At Umatilla we gathered twice with eight tribal elders, including two of their chiefs. We began by asking a series of open-ended questions about historical events that affected the tribes. The conversations were taped, and later transcribed. The authors then compiled the first draft of the Umatilla tribal historical trauma genogram. This draft was brought to the second meeting for review, input, and approval. In both instances the discussions were lively with the tribal elders fully engaged. This process was replicated at Klamath with very similar results. One difference at Klamath was that we held separate meetings for Modoc, Klamath, and Pai-ute tribes. This was done in recognition of their unique and sometimes antagonistic histories.

The Umatilla Tribes

The Confederated Tribes of the Umatilla Indian Reservation (CTUIR), with about twenty-five hundred enrolled members, is home to the Walla Walla, the Umatilla, and the Cayuse. Prior to the arrival of whites, the tribes numbered about eight thousand and lived on the Columbia River around the confluence of the Yakama, Snake, and Walla Walla Rivers. Intertribal trade was a defining activity for the CTUIR tribes. Several large ancient trading locations (Wallula, Wascopum) lay within their territories, and the area tribes served as important middlemen along well-established intertribal trade routes between the Plains peoples to the east and the Coastal peoples to the west.

In part because of their prominent role in trade, the CTUIR had relatively early contact with Europeans. Spaniards had traveled up the coast as early as 1770s, and Russian and French traders seeking beaver pelts entered into local trade relationships with Native people by the early 1800s. In 1817–18, the Nez Perce trading fort (renamed Walla Walla in 1835) was established in the heart of CTUIR territory, and families in the area had relatively easy and early access to European goods. Even before the actual arrival of foreigners, however, their presence had impacted the CTUIR people. European-borne diseases had twice swept through the people prior to the arrival of Lewis and Clark in 1805. Of central importance, too, was the appearance of the horse in trade from the south. Very quickly, the area tribes became known for their huge herds of horses, as well as for the speed and endurance of the Cayuse and Appaloosa breeds they raised.

In the Treaty of 1855 (ratified in 1859), the CTUIR ceded 6.4 million acres of land to the United States and reserved 510,000 acres for their own use. The treaty, however, was signed not from their former position of strength—as salmon fishermen, horsemen, and traders—but from a weakened position that followed a quarter of a century of rapid and overwhelming changes brought on by the Euro-American invasion of the Columbia River basin. As the beaver trade declined, other immigrants made their way into the area. Among the first was the Protestant missionary Marcus Whitman and his entourage, who arrived in 1836 with the idea of eradicating Native practices and instilling in the Indians both "civilization" and "true" belief. He, his family, and a couple of other visitors were killed eleven years later in reaction to the perception that Whitman was behind many of the illnesses afflicting the tribes and that he was implicated in the increasing numbers of American immigrants flowing into CTUIR lands. The transformation of the area during this period is almost unimaginable: in 1843, about nine hundred Euro-Americans immigrated into the newly acquired Northwest Territories; in 1844, the number had increased to about twelve hundred; and by 1847, the year of Whitman's killing, about forty-seven hundred were thought to have immigrated to the area. The Whitman "massacre," as it came to be known among Euro-Americans, triggered overt hostilities between Indians and whites (the "Cayuse War") that were brought to close three years later only with the sacrifice of five young Cayuse men who were hanged for the Whitman killings in Oregon City.

The century following the signing of the 1855 treaty nearly destroyed the tribes. Federal and local agents made continual efforts to acquire the prime agricultural lands held by the tribes, eventually reducing tribal holdings to fewer than 160,000 acres. With legally enforced policies of assimilation, traditional ceremonies disappeared from public life. The authority of leaders was destabilized with outside interference. Children were educated in non-Indian institutions antagonistic to Indian history and culture. Hunting and fishing were jeopardized as waters were diverted and fences were erected by farmers, ranchers, and other interests. Moreover, Indians often faced arrest for fishing "out of season." The late 1940s and 1950s were especially devastating, with the eradication of the last horse herds, the flooding of Celilo Falls, the political emasculation of the traditional headmen, and the legalization of alcohol on the reservation. Prior to the era of self-determination, the CTUIR had fallen into extreme poverty and social disarray.

The picture today is much brighter. The CTUIR has approximately twenty-five hundred enrolled members, of whom about half live on the reservation. Even though 48 percent of reservation lands are still held by non-Indians, tribal holdings are increasing, and land acquisition is an established priority. The CTUIR provides over one thousand jobs locally, about half through the tribal government and half through the Wildhorse casino and resort (complete with golf course) and the nearby Tamastslikt Cultural Institute. About 40 percent of the jobs are held by tribal members. If Indians from other tribes are included, Native Americans make up 52 percent of employees. In the last decade, the unemployment rate has been lowered from 37 percent to 17 percent.

The Klamath Tribes

The Klamath Tribes include people from three distinct groups: the Klamath, the Modoc, and the Yahooskin Band of the Snake Indians. Oral histories indicate that the Klamath peoples inhabited a wide area on the eastern slopes of the Cascades and in the adjoining desert areas, from the Deschutes River headwaters in the north to Mount Shasta in California. Archaeological evidence places the Klamath peoples in the area for at least ten thousand years prior to first contact with Euro-Americans in 1826. In 1864, the Klamath Tribes ceded twenty million acres of their lands to the U.S. federal government, reserving their hunting, fishing, and gathering rights and demarcating for use as their homeland about two million acres abounding in forests, rivers, lakes, marshlands, and meadows. In general, members of the Klamath Tribes fared well in the reservation period, pursuing their livelihoods in cattle ranching, timber industries, and freighting.

By the 1950s, the Klamath Tribes were not only economically self-sufficient but were among the wealthiest tribal nations within the borders of the United States. In 1954, however, the Klamath Tribes were "terminated" from federal "protection," stripping the tribes of a land base and the protections that come from having a legally recognized government. Although tribal leaders were able to regain federal recognition in 1986 through the passage of PL 99-398 (the Klamath Indian Tribe Restoration Act), the Klamath Tribes still do not possess reservation lands, apart from a few scattered parcels used for cemeteries. Nonetheless, many, if not most, of the approximately thirty-five hundred enrolled tribal members reside on or near their traditional homelands in southern Oregon.

The social and cultural setting for the Klamath people is indelibly marked by conditions produced when their lands and lives were hit by the tidal wave of the Euro-American invasion of the Northwest in the early to mid-1800s. The backdrop for contemporary Klamath life reveals a devastating history of disease, settler violence, broken promises, confinement, and heavy-handed strategies on the part of the federal government to destroy Klamath languages, traditions, and knowledge. This history resembles that of many western tribes in several respects. Unlike other native peoples in this part of the country, however, the Klamath as a whole were protected for a time from the influx of foreigners by virtue of their relative isolation and inaccessibility. Perhaps more striking, however, is that despite the radical changes and losses wrought by the coming of the whites, many of the Klamath not only survived but did well economically. In large part these successes might be traced to a confluence of factors: traditional values emphasizing hard work and family pride; ownership of the natural resources to respond to market demands for timber; comprehensive knowledge of (and respect for) the lands, animals, and plants; and tribal retention of reservation lands that were not distributed to individual tribal members through the Allotment Act. The tribal retention of reservation lands during this time stands in contrast to the experiences of many, if not most, other western tribes, who lost significant portions of their reservation lands when "excess" lands were opened in the early 1900s to white homesteaders. The continued ownership of the forests, marshes, and fields by the Klamath Tribe provided jobs, per capita payments, and a safety net for tribal members who lost their personal allotments through inexperience, misunderstandings, trickery, or hardship. The force and significance of the 1954 termination of the Klamath Tribes is exposed against this history of hardship, endurance, and tribal adaptation. In turn, much of the significance of the ongoing politics and hard feelings of everyday life in Klamath communities is visible against the lingering effects of termination.

The genograms draw a visually compelling picture of the many prolonged and repeated losses and traumas suffered by Native Americans. Figures 10.1 and 10.2 show the historical trauma genograms produced by elders at the two tribal sites. The genograms produced in our gatherings have made their way back to their respective communities. In one tribal site, the genogram hangs in their museum. At the other, the genogram is displayed in the tribal government building. Both genograms were used in the HOWS conference series.

Lessons Learned

Historical traumas are generally known in these communities, and tribal elders participating in the project easily reconstructed the histories of events and traumas. Despite being well known, however, the events evoke strong emotional reactions when they are elicited.

As noted above, tribal consultants produced rich histories of the losses and traumas that had been suffered by their tribes. One might imagine that

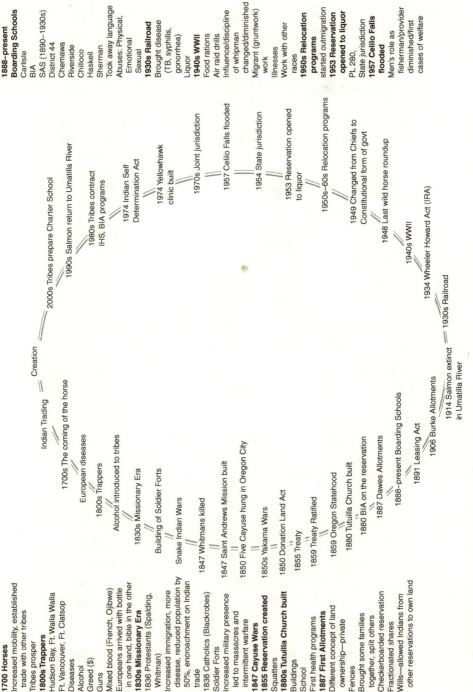

Figure 10.1. CTUIR tribal historical trauma genogram.

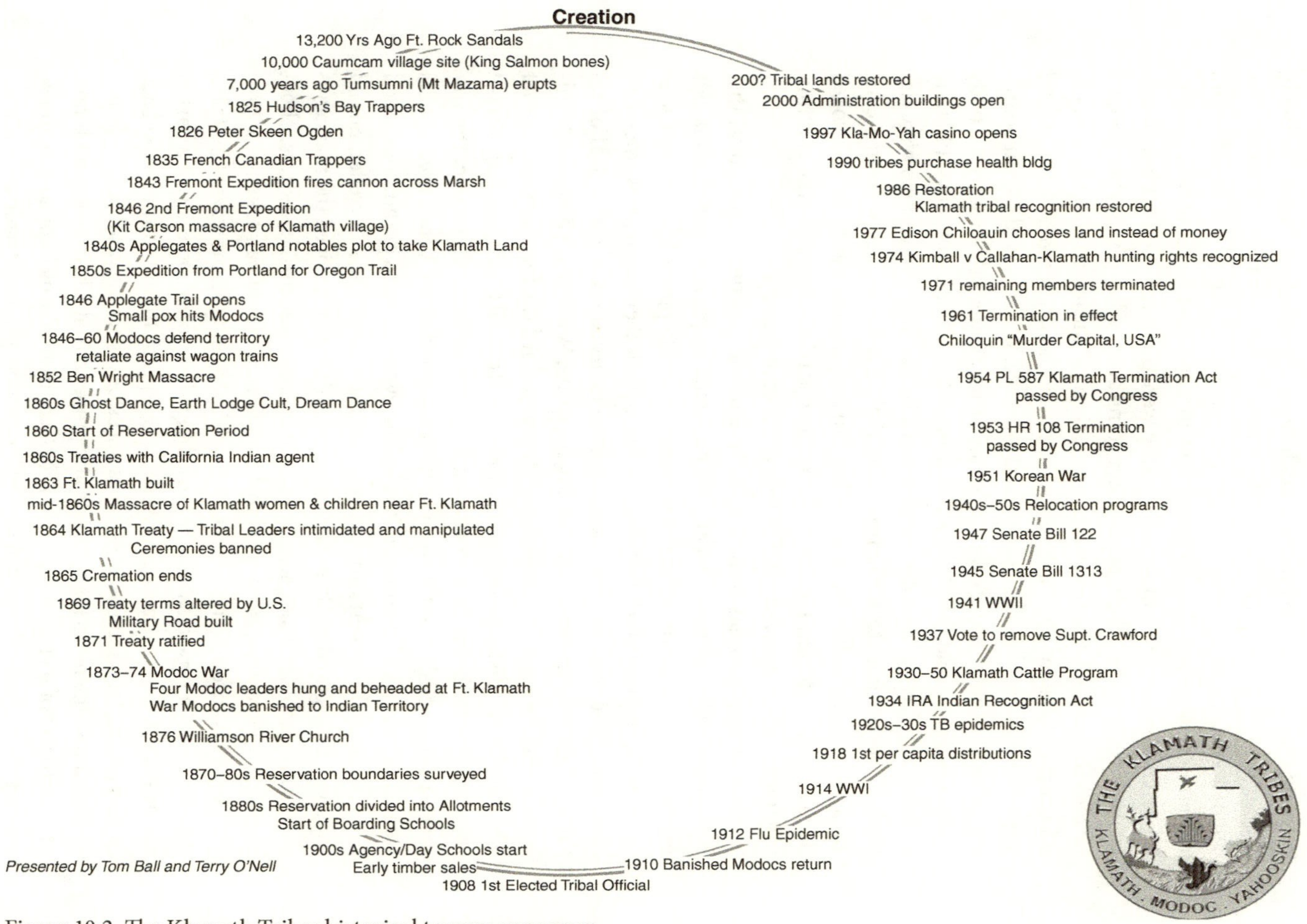

Figure 10.2. The Klamath Tribes historical trauma genogram.

it would prove difficult to pull together historical events from before the living memories of the consultants. Nothing could be further from the truth. The elicited historical traumas, while not everyday fare for conversation, nonetheless were well known to our consultants. Despite being well known, however, the emotions upon their telling were often raw. One female panelist wept as she talked about her brother going away to boarding school, where he took ill and died. She never saw him again, and she talked about how much it hurt to think about his separation from their family when he was sick and when she thought about his unattended gravesite. When a child died at boarding school without "money on the books," the schools did not send the body home for burial, and the child was buried at the school. Not only did many of these children lack proper Indian burials, but family members were denied the opportunity to properly send off their loved ones. This woman's tears, shed seventy years after the death of her brother, and the way her tears evoked deep empathy and similar stories from other participants reveal the continuing impact of unresolved grief in this tribal community.

This example comes from the lifetime of the consultant, but equal distress attended the telling of events that happened in previous generations. For example, there was the telling of a massacre that happened two generations prior to the lifetime of the panelist. In this historical event, many women and children of the tribe camped near a fort in expectation of the arrival of rations, while the men were out hunting for game. When the women and children saw a small herd of cattle being driven toward the fort, they assumed it was time for the disbursement of their rations. They all began running toward the fort, despite being told to stay back by the soldiers. Of course, the soldiers spoke English, and the women and children did not. When their shouts went unheeded, soldiers opened fire, killing everyone but a grandmother and her granddaughter. Tears streamed down the face of the storyteller, an old woman whose grandmother was that small child who survived the massacre.

To give another example, one man told, with undeniable distress, about chancing upon a museum display that contained a lock of hair taken as a "trophy" from his ancestor's body after his death by hanging. In the ways of his tribe, the remains of a person should be buried together. So, to come across a part of his ancestor, not buried, and displayed so disrespectfully, instantly brought back to him the brutal circumstances of his ancestor's lynching death and the continuing impediments to his complete and proper burial. This participant is now in the process of trying to "prove" his descent from his ancestor so he can use existing laws (Native American Graves Protection and Repatriation Act) to repatriate the hair with the rest of his ancestor's remains. He has also taken spiritual measures to help himself after this deeply disturbing encounter.

The context for historical trauma is the whole tribal story, starting with creation and moving forward through the generations.

When we entered these communities we intended to gather information from the elders about the many historical traumas experienced by the tribes. Our focus was squarely on the traumas. At both sites, however, we were given clear instruction to start our genograms not with the coming of the white man but with the true starting point—creation. The tribal consultants also directed us to draw the history in a circle, rather than in a linear form, and to place the events on the circle in a counterclockwise direction, the sacred direction for these tribes. Historical traumas, they told us, are part of the larger story of the tribes, and that story is grounded in spiritual truth. This story does not deny the possibility that biochemical effects accompany the experiences of trauma but emphasizes instead larger systems: families, tribes, cultures, and spiritual beings.

The findings from this work provide ample evidence that multiple historical traumas permeate the tribal histories of both the Umatilla and Klamath peoples. A quick review of recorded events reveals their association with some form of loss: of life, of land, of freedom, of a way of life, of culture, of spirituality. For the Umatilla, two such losses were especially formative: the loss of horse culture is instantiated in the importance of the last Wild Horse Round-Up and the loss of self-sufficiency through fishing in the flooding of the dam constructed on the Columbia River. For the Klamath, the genogram is marked instead by the incessant and endless machinations of non-Indians to dispossess the Klamath of their land, tree, and water resources, and the culmination of these shameful dealings in termination and the complete loss of their reserved treaty lands.

While there is some similarity and overlap between the losses elicited at the two sites, the story of historical traumas at each site was culturally and historically unique.

After compiling the information from the meetings, it became clear that different narratives surrounded the meaning of historical traumas at each of the two tribal sites. For the Umatilla tribal consultants, the story was told around two central concepts in their culture: *tamanwit*, the natural law that orders all of life, and *tichum*, the knowledge that all of life is intertwined. Before the coming of whites, *tamanwit* and *tichum* fit together in the values of hard work and cultivating a good heart. Good hearts are generous, thankful, and respectful and are seen in the morning prayers of thanks for life, in the first salmon or first roots ceremonies, and in the well-known hospitality of the people. With the losses and traumas of contact, the people became overwhelmed with fear and unresolvable grief. Keeping a good heart is hard when fear, grief, shame, and anger are natural reactions to history and to the ongoing situation. Generosity, thankfulness, and respect are hard to maintain when greed, racism, and alcohol are always around. Historical traumas have hurt the spirit of the people, but their spirit is getting stronger and stronger: fish are coming back to the rivers; the people have voted to respect an important burial site against the dictates of economic development; and a respected language program is in place. The consultants from the Umatilla tribes emphasized that one way to keep spirit growing is to remember history, not as it is told by those who tried to destroy them, but as they know it. They can look for ways to bring help to those who are still hurt and teach the children pride, not shame. As the wounds are healed and the hurting brought to an end, good hearts and hard work will be restored to the people. There was a moral running through the story told at this tribal site: *tamanwit* and *tichum* have the power to bring the people back to health.

For the Klamath tribal consultants, the story centered around their primordial relationship with the land, its near destruction, and the imperative to return to their sacred responsibility of caring for the land and being cared for by the land. Panelists emphasized that the people of the Klamath Tribes have always been in this land, citing the thirteen-thousand-year-old sandals uncovered by archaeologists in an area cave, noting tribal knowledge about the creation of Crater Lake when Mount Mazama exploded about eight thousand years ago, and reminding listeners that their people have lived here for hundreds of generations. The consultants from the Klamath Tribes repeated various aspects of this story, noting how the land fed them, gave them medicines, clothed them, and protected them. They noted that their Creator, *Gmok'am'c*, told their ancestors when and where to find the plants, fish, and animals that sustained their families, noting, too, that they had a responsibility to take care of the land, to clean out the springs, to be respectful not greedy, to give thanks for these gifts in ceremony. The panelists summed up this all-encompassing relationship stating that the land gave them all that they needed and taught them how to live, and they, in turn, were good stewards of the land. Describing the effects of colonialism and termination, they highlight family infighting, being shunned by other tribes, feeling lost without the tribe, blaming each other, and trusting no one. The panelists acknowledged that the restoration of federal recognition of their Tribal status has helped but that until the Klamath Tribal peoples can once again take their places as the rightful stewards of these lands, the suffering of the people will continue. They said that when they reestablish the immortal connections between themselves and this land, their children and grandchildren will be able know their place in the world and to find trust and forgiveness for themselves, each other, and their ancestors. The moral of the Klamath Tribal story was that their grandmother, the land, has been kidnapped, raped, starved, and abused and that the Klamath peoples must get her back and take care of her in the right way.

This investigation of historical traumas reveals itself as a story of suffering and pain but also of survival and resilience; the story is not yet over.

Just as we had to learn that the story didn't begin with the traumas or the coming of the invaders, we also had to learn that the story did not end there either. At both sites, elders reminded us that historical traumas are not only a thing of the past but continue in attacks on treaty rights, the land base, and in acts of racism. However, they also called our attention to recent positive events and consistently expressed hope for the future. At one site, the elders directed us to incorporate recent events such as progress in language and cultural revitalization, the return of salmon to one of their rivers, the success of their new tribal school and recent economic successes. At the other site, elders talked of their sense of the progress the tribes would make as they worked to complete the ongoing process of tribal restoration after the devastation of termination. Their message was, "We have always been here; we are still here; and we're not going anywhere."

Historical trauma genograms document the intergenerational, community, historical and spiritual aspects of Native American experiences of trauma.

Discussion

Historical trauma is both real and extensive. In our introduction we cited empirical studies as well as the conceptual work of some of the leading Native scholars in this field. The two tribal genograms described in this chapter provide visual substantiation of the overwhelming numbers of historical traumas for these two tribes and add to the body of evidence about historical trauma. It is time to recognize the Holocaust of the First Nations peoples of the United States and the rest of the Western Hemisphere. More than 99 percent of the indigenous people of what is now the United States were wiped out. Of the estimated 30,000,000 indigenous people in 1492, there were 237,000 survivors counted in the 1890 U.S. Census. Of the two billion acres of Native land, only fifty million remain in Native control. Compounding the problem, our nation's history books erase this reality. It is time for the true story to be more widely known and to make reparations by providing the time and resources for Native America to come up with their own solutions to the continuing devastation wrought by the Holocaust of their peoples.[4]

The term "historical trauma" might lead some to think that these traumas are "just historical," ignoring two important issues. First, historical traumas can and do refer at times to events that have occurred within living peoples' lifetimes. The federal policies of termination and the boarding school are both clear examples of historical traumas that have happened in the lifetimes of contemporary Native Americans. So, too, is the moving experience of the tribal consultant who unexpectedly came upon his ancestor's remains displayed in a museum. Second, even when events are clearly located in the past they nonetheless continue to elicit emotionally charged reactions. Witness for example the tears of the tribal consultant every time she retold the story of the massacre that her grandmother barely survived over 150 years ago. Based on our experience working with numerous tribes, events from the sometimes distant past often evoke powerful emotional responses. In other words, this woman's tearfulness is not unusual; it is common when Indian people talk about these devastating kinds of events.

Research shows us that PTSD is both cumulative and intergenerational, and in populations that have suffered prolonged and repeated traumas, a set of symptoms exists that is more insidious than PTSD (Herman 1993). We know then that the greater the number of traumas, and the longer the duration of trauma, the more complex and intractable the symptoms. The two tribal historical trauma genograms both show a pattern of repeated and prolonged trauma over many generations. Their experiences are similar to those of most tribes. It should be no surprise to anyone then that Native Americans suffer from so many negative social and health problems.

Let us examine another trauma case when lack of a proper diagnostic category led to much suffering and lack of efficacy. When Vietnam veterans returned home from the war many of them suffered with debilitating symptoms associated with their war experience. They sought help from providers who were unprepared to deal with them and their war trauma; there was no name for what they were going through and therefore no prescribed treatment. These veterans suffered, their families suffered, their communities suffered, and this country suffered as their trauma experiences remained invalidated and, as such, untreated. Providers, bound by laws and ethics, had only existing diagnoses at their disposal, which were inadequate to help traumatized veterans. Clinicians were stuck, trying to put a square peg into a round hole. It took the voices of the veterans, and their allies (many, it must be said, were from the ranks of care providers) to force the realization that the veterans themselves, the people who were suffering, needed to be listened to. The stories of their war trauma needed to be validated. It took too long, but finally in 1980, war trauma as the source of their ongoing and severe distress was validated, and PTSD was added as a recognized mental health disorder to the DSM-III (APA 1980).

The terrible toll this long wait took on the veterans, their families, their communities, and this country is well known. While these veterans suffered sometimes in silence, and sometimes in violence and loud rage, with their terrible nightmares and flashbacks untreated, it exacted a terrible toll on their health and welfare, and on their families. The only relief for many of them was to self-medicate with alcohol and drugs. They were not able to hold onto jobs to support their families; they were prone to violent outbursts that landed them in jail, hospital, or worse, a cemetery. Too often the same fate befell their families. Untreated, their war trauma spiraled into a cycle of repeated traumas, job loss, divorce, estrangement from children and other family members, alcohol and drug abuse, violence, and rage. And until 1980, the veterans were blamed for their symptoms. They were victimized twice. Our country wondered what happened to its sons and daughters, its spouses, its fathers and mothers who had gone off to war whole and came back broken, prone to long spells of silence, violent outbursts, and with a vacant faraway look that was hard to describe, but that every family member of one of these war-affected veterans knew too well.

It took these warriors many more years of further battle, telling and retelling their war experiences, for progress to be made. These were men and women who went to war, came back and were not only untreated and mistreated, but were blamed for their behavior, for being weak-willed. It took the stories of mothers and fathers, wives and husbands, and even those of children, to finally win this battle for the soldiers' souls. They, and they alone, knew that the driving force behind their alcohol and drug abuse, their violence and rage was their war trauma. Beyond their physical wounds, they had been wounded to the very core of their souls. They needed, they demanded, and they finally got a diagnosis that both validated and fit their war experience. For some it was too little, too late. For others, they were finally able to come home.

Can PTSD be found in Indian communities? Are the rates of PTSD higher than in other communities? Is it often a more "complex" type of PTSD? The answer to all these questions, in our experience, is yes. Nonetheless, clinicians working solely within the framework of PTSD will struggle to provide adequate help for their Native American clients. The realities and effects of historical traumas fall outside clinical understandings, and oftentimes outside of clinicians' personal knowledge. For Vietnam veterans, effective diagnosis and treatments happened only after they stood up and demanded that their war traumas be validated as the root of their difficulties. Until PTSD was developed, clinicians working with veterans had to force square pegs (the effects of war trauma) into round holes (a variety of problems such domestic violence, alcohol and drug problems, depression, etc., that were not linked to trauma, leading to a blaming of the person so afflicted). The development and acceptance of PTSD did not occur overnight. It took research dollars, clinical trials, panels to codify best practices, and a host of other important efforts.

In Indian Country, the cause of the widespread difficulties facing individuals, families and communities is also known. The people, and their allies, know what the silent killer is. Like the Vietnam veterans who knew that their war trauma was at the root of their problems, so do the people of Indian Country know what is at the root of their problems. Undiagnosed, invalidated, and unchecked, it continues to exact its toll in lives lost, chronic diseases, alcohol and substance abuse, domestic violence, homicide and suicide, and oftentimes abject poverty: historical trauma and unresolved grief. As Ed and Bonnie Duran stated so eloquently in their book, *Native American Postcolonial Psychology* (1995), if we are serious about healing in Native America we need to stop mistaking the complex symptoms resulting from the repeated and prolonged effects of historical trauma, for PTSD, and call it what it really is: "a chronic reaction to genocide and oppression." It is not depression, anxiety, or any of the other round holes into which the DSM must fit everyone. It is not even complex PTSD.

Historical trauma is not a simple cultural variant of PTSD. It is a diagnosis that comes from the indigenous knowledge base and can be an important part of an indigenous response to the serious difficulties facing many tribal persons. Historical trauma genograms are visual depictions of historical traumas and how they fit into the whole history of individual tribal nations. They might also be powerful and cathartic healing tools. The use of these genograms in tribal counseling programs begs to be tested, measured, and analyzed to see just how helpful they can be. They might also be used to train nontribal personnel who come to work for a tribe to better understand the population with whom they are working. They might also be used as a healing tool at the tribal level, and again, this begs for further research and research dollars.

Looking at all the historical traumas listed by these two tribes, and realizing that other tribes could detail equally long lists, is it any wonder that Native people exhibit so many negative statistics? Ed and Bonnie Duran (1995) say that these statistics reveal a natural reaction to an unnatural situation, much like the reactions of Vietnam veterans to their war trauma. Yet, unlike the Vietnam veterans, and subsequent returning veterans, who eventually got the help they needed, Native Americans continue to be mistreated and misdiagnosed by providers lacking the right tools. The time has come to listen to the people who are suffering, and to heed the work of the scholars who have added to our understanding of historical trauma in the lives of Native Americans. We have come full circle, back to the insights that come from the prayers and meditations of a tribal elder at a planning meeting for a healing conference: that historical trauma and unresolved grief are the silent killers of first nation peoples, and that the solutions must come from them. We are also back to the argument of Gone (2009), who after investigating the meanings of healing for Native clinicians comes to a very similar conclusion: that therapists working with Native populations must start with indigenous ways of understanding, rather than simply bringing in established treatments and modifying them for cultural variations. It is time to stop hammering square pegs into round holes.[5] *Sepk'eec'a.*

Acknowledgments

The authors acknowledge the Northwest Indian Prevention and Intervention Research Center, Oregon Social Learning Center, Grant #P30MH46690, for support for the research on which this chapter is based. We owe special thanks to the participating tribal governments, the Confederated Tribes of the Umatilla Indian Reservation and the Klamath Tribes, for their support of this work. We were so honored, humbled, and privileged to have been allowed access to the tribal elders at both sites. We want to thank the tribes for allowing us access, and we cannot express enough our gratitude to the elders for sharing their stories, their tears, and their Indian humor, sepk'eec'a. We also want to thank Jan Mustoe for her work on creating the file and poster versions of the historical trauma genograms. We owe special appreciation to Danita Herrera, who organized gatherings, posed important questions, and generally kept us in line, all the while keeping her sense of humor. Byron Good encouraged the publication of this work and helped us to refine our discussion. Two colleagues, Dr. Alison Ball and Dr. Phil Fisher, provided comments on a later draft. We also want to acknowledge the millions of Native American people who perished in the American Holocaust, and the courageous survivors who today sometimes struggle but who continue to fight. Last, we must acknowledge those traditional people who possess the indigenous knowledge that will lead us out of the darkness into a reality where our hearts are once again light and happy.

Notes

There is a reason for the informal writing style used in parts of this chapter. If the people who are most affected by historical trauma cannot understand what is written because it uses academic conventions, then the work dishonors the individuals who shared these stories so that their people can heal. It also dishonors the academics who are trying to understand the complexity of historical trauma and its negative impact on Native peoples. To truly understand the issues discussed in this chapter, we must move beyond a purely academic view to a much deeper, spiritual level, where these stories reside.

1. See, for example, Frank 1961; Dow 1986; Csordas and Kleinman 1990; and Kirmayer 1993.

2. For those who may be unaware of this chapter of American history, the tribe was one of over sixty tribes whose tribal status was "terminated" by the federal government, the final step in the push for assimilation/extermination. Although tribal recognition was later restored to the Klamath tribes it was only after a protracted legal battle, and not until after a terrible period of social chaos. Moreover, even though their tribal status was restored, their lands have not been returned.

3. See Fisher and Ball (2002, 2003) for information on tribal participatory research.

4. Diseases, wars, and massacres were the weapons of the first phase of colonization. Then came the oppression phase, a trajectory identified by Amnesty International's Chart of Coercion, a study that outlined the steps needed to be taken to completely dominate a person's mind, body, and soul. The Chart of Coercion mirrors almost exactly the two genograms. The two tribal genograms provide a visual example of the genocide and oppression, of the holocaust of uber proportion that struck all First Nations people, and that continues today: treaties broken almost as soon as they were signed; removal from traditional lands; an early reservation period that resembled prisoner of war camps; forced assimilation aimed at stripping religion, culture, and traditions; children stolen from their families and sent to boarding schools where they were forced to give up their names, their language, their dress, even their long hair, and much worse; the physical, mental, spiritual, and sexual abuses; relocation; termination; and on and on. Today more can be added to this list: the armed conflicts such as Wounded Knee and Oka and others; the conflicts in the Northwest over salmon and water; the continued environmental degradation of our lands; and on and on. Let us make no mistake, colonization has not stopped.

5. Further research questions also include documenting the different kinds and levels of historical trauma symptomatology. As demonstrated in the examples of our consultants, there appears to be a wide range of emotional reaction to these historical traumas. Is this a function of time, whether or not a relative suffered this trauma, whether the person experienced this trauma his or her lifetime: all these are questions further research can perhaps tease out. Are there treatment modalities that work? It is the authors' experience that traditional methodologies work: the canoe journey on the Northwest Coast. In our view, it is important to give the research dollars to those who would research Native American traditions and beliefs for ways to recover, to find the therapeutic answers in Native languages and ceremonies. This is a spiritual wound, and it needs spiritual intervention, an indigenous intervention. Let Native Americans tell their own stories. We often hear from Native Americans, "Let us control our own destiny; then and only then, will we be able to heal and return to good health."

References

American Psychiatric Association
  1980 Diagnostic and Statistical Manual of Mental Disorders, 3rd ed. Washington, D.C.: American Psychiatric Association.
Ball, Thomas J.
  1998 Prevalence Rates of Full and Partial PTSD and Lifetime Trauma in a Sample of Adult Members of an American Indian Tribe. Ph.D. diss., University of Oregon.

Brave Heart, Maria, and Lemyra DeBruyn
  1998 The America Indian Holocaust: Healing Historical Unresolved Grief. Ameri-
      can Indian and Alaska Native Mental Health Research 8:60–82.
Cedar Project Partnership et al.
  2008 The Cedar Project: Historical Trauma, Sexual Abuse and HIV Risk Among
      Young Aboriginal People Who Use Injection and Non-Injection Drugs in Two
      Canadian Cities. Social Science and Medicine 66:2185–94.
Csordas, Thomas J., and Arthur Kleinman
  1990 The Therapeutic Process. In Medical Anthropology: Contemporary Theory
      and Method. Thomas Johnson and Carolyn Sargent, eds. Pp. 11–25. New York:
      Praeger.
Denham, Aaron R.
  2008 Rethinking Historical Trauma: Narratives of Resilience. Transcultural Psy-
      chiatry 45:391–414.
Dow, James
  1986 Universal Aspects of Symbolic Healing: A Theoretical Synthesis. American
      Anthropologist 88(1):56–69.
Duran, Eduardo, and Bonnie Duran
  1995 Native American Postcolonial Psychology. Albany: State University of New
      York Press.
Duran, Eduardo, Bonnie Duran, Maria Yellow Horse Brave Heart, and Susan Yellow
      Horse–Davis
  1998 Healing the American Indian Soul Wound. In International Handbook of
      Multigenerational Legacies of Trauma. Yael Danieli, ed. Pp. 341–54. New York:
      Plenum Press.
Evans-Campbell, Teresa
  2008 Historical Trauma in American Indian/Native Alaska Communities: A Multi-
      level Framework for Exploring Impacts on Individuals, Families and Communi-
      ties. Journal of Interpersonal Violence 23:316–38.
Fisher, Philip. A., and Thomas J. Ball
  2002 The Indian Family Wellness project: An Application of the Tribal Participatory
      Research Model. Prevention Science 3:235–40.
  2003 Tribal Participatory Research: Mechanisms of a Collaborative Model. Ameri-
      can Journal of Community Psychology 32:207–16
Frank, Jerome D.
  1961 Persuasion and Healing. Baltimore: Johns Hopkins University Press.
Gagne, Marie-Anik
  1998 The Role of Dependency and Colonialism in Generating Trauma in First
      Nations Citizens: The James Bay Cree. In International Handbook of Multigen-
      erational Legacies of Trauma. Yael Danieli, ed. Pp. 355–72. New York: Plenum
      Press.

Gone, Joseph P.

2009 A Community-Based Treatment for Native American Historical Trauma: Prospects for Evidence-Based Practice. Journal of Consulting and Clinical Psychology 77(4):751–62.

Hazel, Kelly L., and Gerald V. Mohatt

2001 Cultural and Spiritual Coping in Sobriety: Informing Substance Abuse Prevention for Alaska Native Communities. Journal of Community Psychology 29(5):541–62.

Herman, Judith L.

1993 Sequelae of Prolonged and Repeated Trauma: Evidence for a Complex Post-traumatic Syndrome (DESNOS). In Posttraumatic Stress Disorder: DSM-IV and Beyond. Jonathan R. T. Davidson and Edna B. Foa, eds. Pp. 213–28. Washington, D.C.: American Psychiatric Press.

Jones-Saumty, Deborah

2002 Substance Abuse Treatment for Native Americans. In Ethnicity and Substance Abuse: Prevention and Intervention. Grace Xueqin Ma and George Henderson, eds. Pp. 270–83. Springfield, Ill.: Charles C. Thomas.

Kawamoto, Walter T.

2001 Community Mental Health and Family Issues in Socio-Historical Context: The Confederated Tribes of Coos, Lower Umpqua, and Siuslaw Indians. American Behavioral Scientist 44(9):1482–91.

Kirmayer, Laurence J.

1993 Healing and the Invention of Metaphor: The Effectiveness of Symbols Revisited. Culture, Medicine, and Psychiatry 17(2):161–95.

Manson, Spero M.

1996 The Wounded Spirit: A Cultural Formulation of Post-Traumatic Stress Disorder. Culture, Medicine, and Psychiatry 20:489–98.

Maviglia, Marcell A.

2002 Historical Trauma and PTSD: The "Existential" Versus the "Clinical." Italian online Psychiatric Magazine. http://www.priory.com/ital/frostates2e.htm.

Moffitt, Pertice M.

2004 Colonialization: A Health Determinant for Pregnant Dogrib Women. Journal of Transcultural Nursing 15(4):323–30.

Morrissette, Patrick J.

1994 The Holocaust of First Nation People: Residual Effects on Parenting and Treatment Implications. Contemporary Family Therapy 16(5):381–92.

Stein, Murray D., John R. Walker, Andrea L. Hazen, and David R. Forde

1996 Full and Partial Posttraumatic Stress Disorder: Findings from a Community Survey. American Journal of Psychiatry 154:1114–19.

Struthers, Roxanne, and John Lowe

2003 Nursing in the Native American Culture and Historical Trauma. Issues in Mental Health Nursing 24:257–72.

Tafoya, Nadine, and Ann DelVecchio
  1996 Back to the Future: An Examination of the Native American Holocaust Expe-
    rience. *In* Ethnicity and Family Therapy, 2nd ed. Monica McGoldrick and Joe
    Giordano, eds. Pp. 45–54. New York: Guilford Press.
Walters, Karina L., and Jane M. Simoni
  2002 Reconceptualizing Native Women's Health: An "Indigenist" Stress-Coping
    Model. American Journal of Public Health, 92(4):520–24.
Walters Karina L., Jane M. Simoni, and Teresa Evans-Campbell
  2002 Substance Use Among American Indians and Alaska Natives: Incorporating
    Culture in an "Indigenist" Stress-Coping Paradigm. Public Health Rep 117(Suppl. 1)
    :S104–17.
Weaver, Hilary N.
  1998 Indigenous People in a Multicultural Society: Unique Issues for Human Ser-
    vices. Social Work 43(3):203–11.
Whitbeck, Les B., Gary W. Adams, and Dan R. Hoyt
  2004 Conceptualizing and Measuring Historical Trauma Among American Indian
    People. American Journal of Community Psychology 33(3–4):119–30.

CHAPTER 11

Culture, Trauma, and the Social Life of PTSD in Haiti

Erica Caple James

The massive shock experienced by millions in Haiti and the Haitian diaspora during and after the January 12, 2010, earthquake has provoked numerous psychosocial rehabilitation projects in response to this emergency. International medical missions, faith-based, humanitarian relief, and development aid organizations (among others) have inaugurated a variety of trauma treatment programs in Haiti that offer competing and sometimes conflicting interventions. Each also arises from distinct views of the relationship between personhood and embodiment and produces modalities of redressing suffering that are rooted in particular cultures, histories, and clinical perspectives. For example, the Israel Center for the Treatment of Psychotrauma (ICTP) has launched an elementary school–based program, Project Resilience Haiti: Rebuilding Community,[1] which uses cognitive behavioral therapy, eye movement desensitization retraining (EMDR),[2] somatic experiencing,[3] and other therapeutic methods to identify and treat posttraumatic distress in Haitians. In another example, the Unitarian Universalist Service Committee sponsored representatives from the U.S.-based Trauma Resource Institute (TRI),[4] an organization established in 2006,[5] to train Haitian caregivers in "somatic trauma-healing techniques."[6] The TRI's trauma resiliency model (TRM), assumes that trauma is a universal physiological phenomenon and claims that its treatment—an amalgam of somatic-based therapies like Jane Ayres's sensory integration theory, Eugene Gendlin's focusing, and Peter Levine's somatic experiencing—has been substantiated by current research about the brain.[7] Another psychosocial intervener after the earthquake—the

Center for Mind-Body Medicine, founded by James S. Gordon, M.D., in 1991—launched a local version of its Global Trauma Relief (GTR) program in Haiti. GTR "pioneers," as its website describes them, train "local healthcare professionals and educators to teach children and adults simple, powerful self-care and self-awareness techniques that can relieve stress and suffering, using the Center's unique small group model."[8] According to Dr. Gordon, the goal of the program is "to create an organization that will respond as Doctors without Borders does to the physical . . . to the psychological and emotional needs of whole countries."[9] Underlying these globalizing mental health treatment ventures is an assumption that trauma, and specifically posttraumatic stress disorder (PTSD), are universal conditions that can be ameliorated through each brand of treatment.[10]

As I have documented elsewhere (James 2010), the inauguration of mobile mental health therapeutic programs in response to social disruption and states of emergency in Haiti is not a new phenomenon. The rapid propagation of psychosocial interventions in the aftermath of the earthquake suggests that now is the time to return a critical eye to the subject of PTSD and its controversial social life in the troubled nation. Haitian mental health professionals concur with this cautionary stance. In response to the onslaught of requests from "relief organizations, missionary groups, and others with disaster counseling skills" seeking information on how to implement mental health treatment programs in Haiti, Dr. Guerda Nicolas, a psychologist with long-standing experience conducting clinical work both in Haiti and with diaspora Haitians in the United States, warned prospective interveners: "Please stay away—unless you've really, really done the homework. . . . Psychological issues don't transcend around the globe. . . . People fail to recognize that it's not going to work the way you think it's going to work, it's not just an issue of being trained as a psychologist. . . . The kind of treatment model developed for PTSD doesn't integrate folk medicine, it doesn't take into account cultural aspects, and it makes the assumption that people have the wherewithal to avoid traumatic events."[11] Dr. Nicolas's statements raise provocative questions regarding the universality of PTSD and, if the disorder truly does manifest globally, whether cultural, material, and structural conditions are factors that shape its occurrence. A subtle tension implied by this statement (the exploration of which is beyond the scope of this chapter) is the extent to which the development of PTSD is a biological universal or the product of "local biologies" (Lock 1995; Lock and Nguyen 2010)—"the way in which biological and social processes are inseparably entangled over time, resulting in human biological difference . . . that may or may not be subjectively discernible by individuals" (Lock and Nguyen 2010:90).

The DSM's PTSD construct implicitly assumes a set of psychosocial and material conditions that may produce individual behaviors of avoidance of contextual and environmental triggers (among other responses). For many in Haiti, however, avoidance of settings or contexts that evoke past traumas may be difficult, if not impossible, because of complex phenomena comprising *ensekirite*. Since the late 1980s, the term "ensekirite" (Haitian Creole for "insecurity") has indexed the ontological uncertainties and dangers of an everyday political, criminal, and interpersonal violence that has flourished amidst growing risks of environmental and infrastructural harm (James 2008, 2010). In my usage of the term, ensekirite describes the experience of living at the nexus of multiple uncertainties[12]—political, economic, environmental, interpersonal, physical, and spiritual—and as I will discuss later, ensekirite is mediated through the body.

Given such circumstances, what severity of symptoms and evidence of debilitating experience meet criteria for PTSD, especially in contexts in which ruptures in daily life are routine? Although imported brands of trauma therapy may prove efficacious in ameliorating the struggles of Haitians in the aftermath of psychosocial ruptures, there may also be impediments to effective treatment that result from reliance on the DSM's PTSD criteria to diagnose traumatic sequelae. For example, Dr. Nicolas's work with Haitian immigrant woman has shown that cases of severe depression have been missed because patients did not display disturbances of weight, sleep, attention, or mood that met DSM criteria. According to Nicolas, "You can have a Haitian who is very, very depressed and they get up in the morning, they take care of their kids, they still get dressed, they go to work . . . [b]ut they still have this sense of emptiness that they cannot describe."[13] The example of the "underdiagnosis" of depression among Haitian immigrant woman in the United States raises questions of whether the DSM's PTSD diagnosis might also be underdiagnosed, not only among Haitian immigrants but in Haiti itself—especially given the variability and specificity with which trauma manifests cross-culturally, and the routine occurrences of ruptures of varying magnitudes that are characteristic of ensekirite.[14]

In this essay, I raise questions about the PTSD diagnosis and its social life in Haiti. I argue that the efficacy of mobile modalities of mental health treatment depends on the extent to which these models take into account how Haitian traditional understandings of personhood, embodiment, and trauma are complex and dynamic. Customary or vernacular methods of care for emotional and physical distress can provide a language through which many Haitians understand and express their trauma. Nevertheless, even these culturally based methods of care may fail to repair the ruptures wrought by devastating social experiences. Organized efforts to address and redress psychosocial trauma must also respond to the phenomena of ensekirite. It is important to note, however, that just as the PTSD diagnostic criteria have changed (see Good and Hinton, the Introduction to this volume), the contours of ensekirite and its psychosocial sequelae have also transformed over time. As the stories in this chapter demonstrate, the conditions of rupture that occur cyclically in the nation may provoke the irruption of past traumas (and affect the experimental or improvisational manner of its treatment) in unanticipated ways.

This essay is a meditation on more than twenty-seven months of field research I conducted in Haiti between 1995 and 2000, tracing the international-, national-, and local-level responses to traumatized victims of human rights abuses from the 1991 to 1994 coup periods. In 1996, I was invited to volunteer[15] at a women's clinic that Haitian and U.S.-based women's rights organizations had founded that year in Martissant, a highly populated *bidonvil* (shantytown) just outside Port-au-Prince. I worked there regularly until spring 1999. Between 1998 and 1999, I also trained with Haitian mental health practitioners at the Mars/Kline Center for Neurology and Psychiatry at the State University Hospital to understand better the subjective experience of psychosocial trauma in Haiti. Moreover, between 1997 and 2000, I worked at the Human Rights Fund, a political development assistance program funded by the United States Agency for International Development that housed a rehabilitation program for torture survivors and their dependents. In addition to providing a number of other medical, legal, and social services to victims and their dependents, the Rehab Program, as it was called, held therapy groups for its beneficiaries in which I participated. I also analyzed hundreds of client dossiers that represented the traumatic experiences of nearly twenty-five hundred beneficiaries of the program.

Throughout these ethnographic fieldwork and therapeutic activities I witnessed how ensekirite was becoming both a material and ghostly presence that affected many people physically, emotionally, and even spiritually. Acts of violence were visible but complex—simultaneously displaying motives of personal vengeance, economic profit, and political threat. I also learned that ensekirite indexed the uncertainties and risks of life in a nation hampered by a succession of natural disasters, and technological and industrial accidents—routinized ruptures that make the resumption of normal life difficult, if not impossible. In response to such conditions, numerous international (and national) mental health interveners like those described above attempted to redress the long-term effects of psychosocial trauma in everyday life, but to varying degrees of success.

In the remainder of this chapter, I describe the relationship between ensekirite and psychosocial trauma as articulated in a variety of therapeutic contexts in which I was a participant in the late 1990s and analyze how the dynamics I observed challenge conventional understanding of PTSD and its contemporary treatment in Haiti. I have selected two cases from my fieldwork that have troubled me in the years since I left Haiti. Each in different ways illustrates the complex experiences of ontological insecurity and the disordered subjectivities that such states may produce. The story of a young man whom I call Jean-Robert Paul, whose parents were targeted for political violence during the 1991–94 coup years, provides context for conceptions of personhood, embodiment, and emotion in Haiti. Not only does his case illustrate how the experience of ontological insecurity may fracture individual subjectivity, it also shows some of the unintended negative consequences of improvisational treatment that well-intentioned national and international interveners provided to Haitians both within and across national borders.

A second story, of a woman whom I call Odette Jean, raises several questions about the subjective experience of trauma, the ways in which PTSD may or may not manifest, and the efficacy of mobile mental health interventions currently being implemented in post-earthquake Haiti. Through these examples this chapter offers the following main points: First, interventions focused on the psychosocial effects of the earthquake must also track the ways in which traumatic experiences sustained during past periods of acute ensekirite (and as a result of human-authored, rather than natural disaster) may complicate how trauma manifests in response to subsequent ruptures in routine. Second, either in cases of human-authored or natural disasters, the lack of knowledge about missing persons and the inability to observe customary mortuary rites for those lost and presumed dead are among the most devastating experiences for Haitians, which, when unresolved, can contribute to posttraumatic stress.[16] Third, there remains a risk that in acknowledging the cultural and temporal specificity of Haiti trauma in climates of ensekirite, Haitians may be viewed as not meeting criteria for PTSD and be denied treatment that would provide a standard of care in settings of greater security.

Conversely, under conditions of social instability and rupture, international (and even national) interveners implementing a variety of brands of mobile trauma therapies may inadvertently perpetuate a situation in which care is experimental, unregulated, and unsustainable—placing further at risk already vulnerable Haitians. Finally, psychosocial treatment programs focusing on acute *individual* traumatic suffering will not be effective in the long term unless *collective* security—political, economic, and social—is established and sustained in Haiti.

Ensekirite and Trauma in Haiti

Between 1957 and 1986, the Duvalier dictators inculcated a climate of terror in Haiti by deploying the military to target particular kinds of violence against individual enemies of the state and civil society associations. The *tonton makout*—armed paramilitary forces that mobilized the baneful power of the occult to threaten, extort, and repress fellow citizens—instilled fear in and controlled communities across the nation (Trouillot 1990). The methods of "necropolitical" terror (James 2010; Mbembe 2003)—acts that subjugated life using the power of death to violate moral, social, and physical boundaries— were rape, disappearances, murder, display of corpses, and other egregious acts. This style of violence was first used systematically during the presidential administration of physician and ethnologist François "Papa Doc" Duvalier (1957–71) and continued under the reign of his son, Jean-Claude "Baby Doc" Duvalier (1971–86), until his ouster and exile in 1986. Between 1986 and 1990, reciprocal violence occurred between members of a reactionary military that reproduced "Duvalierism without Duvalier" with impunity, and the militarily weaker prodemocracy sector—some members of which attempted to "uproot" (*dechouke*) individuals known to be Duvalier loyalists or tonton makout. During this period Haitians began to use the term "ensekirite" to characterize the violence throughout the nation, but especially to connote how the repression was especially acute for the poor who remained targets of Duvalierist forces.

Despite the overarching atmosphere of fear and uncertainty, on December 16, 1990, Haitians elected to the presidency former priest Jean-Bertrand Aristide, a staunch advocate for political and economic justice who gave voice to the frustrations of the poor. Hopes for democracy were short-lived: on September 30, 1991, the Haitian military usurped power and forced Aristide into exile after less than eight months in office. During the three years of ensekirite that followed, the coup apparatus—composed of members of the army, civilian paramilitary attachés, and *zenglendo* (armed bandits or criminals)—deployed necropolitical violence on a widespread scale in attempts to destroy systematically the physical, social, kinship, and moral foundations of their opposition. While the international community debated whether or not to intervene militarily to restore democracy, the strategies of detention and disappearances, gang rape, repeated rape and forced incest, murder and mutilations of corpses, and theft and destruction of property, were directed against those individuals and neighborhoods held to be loyal to President Aristide. The U.S.-led Multinational Force (MNF)—a coalition of military units from twenty-eight nations authorized by U.N. Security Council Resolution 940—intervened in September 1994 to restore Aristide to the presidency (on October 15,1994), thereby inaugurating the postcoup era of "democracy." During this time of entrenched economic stagnation, ensekirite continued unabated but in altered form. It began to refer to the proliferation of political, criminal, and gang violence that could occur at any moment and without a predictable pattern, as well as to the everyday crimes the political motivations of which were less clear. The combination of these forms of violence and social and material uncertainty hindered the nation's attempts to consolidate democracy, rule of law, and sustained economic growth.

The climate of fear inculcated by state-sponsored violence and the widespread material fragility of life in contemporary Haiti is but one aspect of a broader, collective sense of "ontological insecurity" (Giddens 1984) that especially characterizes the life of the poor. In his complex structuration theory, the sociologist Anthony Giddens defines ontological security as "confidence or trust that the natural and social worlds are as they appear to be, including the basic existential parameters of self and social identity" (1984:375). The *sense* of security generated by the routinization of daily life is integral to and engenders the existential foundations of self and body, social action, and, ultimately, the reproduction of the structure of society. As the foregoing discussion shows, the reality of ensekirite in Haiti, especially among the poor, is that there can be no presumption of stability, security, or trust for the individual or collective group. On the contrary, "ontological insecurity" (Giddens 1984:62) forms the existential ground of day-to-day life in Haiti, where disruptions and fluctuations in social institutions and practices may be the norm. In post-earthquake Haiti, even the sense of security that the physical geography may have once provided (despite recurring fluctuations in the sociopolitical sphere) can no longer be presumed.

To some extent, PTSD, a psychiatric diagnostic category utilized in Haiti only relatively recently, has been useful to describe the profoundly disruptive impacts of ensekirite and can assist in describing what for many Haitians has been a paradigmatic shift in the mode of being-in-the-world. But PTSD still fails to capture the complex effects of ongoing uncertainty in Haiti. In my discussions and physical therapy with women of Martissant, their suffering corresponded to continual stressors, rather than a single etiological traumatic event from which there was now a "post"—as is commonly conceived of PTSD (Basoglu 1992; Herman 1992; van der Kolk et al. 1996; Marsella et al. 1996; Young 1995).

Furthermore, the conception of trauma or the traumatic memory as residing in the individual sufferer and originating in the past was belied by my experience of everyday life in the Martissant bidonvil. There the literal ghosts of the past are very present in mundane reality and irrupt into conscious awareness from both within and without the individual (James 2008). States of ensekirite force us to ask the following question: when ruptures in the fabric of social life are routine, of what use is a concept of posttraumatic stress? What threshold or boundary exists between normal mourning and grief and pathological responses to traumatic events? When ruptures become routine, what possibility is there for sustained hope, or for a sense of ontological security? In what social institutions or actors can Haitians invest as guarantors of public health and security?

The Social Life of PTSD in Haiti

The DSM's PTSD construct has been influential in the development of what I have called elsewhere the "political economy of trauma" (James 2004). PTSD was exported to Haiti in the 1990s through multiple international humanitarian relief efforts following both human-authored and natural disasters. During my ethnographic study of rehabilitation programs aiding survivors of organized violence, I learned how trauma treatment practices transformed the political subjectivity of both providers and recipients of care. Haitian psychiatrists and psychologists who had trained abroad adopted the DSM-IV PTSD diagnostic category in their clinical work and teaching at the State University Hospital's Mars/Kline Center for Neurology and Psychiatry. In our discussions between 1998 and 1999, many clinicians felt the PTSD category was superfluous and claimed that its features could be encompassed by depression and anxiety. Many also felt that the diagnosis failed to address the particular cultural ways that Haitians experienced emotional distress after a shock. In a context in which international humanitarian aid organizations wielded and continue to possess tremendous power over Haiti and its citizens— a form of humanitarian governance that has expanded exponentially since the earthquake—Haitian mental health practitioners deployed PTSD to demonstrate their own clinical competence (Good 1995, 1999) and to access both national and international resources for the public and private institutions with which they were affiliated. The technologies of trauma used to aid Haitians to render inchoate experiences of victimization discursive and legible contributed to the commodification of their suffering. An unintended consequence was that formerly independent activists (*militan*) adopted new identities as patient-clients of the aid apparatus.

This political economy of trauma notwithstanding, the PTSD construct can provide tools for understanding the extreme suffering of Haiti's victims. Some Haitians manifest posttraumatic stress in ways that resemble biomedical conceptions of PTSD; however, their so-called symptoms are frequently interpreted through other moral meaning systems. For example, one woman with whom I worked closely between 1997 and 1999 in administering a Haitian Creole translation of the Clinician-Administered PTSD Scale remarked that she frequently saw *vizyon* (visions)—a term that typically refers to religious visions—on a "screen" in front of her. These images, however, were of her own victimization by members of the coup apparatus rather than of explicitly religious content. That religious discourses would provide a structure or framework through which to interpret extraordinary experiences is not surprising. Proponents of evangelical Protestantism have traced the roots of Haiti's individual and collective traumas to historical involvement with the widespread religion of *Vodou*, from the purported diabolical pact that Haitians made with Satan in 1791 to attain the powers required to overthrow French colonial forces (McAlister 2012) to contemporary practices of ancestral and family religious traditions. Understandings of suffering arising from and linked to the epistemology of the Vodou tradition may also identify the ultimate etiology of affliction in the moral realm, for example, the failure to uphold kinship and other spiritual obligations, or—particularly with respect to the baneful practices of sorcery—as the result of another individual's jealousy or malediction (Brodwin 1996; Farmer 1992; James 2012). In these cases, conversion to Protestantism has become a means by which some Haitians sought psychosocial healing, and economic and spiritual security, as well as immunity from vulnerability to others' occult practices (Conway 1978).

As I observed during my fieldwork, these religious perspectives operated alongside the secular theodicies of feminism and human rights. Haitian *viktim*—self-named "victims of human rights abuses"—whom I encountered at the women's clinic and Human Rights Fund reinterpreted the ultimate causes of their suffering through a political lens as the result of gender inequalities and a predatory state. But these secular interpretations were often insufficient to mitigate the ongoing subjective experience of trauma.

Personhood, Embodiment, and Emotion
in Traditional Haiti

My understanding of Haitian traditional conceptions of embodiment derives in no small part from the clinical and therapeutic work in which I participated among the poorest residents of Port-au-Prince and the provinces and from analysis of the testimonies and other documentary evidence contained in the case files at the Human Rights Fund.[17] From these qualitative and archival methods I learned that several cultural components influenced the subjective experiences of emotion, illness, and suffering: the religious beliefs and ritual practices of Vodou—comprising a mélange of European Catholic, Masonic, indigenous, and African traditions that fused during the colonial period; the crafts of bonesetters (*doktè zo*), midwives (*fanm saj*), and other manual therapists; and, in many cases, the theologies of the evangelical Protestant denominations that understand everyday life in Haiti as subjected to the struggles between unseen forces.[18] I also came to understand that many Haitians experienced the circulation of substances like blood, heat, and cold in the body; the unpredictability of environmental forces; the acts of invisible spirits and ancestors; and the benevolent and malevolent magical practices of occult actors, as factors affecting the relationships between psyche and soma.

In Haitian traditional culture, the "self" or "person" is located at the nexus of relationships among the living, the ancestors, and the divine spirits (*lwa*) (Brown 1989:257; 1991). In order to maintain balance among the person, family, and larger community, individuals must honor the duties and obligations that accompany each relational linkage between the living and the dead. Although personhood and identity are indelibly tied to the lwa for ritual practitioners of Vodou (Dayan 1991:50), I found that even for Haitians who did not explicitly admit to or describe service to the divine spirits, their understandings of the embodied self were inextricably linked to the folk religion's theology. The embodied person comprises multiple parts. The *kò kadav* is the material body. It is separable from the complex soul and decays after death (Brown 1989:265–66; Dayan 1991:51). The *gwo bonanj* (the big guardian angel), is a nonmaterial "metaphysical double of the physical being" (Deren [1953] 1970:226) that detaches from the body during sleep (Brown 1991:351–52; Dayan 1991:51; Deren [1953] 1970:25–26; Larose 1977:92; Métraux [1959] 1972:120, 303) and in the course of ritual spirit possession— returning after the lwa has completed its intended action (Bourguignon 1984:247). An individual experiencing emotional distress may say that his or her "big guardian angel" is upset (Brown 1989:264). Vulnerable to sorcery and magic, the gwo bonanj can be especially defenseless at death, when it may become a "disembodied force wandering here and there"—a *zonbi*[19] (Larose 1977:93). Somewhat like the lwa, the detached zonbi can possess individuals; but rather than manifesting in a circumscribed ceremonial context, the zonbi acts as an unruly and malevolent force seeking a permanent home until it can be detached through ritual means. A captured zonbi can also be sent by a relative to avenge an injustice before the mortuary rituals have dispersed it (Larose 1977:95; McAlister 2002:102–11). In addition to the gwo bonanj, the *ti bonanj* (little good angel) is a force that is deeper than consciousness, acts as a conscience, and can enervate the individual in times of stress (Brown 1989:265; Deren [1953] 1970:26; Larose 1977:94). The *nanm* is the animating force that disappears after corporeal death (Brown 1989:264). Finally, the *zetwal* (star) is a celestial component of the self that resides outside the body and relates to the person's destiny.

The seat of the gwo bonanj is the head (*tèt*), an important component of Haitian ethnophysiology that links psyche and soma, as well as the material and spiritual dimensions of many emotions, illnesses, and diseases. Disorders of the tèt give rise to a number of bodily afflictions like *tèt fè mal* (headache, migraine), *tèt vire* (dizziness, vertigo), and others to be discussed below. As a result of a variety of psychic, social, spiritual, and material (etc.) imbalances, the tèt may become the repository of excess bodily substances or forces: "When an individual is worried, his or her head is said to be 'loaded.' In excitement, the head heats up; when the head cools, the individual becomes calm, also sad" (Bourguignon 1984:262). The substance that regulates the circulation of hot and cold in the body is *san* (blood); imbalances in its flow render individuals vulnerable to illness (Laguerre 1987:70). Foods that one eats, individual acts, and environmental and the aforementioned spiritual factors influence the balance of heat and cold in the blood (Laguerre 1987:70–71). The permeable boundaries of this embodied self render subjectivity and life itself as relational, but also subject to the precarities of local behavioral ecologies (or local biologies).

The foregoing discussion presents an image of an embodied subject whose social relationships and environment are also constitutive aspects of subjectivity, of the self, and of personhood.[20] For Haitians who become possessed by divine entities while serving the spirits, or furthermore, who are slain in the Holy Spirit in Protestant and Catholic charismatic worship services, dissociative states are not necessarily alien or pathological; rather, they are desirable. However, ruptures in the linkages among the individual, community, ancestors, and the lwa can cause emotional disorders, illness, and other material and spiritual problems, not only for the individual, but also for the extended family, both living and dead.[21] Given these complexities, how do Haitians define trauma? How should it be treated? Does the narration of suffering necessarily facilitate healing at either individual or collective levels?

I raise these questions knowing that I cannot answer all of them in this short essay but offer now the case of Jean-Robert Paul as one that offers some troubling answers. In this example, Jean-Robert is situated at the nexus of the encounters among Haitian traditional understandings of emotional and physical distress (and their remedy), and a bricolage of pharmacological treatments proffered by international biomedically trained clinicians in the United States and their expatriate and Haitian counterparts in Haiti.

Jean-Robert Paul

I met Jean-Robert in 1998 at the Human Rights Fund Rehabilitation Program, "the Fund," as the program was called informally. He was a twenty-one-year-old man who worked now and then as a groundskeeper, primarily to "hang out" with staff in the *lakou* (courtyard) inside the walled campus. Of slight but not frail build, he had a mischievous grin and sunny disposition, always smiling at me when I arrived each day. At times he was the object of ribbing, especially when he tried to banter with the armed private security guards and drivers who congregated on the verandah at the entrance to the gingerbread-style building. Jean-Robert had been a beneficiary of the Rehabilitation Program since April 1997. He was considered an indirect victim of politically motivated violence because his parents, pro-Aristide activists, were direct victims of human rights abuses. They had been murdered in 1994, just prior to the restoration of constitutional order. Gaining beneficiary status provided Jean-Robert a small stipend, housing assistance, medical care, and other social support.

However, Jean-Robert may also have had a liminal status at the Fund because he was also perceived to be *fou* (insane). When I inquired about him at the Mars/Kline Center for Neurology and Psychiatry and among the facilitators of the therapy groups for viktim at the Fund, both the international and Haitian mental health specialists had labeled him schizophrenic. They told me that his memories of the circumstances engendering his beneficiary status were disjointed and tremendously distressing. I would eventually witness directly what I interpreted as the irruption of the traumatic past into the present. The incident caused me to question further the concept of PTSD and how it might manifest in cross-cultural contexts.

One day inside the Human Rights Fund building, Jean-Robert suddenly became angry and aggressive toward staff members. He had come to request additional financial support, but at the time program funds were diminishing. The program director denied his request and in response, Jean-Robert became agitated. Then, something shifted, transforming Jean-Robert's usual demeanor and seemingly allowing another "persona" to speak the frustration of his condition. This shift was alarming, a stark contrast to his customary "presentation of self in everyday life" (Goffman 1959). His face changed, becoming taut and drawn with tension. His gaze no longer focused on the physical space around him. Rather, he seemed to be peering into the distance, perhaps recalling the past, but not seeing those of us physically near him. He started breathing heavily and was clenching and unclenching his fists. He began speaking strongly and with a deeper voice that was quite different from his usual soft-spoken tone. It was one with eloquence and passion, but also pathos. He said, "Look at me. Look at my body. Look at how I've shrunk in size. I used to be a man. I don't have anywhere to sleep. I don't even have a bed." The two nurses who staffed this program quickly approached Jean-Robert to calm him down. One wiped his forehead, attempting to cool him down. He seemed shaken by the force of emotion that had overcome him and by his own utterances, but was eventually soothed, returning to the placid individual to whom I had become accustomed.

Later, the nurses explained that his head (tèt) had become hot (cho) and that their ministrations had been meant to reverse the flow of excess blood to the head that caused his outburst. Building on the discussion above of traditional understandings of embodiment in Haiti, the condition of tèt cho (hot head) or move san (bad blood) (Farmer 1988), could cause endispozisyon (indisposition)—spells of falling out or fainting and weakness—as well as other disordered states. Jean-Robert's condition of tèt cho was common among the Rehabilitation Program clients. Many Haitian mental health practitioners told me that a heightened emotional state and propensity to eruption in aggression was characteristic of viktim, a pattern that accords with DSM-5's criteria for PTSD. However, the moment Jean-Robert's behavior and speech changed also resembled the way that the lwa, the Haitian Vodou spirits, entered the head of a supplicant and began communicating through the devotee's body. Although in ritual circumstances the entrance of the divine spirits is desired (Brown 1991), in this case, possession by the specter of a traumatic past was an unwelcome intrusion, despite its prophetic, revelatory nature. But such a manifestation of distress might also be interpreted through the DSM-5's description of dissociative reactions.

Jean-Robert's status in relationship to this U.S.-funded trauma treatment program raises larger questions about the moral and political economy of PTSD in Haiti that I can only gesture toward here. How had Jean-Robert become the ward of an international nongovernmental organization and a patient of international and national psychologists, psychiatrists, and other humanitarian aid workers in Haiti? What happens when a succession of biomedically trained caregivers attempt to treat conditions with which they possess little familiarity and experience, not to mention, cultural competency, and the care is perceived as harmful rather than palliative?

Jean-Robert's past can be reconstructed only in part. Its ghostly traces existed in fragments contained in his "trauma portfolio"—the case file containing affidavits and medical records documenting his past experiences of rupture—and in the memories of the caretakers who had provided him asylum. As mentioned above, in June 1994, just prior to the restoration of democratic order by international military intervention, the young man became what the Rehab Program characterized as an "indirect" victim of organized violence. He had been seventeen years old, an only child, and residing with his family in a small, isolated coastal town near the westernmost tip of Haiti's southern peninsula. On that fateful day in June, members of the military murdered Jean-Robert's parents on the street in a quintessential example of necropolitics. One of his psychologists told me that soldiers wielding ma-chetes beheaded his parents directly in front of him. The killing ruptured the ties between him and his natal family, and subsequently, to his country.

After the decapitation of his parents, Jean-Robert fled Haiti with hopes of attaining asylum in the United States. I do not know if he was able to per-form customary mortuary rites to lay the souls (zonbi) of his parents to rest or if he left immediately. Customarily, funerary rites would have included more than a week of activities immediately after death and would comprise a "wake, funeral (in a chapel, if possible), procession to the cemetery, and burial" after which "the nine-day mourning period begins, in which relatives and neighbors of the deceased gather nightly to mourn, chant Catholic texts, socialize, recreate, and cajole the dead (with food) to take leave of the living for the world of the ancestors" (Richman [2005] 2008:124).[22] As I have docu-mented elsewhere (2008, 2010), the failure to perform customary mortuary rites—whether from lack of the body or of means to conduct these time- and resource-consuming practices of sociality—could be devastating socially, emotionally, and spiritually. Angry spirits can even torment survivors, leav-ing what one woman with whom I worked described as stigmata on her body after nightly struggles with the spirit of her deceased husband (James 2008).

It is doubtful that the then seventeen-year-old young man, fleeing for fear of further persecution, had the financial means or the time to arrange these mortuary practices. Jean-Robert most likely left immediately after the mur-ders to seek sanctuary outside Haiti. What is certain is that he disembarked on a perilous journey by boat with hopes that refuge lay in the United States. Such sea journeys are hazardous and frequently result in interdiction, im-mediate repatriation, or even death by starvation or drowning. Jean-Robert was fortunate to have landed in south Florida, but he was apprehended and then detained at the notorious Krome detention facility in Miami while his asylum request was pending. In the 1980s, the conditions at Krome were de-plorable, leading one writer to compare the adult facility to a "theater of the absurd" and to a concentration camp (Nachman 1993:251, 254). Conditions in the early 1990s provoked hunger strikes among inmates and protests by human rights activists outside its walls.[23] But as an unaccompanied minor, Jean-Robert did not remain there long. In September 1994, he received asylee status and was sheltered in a program for unaccompanied minors in Boston, Massachusetts. There he began to unravel.

Jean-Robert's trauma portfolio provides some information about the onset of psychosis. After arriving in the U.S., he began recalling how his parents had been murdered, and a note in his case file says that from that moment of recall his "disorder was unleashed" (*la maladie est déclenchée*). He suffered visual and auditory hallucinations and paranoid thinking and was violent toward others. Psychiatrists diagnosed "subchronic schizophrenia" and prescribed antipsychotics and antidepressants. During one acute psychotic episode, Jean-Robert was hospitalized and injected with antipsychotic and antispasmodic drugs. Presumably, he had not been compliant with his treatment and the injections ensured that his symptoms would be managed. Jean-Robert felt that the medications were too strong, and he reported that they "hit him in the head." That he experienced medical treatment as blows suggests that their intent was to pacify and subdue him, rather than to relieve his suffering.

In October 1996, despite receiving political asylum, Jean-Robert was repatriated to Haiti. Upon his arrival in Haiti the United Nations International Civilian Mission processed Jean-Robert's case without providing treatment; its victim assistance services had been suspended earlier that year. His trauma portfolio was next transferred to Médecins du Monde (Doctors of the World), whose Spanish psychiatrist examined him and diagnosed schizophrenia, but otherwise good health. She proposed psychotherapy and a new course of antianxiety and antipsychotic medications.

Throughout these travails and shifts from one institution and organization to the next, Jean-Robert had not asked for treatment but rather, amelioration of the structural conditions that prevented him from living. His report states that as he was unemployed and that he desired social assistance and return to the United States. Unfortunately, in 1997 Médecins du Monde also ceased providing treatment to victims of human rights abuses. Jean-Robert was next transferred to the Human Rights Fund, receiving eligibility in April of that year. In 1999, a few months after I witnessed Jean-Robert's dissociative outburst, the Rehabilitation Program would also cease providing services, leaving its beneficiaries to seek support from the fragile Haitian state or to negotiate the cycles of insecurity on their own.

How are we to interpret the fragments of Jean-Robert's case? Certainly, these rehabilitative measures transformed Jean-Robert's disordered subjectivity in both positive and negative ways, offering care on the one hand and a measure of security, but also the "pharmaceuticalization" of self and bodily experiences on the other (Biehl 2010). Nonetheless, the national and international charitable, human rights, religious, and medical groups intervening to aid Haitians during its persistent states of emergency had limited capacity to provide sustainable assistance. As each organization lost funding, it transferred its collective trauma portfolios and the work of care to other organizations with means. Unfortunately, Haitians with chronic disordered conditions received less social and material support to rebuild their lives and find paths toward sustainable security. But it is important to note how many of these institutions medicalized, and in large part, depoliticized the grief and feelings of loss (and righteous indignation) that Jean-Robert suffered when he desired social support, the right to work, health, justice, and security.

Odette Jean

My work with Odette Jean raises additional provocative questions about how to address complex posttraumatic stress in situations of chronic insecurity and the gendered ways in which Haitian trauma and mourning manifest and are mitigated. In February 1999, I interviewed Odette, then a fifty-eight-year-old woman, in the clinic at which I had voluntarily been providing physical therapy to rape survivors and other women patients. In the small room where we worked, Odette spoke about the violence in the neighborhood as a component of her life story. A few days prior to our meeting a brutal murder had taken place in the mountains above the clinic. Odette heard about the killing from other women who lived near the murder site—a section of the deforested mountain called the Zòn (zone) Siyon. During the coup years, the *siyon,* an open-air evangelical Protestant church, had sheltered many internally displaced Haitians. The mountain was now freckled with makeshift shacks and one-room cinderblock homes with tin roofs, where large families of squatters had built permanent homes.

Odette described how gang members killed the young man, the son of a friend of hers, for unknown reasons. The murderers drowned him, submerging his head in an oil drum that stored rainwater. Residents of the neighborhood were too frightened to bury the body or to report what had happened to the police, as the perpetrators lived in the same neighborhood. Eventually, a couple of women who were also clients of mine went to the police to report the death, and the young man was eventually buried. The story was extremely distressing for Odette because it reminded her of when her own family members were attacked roughly eight years prior to our interview while living in the same vicinity.

Although I had heard many disturbing stories about violent crime in Martissant during and after the coup years, and witnessed its effects on the women I saw at the clinic, what struck me on this occasion was *how* Odette recounted the story. At the time her words came in halting fragments and erupted into the narrative of the recent murder in disjointed elliptical phrases. She then slipped into a description of her embodied shock (*sezisman*) and feelings of resignation after her own past losses, then a few words later returned to the story of the recently drowned young man. Odette appeared to be moving in and out of intrusive memories, at times whispering and gazing off at a distance then returning to the present. I then asked her if we could use a diagnostic interview schedule, the Clinician-Administered PTSD Scale for DSM-IV (CAPS) (Blake et al. 1998)—in which I had received training in 1998 at the National Center for Posttraumatic Stress Disorder from the authors of the instrument—as a means to provide a structure through which to approach these distressing biographical details.[24] She agreed, and over the course of a two-hour interview we attempted to reconstruct some tragic events of her life history. Throughout the interview, the events of 1990—when her family members were raped, murdered, and disappeared, and her house was destroyed—and the murder in 1999 of the young man, erupted into the narrative, as did descriptions of the bodily suffering such events caused her. These traumas were the center around which her narrated life history pivoted.

Odette was born in Aux Cayes du Fonds in the southern peninsula of Haiti. Her mother died from an unnamed illness and her father took care of her and her brother until he remarried. When her father died, her stepmother mistreated her and forced her to work from morning until night, denigrating her verbally, and withholding food, soap, and clean clothing. Like many young women who lived in perilous domestic conditions Odette escaped to the capital at the age of sixteen to seek a better life. She began living in the slums of La Saline and later found some security working as a maid for a French family. At around twenty years of age, she fell in love with a young man and became pregnant; however, the young men left her as soon as he learned of the pregnancy. (It's not clear whether she was still working for the French family at this point and was ejected from the household or if she was living on her own.) She described being homeless during her pregnancy and malnourished, and she lacked funds to pay for medical care for the delivery. The General Hospital charged 10 gourdes at the time (approximately US$2) and she had no means of obtaining the sum. So when Odette went into labor, she spent four days attempting to deliver the child on her own without support. Upon returning to the hospital she was admitted and the doctors attempted to remove the child from her body alive, but her little boy had already died.

In the years after this loss, Odette went on to have five more children and described some success as a *madanm sara*, a market woman. She was living with her brother, a sister, and three of her children until that fateful day when her family was attacked because of their prodemocracy activism. Antidemocratic forces in her neighborhood had pressured them to vote against Jean-Bertrand Aristide, but her family remained loyal.

Odette could not give me the exact date of the tragedy that befell her family but stated that the attacks came prior to Aristide's taking power in 1991. As previously discussed, the necropolitical style of violence resembled what would later become a systematic and widespread pattern of terror used against poor Haitian activists both during and after the coup years. Not long after Aristide was elected president, members of the coup apparatus murdered one of her sons at the local market. Others entered her house, burning birth certificates and other identification cards, destroying all that she owned. Her daughter was gang raped. Another son fled the house. During the course of the attack, Odette also escaped and stayed in the unpopulated wilds of the mountains and ravines south of the squatter settlement. Although on October 15, 1994, the U.S. and UN military forces restored constitutional democracy, the intervention failed to disarm the coup apparatus fully. Many of the prodemocracy majority continued to live in the same neighborhoods as their still armed perpetrators. The political and criminal insecurity that ebbed and flowed as a result contributed to Haiti's ongoing economic stagnation and instability. Eventually she returned to living in the Martissant area, but at a much lower elevation than the Zone Siyon.

Odette felt deep remorse about not having prevented her daughter from being raped. Her daughter had become pregnant from the rape and had had a little girl, whom she had abandoned. The girl now lived with another family in the area. The little girl knew that Odette was her grandmother and occasionally approached her to ask for food or other support. This inability to help her granddaughter, because of her own poverty and ambivalent feelings, caused her tremendous suffering.

Most distressing was her son's disappearance. Odette had not heard from or seen the young man in almost ten years. He was presumed dead. It was the lack of knowledge about this missing son that tormented her. Not only was she unable to perform roles as parent and grandparent as would be expected in this moral economy, the absence of his body prevented the fulfillment of customary mortuary rites enabling his soul's passage from living kin to the realm of the ancestors. But while describing how these distressing events dominated her thoughts—a pattern of uncontrollable rumination that Haitians called *dominasyon*—she abruptly returned to describing the conditions of insecurity in 1999, which included gang members who controlled when and how residents of the zone moved through public space.

She also told of her suffering from *tansyon* (literally, "tension"), a condition similar to high blood pressure, referring to a disorder of the blood that resulted from emotional distress. Throughout the interview she stated that she had problems in her head (*mwen gen pwoblèm nan tèt mwen*), and that since the recent murder of the young man was so close to where she once lived, it was as if the murder of her friends' son was also a loss for Odette to bear. It reminded her of how she fled her house when the attack occurred during the coup years and of her inability to protect her children.[25]

As I moved through the CAPS symptom checklist, Odette's negative responses to questions asking whether she experienced hypervigilance, negative affect, feelings of emotional isolation, startle response, or dissociation were surprising to me. Her ruminations on failing to fulfill expected kinship roles could easily be labeled survivor's guilt; she felt profound remorse because of her inability to take care of loved ones. She deliberately chose to reside in an area more distant from the site of her family's attack, as much to avoid the perpetrators who continued to patrol the zone as to avoid triggering horrific memories of that day. Was her posttrauma experience PTSD? Although she did not verbally state having symptoms that corresponded exactly to the DSM-IV criteria, she was among the most troubled individuals whom I encountered in therapeutic contexts in Haiti and seemed unmoored in time, space, and speech. Perhaps, like the women Dr. Nicolas described above as living with unrecognized depression, the traumatic sequelae of the ruptures Odette exhibited could not be captured as PTSD using the CAPS diagnostic instrument.

It may also be that her efforts to find relief through faith—a source of sustenance and resilience for many Haitians, but especially for women who had been targets of violence (Rey 1999)—provided means for coping with the unwelcome memories of her own losses amidst the ongoing insecurity of the zone. To a question that asked about intrusive memories, Odette said that for her the best way to survive was by forgetting. She said, "If you remember, you can't live." These unwanted memories were described as an oppressive domination (dominasyon), and were said to hit her head (*frape tèt ou*). Too much rumination on the past (*kalkilasyon*) would kill her. Instead, her salvation lay in becoming another person through her faith in God and through religious conversion. By forgetting the past and what she could not control in the present, she had begun centering herself in the conversion experience, exercising agency, and perhaps, a modicum of control, through the disciplines of prayer and fasting for others, for Haiti, and for the world. Although Odette's life history contained a seemingly incessant chain of deeply distressing events, her strategies for survival and hope challenge contemporary conceptions of posttraumatic stress that would view avoidance of distressing thoughts as pathological, and would pose treatments that would encourage greater confrontation of and engagement with traumatic memories.

How should we interpret the fragments of this story, especially in light of the collective trauma that Haiti suffered on January 12, 2010? On that fateful day over two hundred thousand people died during the earthquake, and many were buried in mass graves without the mortuary rites that would be customary in Haitian culture. Odette's case suggests how the lack of knowledge of those who are missing may also traumatize thousands of Haitians over time, but especially those who are most vulnerable, the poor. Furthermore, about five thousand inmates escaped from damaged prison facilities and remain at large (BBC News),[26] and many have resumed former careers in fomenting ensekirite through violent crime, extortion, and patrolling of social space both within and outside the internally displaced persons camps. In the years after the earthquake, Haiti has confronted the resurgence of gang violence and sexual violence and the concomitant spread of infectious disease, especially in the camps. There has been an exponential increase of kidnappings of both Haitians and international humanitarians by these nonstate actors. Another unanticipated disaster is a devastating outbreak of cholera carried to Haiti by UN troops from Nepal.

The most pressing task at hand continues to be how to meet the basic needs of Haiti's citizens while also creating and sustaining collective security—a prerequisite, I argue, for aiding Haitians to come to terms with traumatic losses. As they had done during and after the 1991–94 coup years, and as described above, a plethora of organizations have established trauma treatment programs and other mental health initiatives around the nation. Although the various trauma treatment modalities that are currently being offered to Haitians may provide tools that aid in resolution of the psychosocial sequelae of ensekirite, one wonders whether and how successful imported brands of therapy may be in the long term, especially if their techniques do not take into account traditional conceptions of embodiment and the complex self/soul. In addition to this, are the interventions offered sustainable—inculcating in patient/clients durable practices of self-care that may be employed to mitigate past and future ensekirite?

Effective programs must focus their interventions beyond the immediate effects of the earthquake in Haiti. These programs must be comprehensive, accounting for the ongoing effects of routines of rupture in the past, as well as current structural socioeconomic challenges. Nevertheless, international relief funds only trickle into Haiti and have limited effects on the lives of those most in need. But as both Jean-Robert and Odette's examples suggest, by focusing on treating trauma or PTSD to the exclusion of remedying ontological insecurity in Haiti, clinicians, mental health practitioners, missionaries, and other interveners may be medicalizing or pathologizing forms of mourning and grief that are becoming routine given Haiti's ensekirite rather than addressing its historical and (infra)structural roots. Without collective security, how effective can these programs be? Will they merely expand and sustain the political economy of trauma in Haiti, one in which the treatment of trauma aids the interveners as much, if not more, than Haitians?

Notes

1. The ICTP website asserts, "Children in Haiti are suffering from post traumatic distress that manifests itself both in psychological symptoms such as fear and anxiety as well as day to day functioning in school. Our resilience building interventions have been implemented in post-war and post-disaster environments in different cultures and countries and will be adapted to the language and culture of Haiti." See their website at http://www.traumaweb.org/content.asp?PageId=434&lang=En, last accessed January 29, 2014. Treatment modalities are described here: http://www.traumaweb.org/content.asp?pageid=113, last accessed January 29, 2014.

2. See http://www.emdr.com/, last accessed January 29, 2014.

3. See http://www.traumahealing.com/somatic-experiencing/, last accessed January 29, 2014.

4. According to the TRI's website (http://traumaresourceinstitute.com/trauma-resiliency-model-trm/, last accessed January 29, 2014), "Trauma Resiliency Model (TRM) Training is a program designed to teach skills to clinicians working with children and adults with traumatic stress reactions. TRM is a mind-body approach and focuses on the biological basis of trauma and the automatic, defensive ways that the human body responds when faced with perceived threats to self and others, including

the responses of 'tend and befriend', fight, flight and freeze. TRM explores the concept of resiliency and how to restore balance to the body and the mind after traumatic experiences. When the focus is on normal biological responses to extraordinary events, there is a paradigm shift from symptoms being described as biological rather than as pathological or as mental weakness. As traumatic stress symptoms are normalized, feelings of shame and self-blame are reduced or eliminated. Symptoms are viewed as the body's attempt to re-establish balance to the nervous system."

5. See http://traumaresourceinstitute.com/history/, last accessed January 29, 2014.

6. http://www.uusc.org/content/trauma-recovery_group_continues_work_haiti.

7. See http://traumaresourceinstitute.com/history/, last accessed January 29, 2014.

8. See http://cmbm.org/global-trauma-relief/about-gtr/, last accessed January 29, 2014.

9. See *Healing Trauma, Restoring Hope*, http://cmbm.org/global-trauma-relief/the -campaign/, last accessed January 29, 2014.

10. Although the outpouring of assistance to the nation and its people is laudable, a troubling dimension of the expansion and proliferation of these treatment programs is the possibility that Haitian trauma—whether individual, collective, or even national— poses, for those who consider themselves mental health pioneers, a terrain that is ripe for cultivation and transformation through experimental measures, the efficacy of which may not be tracked or regulated by the state (Petryna 2009).

11. See http://www.huffingtonpost.com/erin-marcus/ptsd-manifests-differentl_b _580825.html, last accessed January 29, 2014.

12. While it has become common to refer to the term "structural violence" in order to explain the pernicious effects of poverty, I have found that such a term tends to leave unexamined the complexity of situations of vulnerability that simultaneously involve international, national, and local relations of power, economy, politics, race, gender, and other factors. While naming structural inequalities "violence" can assist in drawing attention to the everyday misery of the disenfranchised individual, community, or nation, it may do more harm than good by crystallizing violence in a fetishistic manner.

13. See http://www.huffingtonpost.com/erin-marcus/ptsd-manifests-differentl_b _580825.html, last accessed January 29, 2014.

14. On the other hand, the recent influx of international mental health workers seeking to ameliorate trauma in Haitians might also produce an overdiagnosis of the condition.

15. I provided physical therapy service to rape survivors and other patients in my capacity as a practitioner of a mode of manual therapy called the Trager Approach, see http://www.trager.com/approach.html, last accessed January 29, 2014.

16. Hinton et al. 2013 have observed similar responses among Cambodian refugees.

17. As discussed elsewhere (James 2010), trauma portfolios were assembled in several periods—the America's Development Foundation staff members had compiled one archive during the early years of the coup period prior to the inauguration of the first iteration of the Human Rights Fund (HRF) project in 1994. These files were stored on-site but were not in the best condition. With the advent of the new HRF Rehab program in 1997, its program directors, upon questioning the authenticity of another second set of case files that had been assembled under HRFII, launched a new system for documenting cases of prospective beneficiaries to which I had full access. In everyday communications the HRF program was called Fon Dwa Moun (Haitian Creole for "Human Rights Fund") or "the Fund."

18. While none of my clients admitted to serving the spirits, the broad formulation of a sociocentric "self/body" (Becker 1991), which follows, was commonly expressed regardless of their stated religious practice.

19. A sorcerer can capture the gwo bonanj when a person is alive. Although this entity is also called the zonbi, in this case, it can be used to force the material person to whom it belongs to labor for the sorcerer as what has conventionally has come to be understood as the living dead. Note, however, that some scholars of religion in Haiti ascribe to the ti bonanj (little good angel) the vulnerability to capture and forced labor as a zonbi (Davis 1988:187–91).

20. As noted elsewhere (James 2008), Brown describes the consequences of the complex components of identity and body on subjectivity, but especially for ritual practitioners: "for the Vodou worshipper, each person is at the core of his or her being, a multiplicity of beings, a polymorphous entity and that it is only at the periphery of life, in areas less important to that person, that he or she adopts clearly definable, and consistent roles or modes of being" (Brown 1979:23). See also Boddy 1988, Brown 1991, Antze 1996, and Lambek 1996 for discussions of how the expression of alternate selves through either spontaneous possession or multiple personality disorder can be considered creative presentations of self in everyday life, regardless of whether such manifestations are willed or involuntary.

21. Even as they are also sources of blessing and healing, relational obligations are sometimes sources of threat to the self. Illness or misfortune can befall the person who is directly culpable for failure to uphold these obligations (Métraux [1959] 1972:256) or other persons within the community.

22. See also Smith 2001:128–32 for a detailed description of the funerary practices of Haiti's Sosyete Ann Leve Ansanm (Let Us Rise Up Together Society).

23. See Patrick Reyna, "Haitian Hunger Strikers Say They Will Die If Not Released," Associated Press, January 4, 1993.

24. I was testing whether the CAPS for DSM-IV could be used in a cross-cultural context.

25. On how rumination on past and present events (often cast in the trope of "thinking too much"), as well as the experiencing of somatic symptom and cultural syndromes,

are at the core of the trauma presentation in many cultures, see Hinton and Good, Chapter 1 of this volume.

26. Nigel Pankhurst, "Haiti Earthquake: Did Appeal Money Make a Difference?" *BBC News*, January 11, 2012, http://www.bbc.co.uk/news/uk-16283942, last accessed February 16, 2014.

References

Antze, Paul

    1996 Telling Stories, Making Selves: Memory and Identity in Multiple Personality Disorder. *In* Tense Past: Cultural Essays in Trauma and Memory. Paul Antze and Michael Lambek, eds. Pp. 3–23. London: Routledge.

Basoglu, Metin, ed.

    1992 Torture and Its Consequences: Current Treatment Approaches. Cambridge: Cambridge University Press.

Becker, Anne

    1991 Body Image in Fiji: The Self in the Body and in the Community. Ph.D. diss., Harvard University.

Biehl, João

    2010 "Medication Is Me Now": Human Values and Political Life in the Wake of Global AIDS Treatment. *In* In the Name of Humanity: The Government of Threat and Care. Ilana Feldman and Miriam Ticktin, eds. Pp. 151–89. Durham, N.C.: Duke University Press.

Blake, Dudley D., Frank W. Weathers, Linda M. Nagy, Danny G. Kaloupek, Dennis S. Charney, and Terence M. Keane

    1998 Clinician-Administered PTSD Scale for DSM-IV. Boston: National Center for PTSD.

Boddy, Janice

    1988 Spirits and Selves in Northern Sudan: The Cultural Therapeutics of Possession and Trance. American Ethnologist 15(1):4–27.

Bourguignon, Erika

    1984 Belief and Behavior in Haitian Folk Healing. *In* Mental Health Services: The Cross-Cultural Context. Paul B. Pedersen, Norman Sartorius, and Anthony J. Marsella, eds. Pp. 243–66. Beverly Hills: Sage.

Brodwin, Paul

    1996 Medicine and Morality in Haiti: The Contest for Healing Power. Cambridge: Cambridge University Press.

Brown, Karen McCarthy

    1979 The Center and the Edges: God and Person in Haitian Society. Journal of the Interdenominational Theological Center 7(1):22–39.

1989 Afro-Caribbean Spirituality: A Haitian Case Study. *In* Healing and Restoring: Health and Medicine in the World's Religious Traditions. Lawrence E. Sullivan, ed. Pp. 255–85. New York: Macmillan.

1991 Mama Lola: A Vodou Priestess in Brooklyn. Berkeley: University of California Press.

Conway, Frederick J.

1978 Pentecostalism in the Context of Haitian Religion and Health Practice. Ph.D. diss., American University.

Dayan, Joan

1991 Vodoun, or the Voice of the Gods. Raritan 10(3):32–57.

Deren, Maya

(1953) 1970 Divine Horsemen: The Voodoo Gods of Haiti. New York: Documentext.

Farmer, Paul

1988 Bad Blood, Spoiled Milk: Bodily Fluids as Moral Barometers in Rural Haiti. American Ethnologist 15(1):62–83.

1992 AIDS and Accusation: Haiti and the Geography of Blame. Berkeley: University of California Press.

Giddens, Anthony

1984 The Constitution of Society: Outline of a Theory of Structuration. Berkeley: University of California Press.

Goffman, Erving

1959 The Presentation of Self in Everyday Life. New York: Anchor Books.

Good, Mary-Jo DelVecchio

1995 American Medicine: The Quest for Competence. Berkeley: University of California Press.

1999 Clinical Realities and Moral Dilemmas: Contrasting Perspectives from Academic Medicine in Kenya, Tanzania, and America. Daedalus 128(4):167–96.

Herman, Judith Lewis

1992 Trauma and Recovery: The Aftermath of Violence—From Domestic Abuse to Political Terror. New York: Basic.

Hinton, Devon E., Sonith Peou, Siddharth Joshi, Angela Nickerson, and Naomi Simon

2013 Normal Grief and Complicated Bereavement Among Traumatized Cambodian Refugees: Cultural Context and the Central Role of Dreams of the Deceased. Culture, Medicine, and Psychiatry 37:427–64.

James, Erica Caple

2004 The Political Economy of "Trauma" in Haiti in the Democratic Era of Insecurity. Culture, Medicine and Psychiatry (28):127–49.

2008 Haunting Ghosts: Madness, Gender, and Ensekirite in Haiti in the Democratic Era. *In* Postcolonial Disorders. Mary-Jo DelVecchio Good, Sandra Teresa Hyde, Sarah Pinto, and Byron J. Good, eds. Pp. 132–56. Berkeley: University of California Press.

2010 Democratic Insecurities: Violence, Trauma, and Intervention in Haiti. California Series in Public Anthropology. Berkeley: University of California Press.

2012 Witchcraft, Bureaucraft, and the Social Life of (US)AID in Haiti. Cultural Anthropology 27(1):50–75.

Laguerre, Michel Saturnin

1987 Afro-Caribbean Folk Medicine. South Hadley, Mass.: Bergin and Garvey.

Lambek, Michael

1996 The Past Imperfect: Remembering as Moral Practice. *In* Tense Past: Cultural Essays in Trauma and Memory. Paul Antze and Michael Lambek, eds. Pp. 235–54. London: Routledge.

Larose, Serge

1977 The Meaning of Africa in Haitian Vodu. *In* Symbols and Sentiments: Cross-Cultural Studies in Symbolism. Ian Lewis, ed. Pp. 85–116. London: Academic Press.

Lock, Margaret

1995 Encounters with Aging: Mythologies of Menopause in Japan and North America. Berkeley: University of California Press.

Lock, Margaret, and Vinh-Kim Nguyen

2010 An Anthropology of Biomedicine. Chichester, UK: Wiley-Blackwell.

Marsella, Anthony J., Matthew J. Friedman, Ellen T. Gerrity, and Raymond M. Scurfield, eds.

1996 Ethnocultural Aspects of Posttraumatic Stress Disorder: Issues, Research, and Clinical Applications. Washington, D.C.: American Psychiatric Association.

Mbembe, Achille

2003 Necropolitics. Libby Meintjes, trans. Public Culture 15(1):11–40.

McAlister, Elizabeth

2002 Rara! Vodou, Power, and Performance in Haiti and Its Diaspora. Berkeley: University of California Press.

2012 From Slave Revolt to a Blood Pact with Satan: The Evangelical Rewriting of Haitian History. Studies in Religion 41(2):187–215.

Métraux, Alfred

(1959) 1972 Voodoo in Haiti. Hugo Charteris, trans. New York: Schocken Books.

Nachman, Steven R.

1993 Wasted Lives: Tuberculosis and Other Health Risks of Being Haitian in a U.S. Detention Camp. Medical Anthropological Quarterly 7(3):227–59.

Petryna, Adriana

2009 When Experiments Travel: Clinical Trials and the Global Search for Human Subjects. Princeton, NJ: Princeton University Press.

Rey, Terry

1999 Junta, Rape, and Religion in Haiti, 1993–1994. Journal of Feminist Studies in Religion 15(2):73–100.

Richman, Karen E.

(2005) 2008 Migration and Vodou. Gainesville: University Press of Florida.

Smith, Jennie M.

    2001 When the Hands Are Many: Community Organization and Social Change in Rural Haiti. Ithaca: Cornell University Press.

Trouillot, Michel-Rolph

    1990 Haiti—State Against Nation: The Origins and Legacy of Duvalierism. New York: Monthly Review Press.

van der Kolk, Bessel A., Alexander C. McFarlane, and Lars Weisaeth, eds.

    1996 Traumatic Stress: The Effects of Overwhelming Experience on Mind, Body, and Society. New York: Guilford Press.

Young, Allan

    1995 The Harmony of Illusions: Inventing Post-Traumatic Stress Disorder. Princeton, N.J.: Princeton University Press.

CHAPTER 12

Is PTSD a "Good Enough" Concept for Postconflict Mental Health Care? Reflections on Work in Aceh, Indonesia

Byron J. Good, Mary-Jo DelVecchio Good, and Jesse H. Grayman

In November 2005, eleven months after a devastating tsunami and barely three months after the signing of the Helsinki accords, which brought to an end nearly two decades of fighting between the Indonesian military and Gerakan Aceh Merdeka (the Free Aceh Movement or GAM), the International Organization for Migration (IOM) in Indonesia invited us to provide consultation concerning mental health strategies in previously high-conflict areas of Aceh (Aspinall 2005, 2009, Reid 2006, Drexler 2008). By February 2006, we were accompanying IOM research teams into villages of three districts of Aceh to conduct a major psychosocial needs assessment, a survey designed to guide IOM in launching postconflict psychosocial or mental health programs, to which we were deeply committed for more than five years.[1]

The survey we helped lead, which included both quantitative and qualitative interviews, produced an outpouring of stories of violence and torture, enacted primarily by the Indonesian military against civilian communities. In one village, interviewers left in such shock that Jesse Grayman, then working for IOM, arranged for the organization to send a mobile mental health team to this village.[2] On February 15, 2006, we joined a group of Acehnese doctors and nurses, including a brave and committed psychiatrist, and a guide who was a former leader of GAM in the area, in a caravan of four-wheel-drive vehicles, marked with the blue and white symbols of IOM, up into the hills of North Aceh. We passed untended rice fields, overgrown pinang (areca nut) groves, and burned-out remains of houses, schools, and other buildings along the side of the deeply rutted, muddy road, finally stopping in a shabby village center, with a few nearly empty shops where people had begun to gather, expecting our visit. We were greeted with coffee, cigarettes, and small talk, which gradually turned more somber as people began to refer to the events of the conflict. After a short time, we walked to the *meunasah*, an Acehnese village center and prayer house, where we were met by a tall, thin man in his forties, wailing loudly as his friends tried to support him. The doctor preceded him up the stairs to a large, open room, where the two sat down, facing each other, surrounded by a growing crowd of villagers, and opened his clinic. Our scribbled handwritten field notes report the following.

In April 2004, men in black shirts came at 4 A.M. and accused this man of being a spy for GAM. They beat him, bound his hands and legs, tied a plastic bag over his head, suffocated him, hung him on a pole like a goat, beat him many times, smashed his head, and left him for dead. The villagers found him and released him. Since then, he can't sleep, he can't work, he can't take care of his family, and he cries constantly. The doctor took control, grabbed his hands, said a prayer, calmed him, took his blood pressure, and gave him an injection of a sedative. Soon he was sleeping quietly.

Thunder and lightning crashed, accompanying a tropical downpour, as one by one, villagers came forward to tell their stories to the doctor. We sat at the edge, talking with those who had come to talk with the doctor. "How are you?" we asked a man who sat quietly, smiling. His eyes began to water. They came and took everything from his house. The villagers were forced to leave, and when he came back, his house was empty, everything was gone. The chickens were gone, everything was gone. He feels sad, he cries easily, he often sleeps at nine then wakes at twelve, and he has little appetite. He was hit; for a long time he couldn't work. He is now a bit better but still has pain in his body. He looks seriously depressed.

A woman tells her story to the doctor. Her husband was taken in 1990, he was cut open, his heart was taken out. He was killed in front of her and her children. Her child had a gun put at his throat. She has a pain in her heart; she feels sad, easily frightened. She was dragged by the soldiers for two meters, then fell unconscious. She still feels pain in her back. They killed her husband in front of her daughter and her children. Her daughter was covered by a cloth, so she didn't have to see. They cut off his ear and put it in the meunasah. She doesn't know where his head was put. She suddenly makes a joke, and the mood lightens.

A woman approaches the doctor crying, telling how she was tortured, her toenails torn out, beaten. Soldiers kept asking her, where is GAM. She didn't know. Her husband was taken, her house was burned, and still now, she doesn't know where her husband is, though this happened in 2004. He wasn't a GAM member, but he was accused and tortured, as they asked where is GAM, where are the weapons. She was suspected of cooking food for GAM. A second group of soldiers came and asked her, where is the flag of Indonesia? Why don't you report to us? She finally escaped to the forest, where she hid for seven days and nights, afraid she would be beaten again. They came back and burned her motorcycle, saying it belonged to GAM, accused her of cooking rice for the combatants, because she had leftover rice in the house. They commanded her to lie down, then shot a gun near her ear, terrifying her. And so the stories went on, for nearly five hours—until the doctor had had all he could take and asked a man from the local soccer team to massage his shoulders and back. We all relaxed for a bit, then took our leave.

For us, this was the start of a long and deep involvement, in which we took this spontaneous trauma clinic as a model for the development of mental health outreach teams, organized by IOM, staffed by young GP doctors and nurses, mostly Acehnese, and funded by diverse donors, particularly the World Bank. These teams traveled regularly first to twenty-five villages (in the pilot phase of the program), then to another fifty (in phase 2 of the program), where altogether they treated over twenty-one hundred persons identified as having mental health problems, most related specifically to the conflict. We fought to have IOM and the donors support these teams; we worked closely with them, carried out formal evaluations and wrote reports, met with patients to hear stories of suffering and recovery, and have continued to advocate for this model of care, even as donor funds for Aceh have largely disappeared. It is from within this position of advocacy, and as social scientists who conducted a formal evaluation of this program, that we discuss the usefulness of posttraumatic stress disorder (PTSD) as a clinical concept in postconflict mental health work.

Trauma, memory, and PTSD have long been the site of anthropological critique and exploration. From Ian Hacking's (1995) fine work on memory, dissociation, and multiple personality disorder, to Allan Young's (1995) groundbreaking work on the emergence of PTSD in the context of the rehabilitation of veterans of the Vietnam War, from Paul Antze and Michael Lambek's (1996) drawing together of the growing ethnographic writing on trauma and memory, to a strand of writing—represented by that of Arthur

Kleinman and his colleagues—that criticizes PTSD as the medicalization and professionalization of social suffering (Kleinman and Kleinman 1991; Breslau 2004), anthropologists have levied sustained criticism of the psychiatric category PTSD as represented by the American diagnostic and statistical manuals. This critique has been elaborated by ethnographers, psychologists, and psychiatrists in special collections in journals such as *Transcultural Psychiatry* (Zarowsky and Pedersen, "Rethinking Trauma in a Transnational World" [2000]) and *Culture, Medicine and Psychiatry* (Breslau and Guarnaccia, "Cultures of Trauma" [2004]), and in edited books such as Das et al. (2000) and Fassin and Pandolfi (2010). Anthropological analyses of trauma and PTSD have been linked to broader critiques of humanitarian interventions in postconflict settings, particularly those using the rhetoric of trauma, as representing a form of "mobile sovereignty" (Pandolfi 2003, 2008) and the emergence of an "empire of trauma" (Fassin and Rechtman 2009).

Anthropological critiques such as these are embedded in broader intellectual debates about the use of the concept of trauma to promote humanitarian governance and in more specific studies of the cross-cultural validity of the concept of PTSD. On the one hand, critiques of "psycho-social interventions" as a "new form of international therapeutic governance" (Pupavac 2001:358; see also Pupavac 2002, 2004, 2012) are part of a larger critical discussion of liberal humanitarianism and responses to complex emergencies, and even broader critical analyses of those theories of economic development that see violence as emerging in settings of poverty, weak states, and underdevelopment and as requiring liberal development aid and the reconstruction of societies as its remedy (Duffield 2001, 2002, 2009, 2012). These incorporate many of the anthropological criticisms of the medicalization and professionalization of suffering in settings of violence and the pathologization of whole populations (Pupavac 2001; Summerfield 2004). A group of human rights activists and psychiatrists involved in humanitarian work for victims of war and torture argue—and here we quote from a 1999 article by Derek Summerfield—that "for the vast majority of survivors posttraumatic stress is a pseudocondition, a reframing of the understandable suffering of war as a technical problem to which short-term technical solutions like counseling are applicable. These concepts aggrandize the Western agencies and their 'experts' who from afar define the condition and bring the cure. There is no evidence that war-affected populations are seeking these imported approaches, which appear to ignore their own traditions, meaning systems, and active priorities" (1999:1449; see also Summerfield 2000, 2001, 2004, 2008).

For Summerfield, the extension of notions of trauma and PTSD to non-Western societies represents forms of psychological imperialism that "risk an unwitting perpetuation of the colonial status of the non-Western mind" (2000:422).

The issue of the cross-cultural validity of the PTSD construct has been submitted to extensive empirical research over the past decade (see Introduction and Chapter 1 of this volume). The best review of this work was undertaken by Hinton and Lewis-Fernández (2011) in the context of debates over the criteria of PTSD in the DSM-5. They conclude that "substantial evidence of cross-cultural validity of PTSD was found," but that issues concerning symptom complexes critical to diagnosis, including the cross-cultural salience of avoidance/numbing symptoms, the importance of local cultural interpretations as shaping symptomatology, the place of somatic symptoms (cf. Hinton et al. [2012]), and the overlap or comorbidity of PTSD, anxiety disorders, and depressive disorders (Hinton et al. 2011; cf. Hinton and Lewis-Fernández 2011) require further empirical research. The research cited by Hinton and Lewis-Fernández, which focuses on symptoms rather than the ontological status of the PTSD construct, is clear. Insofar as the claims that the PTSD construct is limited to Western societies are stated in falsifiable terms rather than purely ideological terms, such claims are not borne out by cross-cultural research. Symptom clusters described by DSM-5 for PTSD are found around the globe.

In this chapter, we do not focus on the broader issues of humanitarian governance and psychosocial interventions for PTSD.[3] We also do not focus narrowly on symptom criteria or the more specific claims about the invention of PTSD in a particular social and historical context or its ontological status across cultures. Instead, we address the issue of the utility of the PTSD concept in clinical or public mental health work in Aceh, and by extension in other postconflict settings.

In this chapter, we propose to elaborate three rather simple claims, which respond to those made by Summerfield (1999:1449), quoted above. First, we provide empirical data suggesting that in the context of postconflict societies with extraordinarily limited mental health resources, "posttraumatic stress" (in Summerfield's terms) is far from a "pseudocondition." To the contrary, what we refer to as "the remainders of violence" in Aceh constitute an extraordinary public health challenge, and critiques such as those by Summerfield serve inadvertently to legitimize the withdrawal of support for the development of mental health services in settings of great need. Second, we argue that while many of the debates about diagnostic criteria and their universality are of little relevance for the development of public mental health care, phenomena that look quite like those described by the technical medical and psychological literature and by current diagnostic systems as PTSD are quite common in the context of clinical work in Aceh. We will suggest that while the focus on criteria over prototypes and the effort to understand psychiatric disorders, particularly PTSD, as "discrete and heterogeneous" conditions (see B. Good 1992) limit the value of the concept, PTSD remains an important clinical concept and target of public mental health interventions. Third, we will describe what findings from our work in the field tell us about the question of whether, in Summerfield's terms, "war-affected populations are seeking these imported approaches," and whether medical and public health interventions for posttraumatic disorders provide benefit to those who are treated.

The research component of the program described in this chapter was not intended to determine whether the specific diagnostic criteria in the DSM-IV are valid for Aceh and Acehnese culture. The research was not basic research, designed to investigate questions critical to PTSD studies, including those about the relationship between symptom measures and diagnostic instruments. Our discussion of whether PTSD is a "good enough" concept refers instead to the question of whether the PTSD construct is a useful concept for identifying persons with mental health problems and organizing their care, particularly in postconflict societies that have suffered widespread violence and in which mental health services are being developed.

Background: The Psychosocial Needs Assessment (PNA) and the Direct Health and Psychosocial Assistance Programs (DHPAP)

Data for this chapter are drawn from the authors' five years of collaboration with IOM Indonesia in Aceh.[4] Beginning in November 2005, IOM conducted a psychosocial needs assessment in three districts, with support from the Canadian government. In February 2006, teams from IOM and Syiah Kuala University carried out a survey, based on a random, stratified survey of 596 adults (seventeen years old or older) in thirty villages in high-conflict subdistricts in three districts along the north coast of Aceh, which had among the longest and most intensive conflict and violence against citizens in all of

Aceh.[5] Research focused on measuring levels of experienced traumatic events (past and current) associated with the conflict; on symptoms of depression, anxiety, and PTSD; on experiences of head trauma (associated with beatings or suffocation); on help-seeking activities; and on local priorities for psychosocial services.[6] Only symptom checklists, not diagnostic instruments, were used in what was intended to be a very rapid needs assessment aimed at guiding IOM's psychosocial and mental health programs. In addition to the quantitative survey, qualitative interviews were conducted with village leaders and randomly selected adults in each village in the study. Data were analyzed in March 2006, and a final IOM report (the Psychosocial Needs Assessment, phase 1 or PNA1) was released in September 2006 (B. Good et al. 2006). Given the magnitude of violence and associated psychological distress documented by PNA1, IOM and the World Bank supported extension of the survey to seventy-five additional villages in eleven additional districts throughout Aceh. This second survey was conducted primarily in July 2006 (ten districts were surveyed in July, one in November 2006), and a total of 1,376 additional adults were interviewed. A second IOM report (PNA2) was released in June 2007 (M. Good et al. 2007). The report grouped districts into six regions representing different geographical and cultural areas of Aceh, which also had differing histories of conflict and violence.

The PNA project found extraordinarily high levels of violence enacted against civilian populations in the villages of rural Aceh. Levels of reported traumatic events were directly associated with levels of symptoms of depression, anxiety, and PTSD, and both were extremely high in this population. The PNA research also found that villagers seldom considered seeking mental health care from the public primary care clinics (*puskesmas*). The primary care system is most commonly associated with maternal and child health care; clinics are often difficult to reach from the more isolated villages; and villagers recalled that during the conflict the military maintained surveillance of the primary care centers. Indeed, the Indonesian military routinely monitored the clinics to catch wounded combatants seeking care and sometimes used the clinics or posts next to these clinics as their bases of operation.

Based on findings of this research, IOM agreed to develop a pilot program that used mental health outreach teams to go into remote, previously high-conflict villages with the explicit mission of providing mental health care and rebuilding the links between these villages and the primary care centers. The IOM mobile mental health teams consisted of general practitioners (GPs) and nurses, working directly for IOM, who were given training and supervision by an Acehnese psychiatrist from Syiah Kuala University and by psychiatrists from the University of Indonesia in Jakarta. Team members worked closely with the local Community Mental Health Nurses (CMHN), who accompanied them into the villages, and village cadre, trained as part of an ongoing World Health Organization project, to take services directly into communities. The IOM teams and local CMHN conducted active case finding in the villages, identified persons with diagnosable mental illnesses, and provided a combination of medications, psychological counseling, and psychosocial group support. Between November 2006 and August 2007, this Direct Health and Psychosocial Assistance Program Pilot Phase (DHPAP Pilot)[7] provided direct mental health care to 581 individuals in twenty-five villages in the district of Bireuen. After eight months, full responsibility for persons still requiring treatment was transferred to local primary care centers. The project was evaluated by external evaluators, who strongly supported the project and verified the quality of care being provided by these teams of nonpsychiatrists. The program developed particularly close working relationships with staff in the district health office and the primary health care centers.

Beginning in November 2007, IOM extended this program to fifty new villages, twenty-five in Bireuen and twenty-five in the neighboring district of Aceh Utara.[8] The DHPAP Extension project provided care to 1,556 persons with significant mental health problems. In addition, IOM livelihood teams provided supportive livelihood training and material (valued at approximately US$300 per client) to 200 of those being treated for mental health problems, with the goal of evaluating the added mental health benefits that would accrue from linking clinical care and vocational support.

The Harvard team was responsible for designing and implementing a formal evaluation of this project. The first 1,137 patients treated were entered into a longitudinal study aimed at evaluating the reduction of symptoms and improvement in social and vocational functioning as a result of the care provided. Patients were interviewed at three times: T1 when entering treatment (February–August 2008); T2 when full responsibility for patient care was transferred to the local primary care clinics (March 2009); and T3 (August–September 2009), six months after the delivery of the livelihood intervention and just a few months before the end of the project. In addition to the quantitative survey questionnaires, qualitative interviews of a small sample of patients were conducted at several times during the course of the program.[9]

Data from the PNA research and the two intervention projects allow us to address the issues raised in the introduction.

Is PTSD a Pseudocondition in Aceh? Trauma-Related Mental Health Disorders as a Public Health Challenge

Mental health problems pose an extremely important public health challenge in low-income societies; this challenge increases very significantly in settings suffering natural disasters or armed conflict. A WHO model estimates that "severe disorders" (psychoses, severe depression, severe disabling anxiety disorders) have a 2–3 percent twelve-month prevalence in a normal population, which increases to 3–4 percent in "disaster" settings, and that mild to moderate disorders, diagnosable conditions deserving mental health services, have a 10 percent twelve-month prevalence, which increases to 20 percent in "disaster" settings, reducing to 15 percent with natural recovery (World Health Organization 2005).

Our PNA research documented extraordinary levels of violence enacted against civilian populations throughout Aceh, particularly in four of the six regions we compared, and these were directly and significantly correlated with extremely high levels of psychological symptoms (B. Good et al. 2006, M. Good et al. 2007). For example, in the two North Coast districts in which IOM later carried out the DHPAP interventions (Bireuen and Aceh Utara), 85 percent and 87 percent of the adult population (respectively) reported experiencing combat or gun fights; 49 percent and 53 percent reported being beaten; 25 percent in each district reported being tortured; 3 percent and 8 percent reported a spouse killed, and 4 percent and 9 percent reported having a child killed. In Bireuen, 68 percent of young men between ages seventeen and twenty-nine reported head trauma—being beaten to the head, strangled, or suffocated (often as part of interrogation). Although rates of physical violence directed at men were higher than those directed against women, women also experienced extremely high levels of direct physical assaults, as well as assaults against their kin and their homes. For example, 20 percent of women (compared with 56 percent of men) reported being beaten, 14 percent (compared with 36 percent) reported being attacked by a knife or gun, and 11 percent (vs. 25 percent) reported being tortured. Violence against civilians—both men and women—was thus extremely widespread in these settings.

It was not surprising, therefore, that the psychosocial needs assessment documented high rates of psychological symptoms. The study used standard scales for depression and anxiety (the Brief Symptom Inventory, or BSI) and for PTSD symptoms (the Harvard Trauma Questionnaire, or HTQ), carefully translated using local idioms, and asked questions about local idioms of distress and trauma-related experiences, including specifically dreams and nightmares (see B. Good et al. 2006 for a description of the instrument developed for the survey). Findings of the PNA research concerning levels of mental health symptoms can be summarized as follows.

First, both PNA1 and PNA2 documented extraordinarily high levels of psychological distress, indicating a significant public health issue. The levels of symptoms were related both to the level of conflict in the region surveyed and to the time in which the survey was carried out. The PNA1 survey, conducted in February 2006, reported some of the highest rates of psychological symptoms in the postconflict literature. For example, using the cutoff score of a mean of 2.5 on a 1–4 scale for the Harvard Trauma Questionnaire, as recommended by Mollica et al. (2004), 51 percent of respondents in Bireuen and 45 percent in Aceh Utara were rated symptomatic for PTSD.

While rates were still high in the PNA2 study, conducted in July 2006, psychological symptoms were significantly lower than in PNA1, even in regions that reported levels of traumatic events similar to those the PNA1 region. Levels of mental health problems were highest in the three regions with the highest levels of traumatic violence experienced. Levels of psychological symptoms were, however, lower in even the highest conflict areas in the July survey (PNA2) than in the February survey. For example, the East Coast region, surveyed in July, had high levels of violence (as measured by the traumatic events scale) comparable to those in North Coast communities surveyed in February, but levels of psychological symptoms were much lower. A rating of "symptomatic for PTSD" (with the mean of 2.5 or higher on the HTQ) was achieved by 8 percent of the total survey population in the East Coast region, as compared with the 34 percent rate for all three PNA1 North Coast districts in PNA1. Extremely high levels of depressive symptoms and anxiety symptoms were also reported in all regions, but again PNA2 scores were lower than PNA1 scores, even in regions such as the Southwest Coast and the East Coast, where traumatic events were similar to those in the PNA1 North Coast region.

Our analyses suggest that the reduction in symptoms from February to July 2006 was due to the advance of the peace process (M. Good et al. 2007).

In February 2006, only six months after the signing of the Helsinki Memorandum of Understanding (MOU), villagers were still extremely anxious that the peace agreement would not last, and many of the perpetrators of military violence had not yet left the region. Our measure of "current stressors" was quite high in February. By July 2006, a kind of euphoria had begun to set in, as the peace process had gone forward without a single breach, and all of the imported Indonesian troops involved in the conflict had left the region. Our measure of current stressors had declined by this time, suggesting that decline in levels of overall symptoms was related to the peace process moving forward, particularly the gradual evacuation of the Indonesian troops involved in the counterinsurgency war, rather than to regional differences and rates of violence.

Second, levels of psychological symptoms were almost equivalent for men and women in both the PNA1 and PNA2 surveys. Given that most population surveys find significantly higher rates of mood disorders among women than men, we interpret these findings to mean that men had particularly high levels of psychological distress and mental health problems, related to higher levels of traumatic violence experienced.

Third, odds analyses indicated that level of traumatic violence experienced by an individual was an extremely high predictor of level of psychological symptoms (demonstrating a clear dose effect [Mollica et al. 2004]). For example, in PNA1, odds ratios for PTSD symptoms being above the cutoff level increased from 1.00 to 4.87, 14.00, and 40.77, as number of past traumatic experiences reported increased from zero to three (assigned an odds ratio of 1.00), to four to seven, eight to ten, or eleven or more events reported. It should also be noted that level of current stressors was also a high predictor of psychological symptoms. PNA2 also found highly significant dose effects of traumatic events on psychological symptoms, but both psychological symptoms and odds ratios were lower in PNA2.

Given the decline in symptoms from February to July 2006, does this suggest that indeed the levels of symptoms reported were simply expected or normal reactions to violence rather than actual mental disorders? In part, yes. Symptom checklists can measure overall levels of distress in an individual or community at a particular time. They are not diagnostic instruments and are not designed to describe the number of persons who are suffering a mental disorder or should be provided mental health services. Such instruments do not, for example, have duration criteria—indicating how long a person has been experiencing such symptoms or where they are in what might be considered a normal recovery process—and reported symptoms of depression, anxiety, and PTSD using such instruments are closely interrelated, indicating overall distress rather than distinct disorders. However, it is our interpretation that the levels of traumatic violence experienced, and levels of closely associated mental health symptoms, are important indicators of the magnitude of the public health challenge. While making no claims to the percent of the population with diagnosable mental illness or those who would benefit from treatment, these data suggested a very significant need for providing quality mental health care in postconflict regions of Aceh.

The community response to newly available clinical mental health services provided a different indicator of the magnitude of the public health challenge. The DHPAP mobile mental health project, launched in February 2008 (two and a half years after the MOU and end of violence), treated approximately 6 percent of the total population of the fifty villages in which the project was conducted—or approximately 11 percent of the adult population. These are clinical data—the number of persons who actually sought care when available in their village, not population-based data. Our interpretation of these data is that whereas the Acehnese are remarkably resilient, and the great majority of people recovered from the distress associated with the violence, a very significant number of people did not recover but developed longer lasting, psychiatrically relevant mental disorders. These represented cases in which symptoms or disorders were clinically significant and not self-remitting and are the disorders that constitute the larger public mental health challenge.

The PNA surveys were not undertaken as pure research but as genuine assessments of the need for services. From a public health point of view, the findings were important. Aceh had suffered not only a devastating tsunami, killing approximately 160,000 persons living along the coast, but civilian communities in the hills had also suffered through an extremely violent conflict—in some regions for nearly twenty years, in other regions for the past five years. In the high-conflict areas, despite the enormous resilience of the population, there were extremely high rates of symptoms of depression, anxiety, and PTSD. For a significant portion of the population—greater than the 11 percent of adults actually treated by the mobile mental health teams—these conditions produced longer-lasting mental disorders. This was, however, a setting in which only four psychiatrists served a population of more than four million people at the time of the tsunami. In a vast province requiring at least a twelve-hour bus ride from the southern borders of the province to the capital, Banda Aceh, in the north, only one psychiatric hospital, four fully trained psychiatrists, and very few psychiatric nurses or clinical psychologists were available to provide care.[10]

Our point in describing the situation in these public health terms is to indicate our view that trauma-related conditions, including depression, anxiety disorders, and PTSD, should be understood and responded to as public mental health problems. The great challenge in postconflict settings with such limited resources is not to treat "trauma" per se or focus narrowly on PTSD, but to develop mental health services that can provide sustainable care for the wide range of mental health problems—organic problems related to head trauma, acute and chronic psychoses, and depression and anxiety disorders, including panic disorder and PTSD—that are certain to be present as remainders of violence in settings of postconflict.

Is PTSD a Culturally Valid Concept in Postconflict Aceh?

But what of the specific PTSD construct, and the claim that it is a pseudo-condition better considered the understandable suffering of war? Our data here are of two kinds. First, we have quantitative data, both from the PNA research and the formal evaluation of phase 2 of the DHPAP program that provided clinical services to members of these communities. Second, we are anthropologists. We carried out interviews with families and village leaders in these communities, as well as with the clinicians who were providing care. We accompanied the medical teams as observers at times, and in particular in November 2008 we and our colleagues interviewed a small number group of patients who had been in treatment for six to nine months, asking about their experiences of care and their symptoms before treatment and at the time of the interview. It was in this context that a local phenomenology of trauma-related illness and PTSD emerged.

An extremely common initial presentation of distress, reflected in our interviews, in clinical interactions, and in the medical records, would begin with a simple statement, *jantung berdebar debar,* my heart pounds.[11] Those diagnosed as suffering a psychiatric disorder would often go on: *Saya sering takut,* I am often afraid. *Teringat,* I have memories that come unbidden to me. *Tidak bisa tidur dengan enak,* I can't sleep well at night; *ada mimpi buruk,* I have nightmares or bad dreams, wake up feeling frightened, and cannot sleep again. *Gelisah,* I often feel restless, anxious, worried. My body feels weak, *lemah*; I lack spirit or energy, *semangat*, so that I am unable to go off to work in the rice paddies or the gardens. In some cases, these symptoms were presented as such—as symptoms—to the physicians or a member of the medical team, with narrative content emerging after several meetings with the clinicians, when a close enough relationship was established to recount horrifying memories, such as those described in the beginning of this chapter. In other cases, the narratives came first, with symptoms essentially describing the embodied response to the events that had occurred. Physicians would then inquire further to determine more specific diagnoses.

In this setting, depression, PTSD, or an anxiety disorder, including panic disorder, seldom appeared as discrete, heterogeneous conditions, as represented in diagnostic manuals. Although this mental health outreach program was conducted two and a half years after the violence had stopped, it was carried out in communities that had suffered years of violence, and any disorder—even schizophrenia or a major depression resulting from the death of a child or spouse in a manner unrelated to the conflict—was caught up in memories of the violence. These had been years of extreme fear and anxiety, of experiences of loss as well as terror. Symptoms of depression, anxiety, intrusive traumatic memories, and sleep disturbances, as well as disabling bodily symptoms, were present in varying degrees in nearly all of the cases treated by the IOM teams. These had also been years of remarkable resilience and a commitment to resistance and struggle, on the part of men, women, and even children (M. Good 2015; M. Good and B. Good 2013). For most, symptoms faded—or were reduced in frequency and severity—after the violence ended, as communities gained confidence that the peace process would hold. Our clinical data, however, indicate that a smaller group of persons developed or maintained more severe, long-lasting symptoms. For many such persons, these conditions were extremely debilitating, reducing their ability to work, to function in the household, or to participate fully in the community.

Despite the ubiquity of symptoms, many of those treated by the IOM teams presented fairly classic clinical pictures of major depressions, generalized anxiety disorder, panic attacks, and somatoform disorders, as well as PTSD. Many presented with relatively high levels of somatic or bodily complaints—pain, stomach problems, heart sensations, loss of energy. Many presented with symptoms indicating mixed depression and anxiety, PTSD with depression or other anxiety disorders (including panic disorder), or one of these disorders with mixed psychotic symptoms. In the case of PTSD, the symptoms of intense, intrusive memories are clearly marked by the Indonesian term *"teringat,"* "to remember" in the sense of memories coming unbidden, in contrast with the term *"mengingat,"* to remember in the sense of an active remembering process. In some cases, individuals described intrusive memories as being linked to acute episodes of extreme fear or anxiety, with symptoms meeting criteria for panic attacks, as well as to nightmares in which these events were vividly reexperienced.

The boundary between acute remembering, often with intense anxiety, and reexperiencing of the kind popularly described as "flashbacks" is often unclear in Aceh. Patients being treated would describe acute, intrusive remembering of terrible events they had witnessed directly, things that had been done to them, or in some cases events they had only heard about when a family member was tortured or killed. Some would describe seeing such events being played out as though on a video—in some cases, even if they had not seen the events directly. Many would describe becoming anxious in specific places in their villages or their homes where terrible events had happened, or in some cases having extremely acute memories be triggered when they were in such settings. And many described avoiding going out in crowds or trying to avoid the places where these events had occurred.

Equally striking was the fact that many people who initially were treated would, at some point early in their care, tell stories of what they had witnessed or experienced as though they had occurred very recently. (Clinicians, as well as researchers, were trained not to request people to retell the stories of their most traumatizing events, given the evidence of the potential harm associated with debriefing. Many persons would, however, talk about what had happened to them at some point in the treatment process or during interviews.) We recall cases in which stories were told to us, or to clinicians (who retold the stories to us), as though they had occurred in the past days, weeks or months, but we or the clinicians would later learn that the events had happened years before, in some especially memorable cases up to sixteen years earlier. Although Indonesian language does not neatly distinguish present and past tense, these stories were told as though in the present, as recent occurrences that were cause for current, ongoing anxiety.

The item on the Harvard Trauma Questionnaire, "feeling as though the event is happening again," is rated as happening "never" by only 22 percent of the patient sample—by only 12 percent of those given a clinical diagnosis of PTSD, but also only 27 percent of those who were not given a PTSD diagnosis. The description of nightmares is often quite similar, suggesting that nightmares are akin to such intrusive memories or flashbacks occurring during sleep rather than waking hours (Grayman et al. 2009; Hinton 2009; Hinton et al. 2009, 2013).

We analyzed the symptom checklist data—of the Harvard Trauma Questionnaire (HTQ)—using the algorithm developed by Mollica et al. (1999, 2004) to determine whether individuals suffered constellations of symptoms consistent with a DSM diagnosis of PTSD. We are quite aware that these were not diagnostic interviews, and no data are available to assess duration criteria. However, this method allows analysis of the copresence in an individual of symptoms that meet criterion B (reexperiencing symptoms), criterion C (avoidance and numbing), and criterion D (arousal symptoms). Following Mollica's method (which counts a symptom as present if it is rated either as 3 or 4 on a 4-point scale), 52 percent of individuals surveyed in Bireuen in PNA1 and 51 percent in Aceh Utara (but only 14 percent of those who were surveyed in Pidie, a neighboring district also surveyed in PNA1) met these criteria for a diagnosis of PTSD. If we increased the severity level of the symptom to a 4, in order to count it as present, the percent of persons meeting these criteria dropped to 26 percent, 25 percent, and 3 percent in Bireuen, Aceh Utara, and Pidie, respectively. In the intervention program we evaluated (DHPAP Extension), the clinicians gave a clinical diagnosis of PTSD to 33 percent of the 1,137 patients in our study at time 1, when initially entering treatment. This would constitute about 3–4 percent of all adults in these villages.

The data presented here cannot provide conclusive evidence for the existence of PTSD—as defined by DSM or ICD criteria—in Aceh. This was not a study of the validity of the PTSD construct in Aceh, seeking answers to the questions raised by Hinton and Lewis-Fernández (2011) in their important review of empirical evidence for cross-culturally validity. The research focused on supporting the public health work, which was the mission of IOM. The data do, however, suggest that trauma-related mental health problems that strongly resemble PTSD present a very significant public health challenge in a setting that has suffered widespread violence and has extremely limited mental health resources. Clinicians on the IOM teams attempted to identify persons who met DSM criteria for PTSD, either as a primary diagnosis or more commonly comorbid with another diagnosis, and found the diagnosis a useful guide for treating patients in these villages.

Describing PTSD as a pseudocondition or a natural response to the ravages of violence misses a critical dimension of PTSD—that it is a condition that persists beyond the expected natural recovery from violence in those settings where the violence has ceased. Such a description tends to devalue the level of persistent suffering and disability experienced by many in postconflict communities and may lead international donors and policy makers to give inadequate attention to the profound mental health needs of such populations.

It is important to add that while classic symptoms of PTSD were present in this population in Aceh, an accurate clinical description requires a notion of complex trauma (see Introduction and Chapter 1 of this volume for a fuller discussion of complex trauma).[12] PTSD as a response to a single, traumatizing event that occurs in the life of someone otherwise secure is profoundly inadequate for understanding persons with prolonged experiences of war or prolonged childhood abuse, which is why there is often such a sharp disjunction between clinical experience in postconflict settings and PTSD treatment protocols. It is also important to note that a focus on PTSD as a discrete and heterogenous condition is often inaccurate and unhelpful in clinical practice. Panic attacks, associated with intrusive memories or flashbacks, are commonly present for those who meet criteria for PTSD in this population, and comorbidity of PTSD, depression, and anxiety disorders, particularly generalized anxiety disorder, may very well be more the norm than the exception (B. Good and Hinton 2009). None of this suggests, however, that PTSD is a pseudocondition. What our work does suggest is that a clinical perspective, joined with a public health perspective, is far more critical to responding to the needs of war-affected populations than narrowly biological or diagnostic perspectives that focus on ever more refined diagnostic criteria rather than on developing interventions that have public health utility in low-resource settings. The challenge of providing mental health care with extremely limited resources for populations profoundly affected by violence remains, unfortunately, marginal for the vast number of researchers in trauma studies, as indicated by research dollars and journal publications.

PTSD: Is There Evidence That War-Affected Populations Seek Western Treatments?

So what about the broad set of claims about trauma treatment as an imposition of treatment forms irrelevant to local cultures, which jeopardize local coping strategies (e.g. Pupavac 2001), or Summerfield's claim that PTSD as a concept serves primarily to "aggrandize the Western agencies and their 'experts' who from afar define the condition and bring the cure," and that "there is no evidence that war-affected populations are seeking these imported approaches, which appear to ignore their own traditions, meaning systems, and active priorities" (1999:1449)?

When IOM began providing outreach mental health services in villages in Aceh that had suffered through the conflict, there was little evidence about what traumatic disorders looked like in this setting, whether people considered these to be conditions that would respond to medical treatment, and whether relatively standard medical treatments—including the use of antidepressant medications, counseling, and psychosocial interventions—would be considered appropriate or would be effective. Some local NGOs worked with torture victims during the course of the violence, despite political repression, and continued this work postconflict. However, the question of the cultural fit of providing diverse forms of mental health care in rural communities was largely unanswered.

The pilot intervention, using outreach teams to provide medical care for persons with diagnosable mental health problems in these high-conflict villages, was inspired in part by the success of the initial visit of the IOM team to a particularly severely impacted village, described in the introduction to this chapter. That initial experience of bringing a mental health team in IOM vehicles to the village suggested that even during the early postconflict period, marked by continued fear of the military, people were anxious to gather and talk with a doctor about illnesses they associated with conflict-related experiences, that they were prepared to tell their stories and describe their symptoms to a medical team, and that they were anxious to find medications that would help relieve their symptoms (M. Good 2010). The DHPAP Pilot project, the nine-month pilot program in twenty-five villages aimed at developing a model of care, built on these impressions. The IOM medical team—consisting of three doctors, three nurses, all Indonesian and all but one of whom were Acehnese—were able to develop methods for case finding; they learned to use village health volunteers (kader), conducted general medical clinics in the villages to screen for persons with mental health problems, and made home visits, during which new cases were often referred. Clinically, the teams gained experience, learned to make clinical evaluations in these village contexts, learned that people would seek medical treatment and would take medications when they were provided, and had the clinical experience of watching many of those they treated recover. The DHPAP Pilot program provided strong evidence that Acehnese villagers who suffered trauma-related mental health problems would indeed seek and make use of treatment, and that the IOM outreach model was a viable means of providing services. What was absent from the pilot study was any strong empirical evidence for the effectiveness of the treatment.

The DHPAP Extension project included an empirical evaluation component, designed to study the effectiveness of these outreach teams when extended to fifty new villages—to determine levels of symptoms and social functioning when persons entered into treatment, to compare levels at times 1, 2, and 3 to learn whether symptoms were reduced and social and vocational functioning improved over the course of treatment, and to learn how those treated evaluated their own response to treatment. The sample consisted of the first 1,137 patients who were treated in the program and agreed to participate in the study. The research was able to follow 1,063 of these patients through to time 3, with only a 6.5 percent loss to follow-up. Unlike the PNA sample, with nearly equivalent numbers of men and women (in the random, population-based sample), the clinical sample consisted of 68 percent women and 32 percent men.

All patients were given an initial clinical diagnosis. When the treating physicians considered it appropriate, medications were provided. Villages were visited on a monthly basis, more often during the initial phase of case finding. Counseling and home visits were part of the usual clinical practice. Support groups were organized in some of the villages, and additional livelihood or vocational support was provided to 200 of the patients. Table 12.1 describes the clinical diagnoses registered by the IOM team for this sample of treated patients at time 1. Generalized anxiety disorder, PTSD, and mixed depression and anxiety made up 90 percent of the treated sample. Of the 1,063 patients who remained in the sample until time 3, 47 percent were given an antidepressant medication, 44 percent were given an antianxiety medication, and only 3 percent were given an antipsychotic medication. Forty percent of the sample used medications for three months or less, and 74 percent of the sample used medications for six months or less. So were the treatments effective? Here we provide four small pieces of data, from a much larger data set, that may be useful to respond to those who question the whole enterprise.

Tables 12.2 and 12.3 provide an overview of the levels of symptoms (divided for women and men) for the PNA2 sample, and the DHPAP patients at time 1, when patients entered treatment, at time 2, which marked the end of the formal IOM treatment, and at time 3, a follow-up five months after time

Table 12.1. Diagnosis of Patients at Time 1 by Gender

Diagnoses	Men		Women		Total	
	% of patient sample suffering disorder	Total patient sample N = 370	% of patient sample suffering disorder	Total patient sample N = 752	% of patient sample suffering disorder	Total patient sample N = 1,122
General anxiety disorder	41%	150	44%	327	43%	477
Mixed depression and anxiety	12%	45	17%	127	15%	172
Depression	4%	15	7%	50	6%	65
Insomnia	4%	15	3%	19	3%	34
Somatoform disorder	10%	37	12%	87	11%	124
PTSD	40%	147	29%	218	33%	365
Psychotic disorders	4%	13	1%	11	2%	24

2 (a total of twelve to eighteen months). The tables indicate percentage of persons in each category who were at or above two cutoff levels for the symptom checklists used: a recommended cutoff level for indicating caseness in international research, and a higher cutoff level we used to identify the more severe cases. The tables reveal two primary findings. First, the clinical sample at time 1 has symptom levels far higher than the normal population distribution in the PNA2 study. Although this would be expected, it indicates that those who sought and decided to make use of medical care, given the case-finding methods employed by IOM, were persons who continued to have extremely high levels of symptoms more than two and a half years after the end of the conflict. Second, the tables demonstrate what the entire outcome study found: levels of psychological symptoms declined dramatically from time of entry into the treatment to the end of the DHPAP outreach activities and continued to drop for the next five months (during which a small percentage continued to receive care from the public primary care clinics). This was true equally for persons diagnosed by the clinical team with anxiety, depression, or PTSD.

Table 12.4 provides data from one of several general questions we asked each respondent at time 3 as the program was ending, concerning their own evaluation (on a 7-point scale) of the change in their symptoms or functioning since they began treatment with the IOM teams. Over 80 percent reported that their symptoms were better, and over 45 percent indicated improvement at the 6 or 7 level on the 7-point scale. Whether measured objectively, using symptom checklists adapted for local cultural conditions, or self-evaluation of whether they had gotten worse or better, the study demonstrated dramatic changes from the beginning to end of treatment, changes that continued into the follow-up period.

We also used a number of measures to try to determine improvement in social functioning, particularly in ability to work. Early in the study we found many people who complained that they were simply not able, not strong enough, or did not feel well enough to work. In this region of Aceh, this usually meant not being able to go to the rice fields or into the forested garden areas to cultivate and harvest a variety of agricultural crops. However, many also engaged in small enterprises—running a coffee shop, baking small cakes and selling them in the market, doing significant handicrafts for cash sales. Of all of the scales and questions we used to evaluate social functioning, a simple set of questions about how many hours a week they could work was most telling. At the beginning of the study (time 1), we asked each individual to

Table 12.2. Symptom Measures for Patients at Times 1, 2, and 3, Compared with PNA2: Women

Symptom Levels	PNA 2 N=1,376	Time 1 N=752	Time 2 N=730	Time 3 N=719
Mean anxiety score "symptomatic" (≥1.75)	46%	90%	69%	60%
Mean anxiety score "high symptomatic" (≥3.0)	10%	45%	25%	12%
Mean depression score "symptomatic" (≥1.75)	40%	76%	57%	43%
Mean depression score "high symptomatic" (≥3.0)	5%	13%	6%	3%
Mean PTSD score "symptomatic" (≥2.5)	12%	28%	15%	8%
Mean PTSD score "high symptomatic" (≥3.0)	4%	7%	3%	1%

Table 12.3. Symptom Measures for Patients at Times 1, 2, and 3, Compared with PNA2: Men

Symptom Levels	PNA 2 N=1,376	Time 1 N=370	Time 2 N=353	Time 3 N=340
Mean anxiety score "symptomatic" (≥1.75)	33%	89%	59%	43%
Mean anxiety score "high symptomatic" (≥3.0)	8%	39%	18%	8%
Mean depression score "symptomatic" (≥1.75)	31%	68%	49%	28%
Mean depression score "high symptomatic" (≥3.0)	3%	9%	3%	4%
Mean PTSD score "symptomatic" (≥2.5)	8%	22%	13%	7%
Mean PTSD score "high symptomatic" (≥3.0)	3%	7%	3%	2%

indicate how many hours of work he or she usually did before becoming sick, and how many could be done when they became sick (with this mental health problem). The whole sample, including men and women, young and old, reported a mean of twenty-eight hours that they estimated they worked before the illness. (Recall, this was during the conflict, when the military would not allow most villagers to go to their fields.) They reported that

Table 12.4. Response at Time 3 to Question: Since you received treatment by IOM, have your mental health symptoms (from stress or trauma) become worse, stayed the same, or gotten better?

	Percent	*N = 1,063*	*% worse, same, better*
Much worse	0%	0	1%
Somewhat worse	0.3%	3	
A little worse	0.8%	9	
The same	16%	167	16%
A little better	37%	388	83%
Better	38%	406	
Much better	9%	90	
Total	100%	1,063	100%

when they were ill, their ability to work declined to a mean of ten hours per week. When asked at time 3, at the end of the twelve-to-eighteen-month follow-up, how many hours per week they were able to work, this treatment sample reported a mean of forty-one hours per week! This and other measures indicated a dramatic recovery of ability to work associated with the mental health intervention.

This study did not have a control group. It was a prospective observational study, not an experimental study. We know that the peace process continued to unfold during this time, that social and economic conditions continued to improve along with security. However, this study began enrolling patients only in February 2008, two and a half years after the August 15, 2005, peace agreement, and approximately two years after most of the military forces began leaving the region. This program identified persons who had not recovered up until that time. It is our interpretation that the medical intervention played a critical role in the recovery of many of those treated by the combined IOM and Ministry of Health teams.

Our qualitative interviews and observations of cases supported this interpretation. It is quite remarkable to hear persons with trauma experiences describing terrible events that happened in the quite distant past—in some cases more than fifteen years earlier—as though they occurred in the past week. It is also remarkable—and gratifying—to watch recovery processes, as individuals who had previously discussed such terrible events with an extreme sense of present temporality begin to discuss these same events as genuinely part of the past. In brief meetings in July 2010 with persons we had interviewed in 2008 as part of the qualitative evaluation, many made clear not only that the symptoms they described were now very much in the past, but that they had no interest in discussing with us the terrible events during the conflict that they had worked through early in their treatment and in some cases had discussed with us in detail in earlier interviews. We were thus able to observe individuals who had clearly been disabled, unable to leave their houses to work, return to full activity.

It is not possible to determine exactly what accounted for the recovery. Our PNA1 data indicated a wide variety of local, cultural, and religious strategies individuals used to try to "overcome bad experiences related to the conflict" (B. Good et al. 2006:46–49). Nearly all of those who reported having such bad experiences reported using prayer to overcome them; high numbers (56 percent and 37 percent in Bireuen and Aceh Utara) reported talking with friends and family members as a strategy; an almost equal number reported consulting a religious specialist or seeking medical help; and the other most common strategy reported was "trying to forget about the experience." Community rituals (*peusijeuk*) were held for returning combatants or political prisoners in many villages (39 percent of respondents in Bireuen reported participating in such a ritual, 17 percent in Aceh Utara). Mental health problems were treated by attending prayer groups (*pengajian*), and the religious description of surrendering to God (*pasrah*) with sincerity (*ikhlas*) was often referred to (though this seems to have been more difficult to achieve in the context of the conflict than of the tsunami—cf. Samuels 2012:133–46).

The IOM project was not, in reality, what Summerfield (1999:1449) described as "imported approaches, which appear to ignore their own traditions, meaning systems, and active priorities." There is no evidence that medical care "jeopardizes local coping strategies," as suggested by Pupavac (2001:358). These were Acehnese doctors and nurses, coming to listen to the complaints and stories of Acehnese villagers, themselves participating in the same religious traditions, who came providing medications they said would be helpful. Some had themselves experienced similar traumatic violence. Providing such medical care, making visits to homes and listening sensitively to what people have suffered, and organizing support groups is not an imported Western model of care. Indeed, medications are highly valued and given local meanings. For persons with PTSD, nearly all of whom had severe sleep disruption, the use of fairly sedating antidepressant medications (such as amitriptyline, which is the only such medication available in the public primary health care centers), may have been effective in helping persons to sleep.[13] All the antidepressants used in the DHPAP Extension project (including SSRIs) may have had some effect in reducing the panic attacks associated with intrusive memories.

Although the medications were apparently useful, and the treatment followed evidence-based practice guidelines (Friedman et al. 2009), we cannot say that the medications themselves were the source of efficacy. It may have been a continued relationship with a small team of doctors and nurses that was particularly significant in enabling many individuals to recover. And the fact of recognition by teams of Acehnese doctors and nurses supported by an international NGO (or in this case an IGO or intergovernmental organization) was also important to these villagers. What we do know is that a large majority of persons treated in this project improved significantly—in terms of symptoms and social functioning, and in their own rating of their mental health—over the course of the treatment. We judge this to mean that the treatment program was highly effective.

Conclusion

We have given only a small hint of what our data suggest. And we have not focused exclusively on PTSD. Indeed, our work argues strongly against a narrow focus on trauma and trauma treatment. Describing immediate psychological responses to disaster or violence as PTSD misses entirely the core of the disorder—the inability to work through trauma in a way that places it in the past, the failure to recover (Shalev 2007). It also argues against narrow debates about symptoms and symptom criteria, to the neglect of a larger public health perspective. On the other hand, our work suggests that PTSD is far from a pseudocondition. It is for many an extremely debilitating condition—a disorder of being unable to put in the past what one desperately wishes to put in the past. And more than this, the care provided by the remarkable young Indonesian doctors and nurses working on the outreach teams makes evident that PTSD, like other trauma-related illnesses, is a treatable condition, that nonpsychiatrist physicians and medical teams can be trained to give high-quality mental health care, and that issues of public commitment and implementation of service models should occupy public health specialists and humanitarian agencies, as well as anthropologists, as much as other aspects of postconflict work. Identifying who can benefit from what kinds of treatments and developing service models that can actually deliver such treatments is of far greater importance than ontological debates about whether PTSD is a real or pseudo condition.

Notes

1. For analyses of this work, see M. Good et al. 2010; M. Good 2010; B. Good 2012; M. Good and B. Good 2013; and B. Good et al. 2015.

2. This description of our initial visit to this village is drawn, in part, from B. Good (2012:529–30).

3. See B. Good et al. (2015) for a discussion of the issue of humanitarian governance. The diagnosis and treatment of trauma-related conditions is only one part of the broader critique of humanitarianism.

4. Authors Byron Good and Mary-Jo Good began as consultants to IOM in 2005, guiding the design of the project. They then continued their collaboration based on a subcontract from IOM Indonesia to Harvard Medical School, initiated in 2006. They took primary responsibility for designing the PNA surveys, analyzing the data (with the assistance of Matthew Lakoma), and writing the PNA1 and PNA2 reports, along with their collaborator and then doctoral student Jesse Grayman, who coordinated the research in the field. All three of us continued to work closely with IOM to develop and evaluate an intervention program to respond to the needs identified in the PNA. The Goods were primarily responsible for evaluations of both the pilot and extension phases of the DHPAP mental health outreach project, described in this chapter.

5. See B. Good et al. (2006) for a full description of methodology of the survey. Sampling was designed to develop a representative sample of adults, households, and villages in high-conflict subdistricts of three districts of North Aceh.

6. See B. Good et al. (2006) and M. Good et al. (2007) for description of the instruments used for the PNA research, including translation and adaptation of widely used instruments and the development of elements of the questionnaire specifically for this survey. The core instruments included a measure of conflict-related experiences, and symptom checklists for depression and anxiety (based on the Hopkins Symptom Checklist 25) and PTSD (the Harvard Trauma Questionnaire), following Mollica et al. (2004).

7. The DHPAP Pilot phase was supported by funds from the Norwegian government to IOM.

8. The DHPAP Extension phase was supported by a World Bank contract with IOM, with funds from DFID, the UK's Department for International Development.

9. Analyses presented here are drawn from B. Good and M. Good (2010).

10. We sometimes remind people that if Aceh were a state in Australia, one would expect there to be 420 psychiatrists, just to indicate the challenge of building systematic mental health care in a setting of so few mental health resources.

11. This analysis reports symptoms in Bahasa Indonesia, or Indonesian language. Local villages in our region spoke primarily Acehnese. The Indonesian terms, here, are translations of Acehnese and the terms used when Acehnese spoke Indonesian.

12. The term "complex trauma" was introduced as early as 1992 by Judith Herman (1992) but continues to carry diverse meanings in the literature. See the Introduction and Chapter 1 this volume, for discussion.

13. The DHPAP Pilot study used only medications identified as essential drugs and available (at least in theory) in the primary health care system. The only antidepressant used was amitriptyline. Following advice of consultants, the DHPAP Extension project added sertraline and fluoxetine to the IOM team's formulary.

References

Antze, Paul, and Michael Lambek, eds.
    1996 Tense Past: Cultural Essays in Trauma and Memory. London: Routledge.
Aspinall, Edward
    2005 The Helsinki Agreement: A More Promising Basis for Peace in Aceh? Policy Studies 20. Washington, D.C.: East-West Center.
    2009 Islam and Nation. Separatist Rebellion in Aceh, Indonesia. Stanford, Calif.: Stanford University Press.
Breslau, Joshua
    2004 Cultures of Trauma: Anthropological Views of Posttraumatic Stress Disorder in International Health. Culture, Medicine, and Psychiatry. 28(2):113–26.
Breslau, Joshua, and Peter J. Guarnaccia, eds.
    2004 Cultures of Trauma. Special Section of Culture, Medicine, and Psychiatry 28:113–220.
Das, Veena, Arthur Kleinman, Mamphela Ramphele, and Pamela Reynolds, eds.
    2000 Violence and Subjectivity. Berkeley: University of California Press.
Drexler, Elizabeth
    2008 Aceh, Indonesia: Securing the Insecure State. Philadelphia: University of Pennsylvania Press.
Duffield, Mark
    2001 Governing the Borderlands: Decoding the Power of Aid. Disasters 25:308–20.
    2002 Social Reconstruction and the Radicalization of Development: Aid as a Relation of Global Liberal Governance. Development and Change 33:1049–71.
    2009 Complex Emergencies and the Crisis of Developmentalism. IDS Bulletin 25:37–45.
    2012 Risk Management and the Bunkering of the Aid Industry. The End of the Development-Security Nexus? The Rise of Global Disaster Management. Jens Stilhoff Sorensen and Frederik Soderbaum, eds. Pp. 21–36. Special Issue of Development Dialogue 58:1–179.

Fassin, Didier, and Mariella Pandolfi, eds.

    2010 Contemporary States of Emergency: The Politics of Military and Humanitarian Interventions. New York: Zone.

Fassin, Didier, and Richard Rechtman

    2009 Empire of Trauma: An Inquiry into the Condition of Victimhood. Princeton, N.J.: Princeton University Press.

Friedman, Matthew J., Jonathan R. T. Davidson, and Dan J. Stein

    2009 Psychopharmacotherapy for Adults. *In* Effective Treatments for PTSD: Practice Guidelines from the International Society for Traumatic Stress Studies. Edna B. Foa, Matthew J. Friedman, and Judith A. Cohen, eds. Pp. 245–68. New York: Guilford.

Good, Byron J.

    1992 Culture and Psychopathology: Directions for Psychiatric Anthropology. *In* New Directions in Psychological Anthropology. Theodore Schwartz, Geoffrey M. White, and Catherine A. Lutz, eds. Pp. 181–205. Cambridge: Cambridge University Press.

    2012 Theorizing the "Subject" of Medical and Psychiatric Anthropology. The 2010 R. R. Marett Memorial Lecture. Journal of the Royal Anthropological Institute. 18(3):515–35

Good, Byron J., and Mary-Jo DelVecchio Good

    2010 Final Evaluation Report: IOM DHPAP Extension Program. Unpublished Ms.

Good, Byron J., Mary-Jo DelVecchio Good, Jesse Hession Grayman, and Matthew Lakoma

    2006 Psychosocial Needs Assessment of Communities Affected by the Conflict in the Districts of Pidie, Bireuen, and Aceh Utara. Jakarta: International Organization for Migration. Available at http://ghsm.hms.harvard.edu/uploads/pdf/good_m_pna1_iom.pdf.

Good, Byron J., Jesse Hession Grayman, and Mary-Jo DelVecchio Good

    2015 Humanitarianism and "Mobile Sovereignty" in Strong State Settings: Reflections on Medical Humanitarianism in Aceh, Indonesia. *In* Medical Humanitarianism: Ethnographies of Practice. Sharon Abramowitz and Catherine Panter-Brick, eds. Philadelphia: University of Pennsylvania Press.

Good, Byron J., and Devon E. Hinton

    2009 Introduction: Panic Disorder in Cross-Cultural and Historical Perspective. *In* Culture and Panic Disorder. Devon E. Hinton and Byron J. Good, eds. Pp. 1–28. Stanford, Calif.: Stanford University Press.

Good, Mary-Jo DelVecchio

    2010 Trauma in Post-Conflict Aceh and Psychopharmaceuticals as a Medium of Exchange. *In* Pharmaceutical Self: The Global Shaping of Experience in an Age of Psychopharmacology. Janis H. Jenkins, ed. Pp. 41–66. Santa Fe, N.M.: SAR Press.

    2015 Acehenese Women's Narratives of Traumatic Experience, Resilience and Recovery. *In* Genocide and Mass Violence: Memory, Symptom, Recovery.

Devon E. Hinton and Alexander L. Hinton, eds. Cambridge: Cambridge University Press.

Good, Mary-Jo DelVecchio, and Byron J. Good

2013 Perspectives on the Politics of Peace in Aceh, Indonesia. *In* Radical Egalitarianism: Local Realities, Global Relations. Felicity Aulino, Miriam Goheen, and Stanley J. Tambiah, eds. Pp. 191–208. New York: Fordham University Press.

Good, Mary-Jo DelVecchio, Byron J. Good, and Jesse Grayman

2010 Complex Engagements: Responding to Violence in Postconflict Aceh. *In* Contemporary States of Emergency: The Politics of Military and Humanitarian Interventions. Didier Fassin and Mariella Pandolfi, eds. pp 241–66. New York: Zone.

Good, Mary-Jo Delvecchio, Byron J. Good, Jesse Hession Grayman, and Matthew Lakoma

2007 A Psychosocial Needs Assessment of Communities in 14 Conflict-Affected Districts in Aceh. Jakarta: International Organization for Migration. Available at http://ghsm.hms.harvard.edu/uploads/pdf/good_m_pna2_iom.pdf.

Grayman, Jesse Hession, Mary-Jo Delvecchio Good, and Byron J. Good

2009 Conflict Nightmares and Trauma in Aceh. Culture, Medicine, and Psychiatry 33(2):290–312.

Hacking, Ian

1995 Rewriting the Soul: Multiple Personality and the Sciences of Memory. Princeton, N.J.: Princeton University Press.

Herman, Judith Lewis

1992 Trauma and Recovery. New York: Basic.

1993 Complex PTSD: A Syndrome in Survivors of Prolonged and Repeated Trauma. Journal of Traumatic Stress 5(3):377–91.

Hinton, Devon E.

2009 Introduction to the Special Section: Nightmares of Trauma Victims—Cross-Cultural Perspectives. Culture, Medicine, and Psychiatry 33(2):216–18.

Hinton, Devon E., Nigel P. Field, Angela Nickerson, Richard A. Bryant, and Naomi Simon

2013 Dreams of the Dead Among Cambodian Refugees: Frequency, Phenomenology, and Relationship to Complicated Grief and PTSD. Death Studies, 37:750–67.

Hinton, Devon E., Alexander L. Hinton, and Kok-Thay Eng

2012 PTSD and Key Somatic Complaints and Cultural Syndromes Among Rural Cambodians: The Results of a Needs Assessment Survey. Medical Anthropology Quarterly 29:147–54.

Hinton, Devon E., Alexander L. Hinton, Vuth Pich, Reattidara Loeum, and Mark Pollack

2009 Nightmares Among Cambodian Refugees: The Breaching of Concentric Ontological Security. Culture, Medicine, and Psychiatry 33:219–65.

Hinton, Devon E., and Roberto Lewis-Fernández

2011 The Cross-Cultural Validity of Posttraumatic Stress Disorder: Implications for DSM-5. Depression and Anxiety 28:783–801.

Hinton, Devon E., Angela Nickerson, and Richard A. Bryant
    2011 Worry, Worry Attacks, and PTSD Among Cambodian Refugees: A Path Analysis Investigation. Social Science and Medicine 72:1817–25.
Kleinman, Arthur, and Joan Kleinman
    1991 Suffering and Its Professional Transformation: Toward an Ethnography of Interpersonal Experience. Culture, Medicine and Psychiatry 15(3):275–301.
Mollica, Richard, L. MacDonald, Michael P. Massagli, and Derek Silove
    2004 Measuring Trauma, Measuring Torture: Instructions and Guidance on the Utilization of the Harvard Program in Refugee Trauma's Version The Hopkins Symptom Checklist 25 (HSCL-25) and The Harvard Trauma Questionnaire (HTQ). Cambridge, Mass.: Harvard Program in Refugee Trauma.
Mollica, Richard, Keith McInnes, Narcisa Sarajlić, James Lavelle, Iris Sarajlić, and Michael P. Massagli
    1999 Disability Associated with Psychiatric Comorbidity and Health Status in Bosnian Refugees Living in Croatia. Journal of the American Medical Association 282(5):433–39.
Pandolfi, Mariella
    2003 Contract of Mutual (In)Difference: Governance and Humanitarian Apparatus in Contemporary Albania and Kosovo. Indiana Journal of Global Legal Studies 10:369–81.
    2008 Laboratories of Intervention: The Humanitarian Governance of the Postcommunist Balkan Territories. In Postcolonial Disorders. Mary-Jo DelVecchio Good, Sandra Teresa Hyde, Sarah Pinto, and Byron J. Good, eds. Pp. 157–86. Berkeley: University of California Press.
Pupavac, Vanessa
    2001 Therapeutic Governance: Psycho-Social Intervention and Trauma Risk Management. Disasters 25:358–72.
    2002 Pathologizing Populations and Colonizing Minds: International Psychosocial Programs in Kosovo. Alternatives: Global, Local, Political 27:489–511.
    2004 Psychosocial Interventions and the Demoralization of Humanitarianism. Journal of Biosocial Science 36:491–504.
    2012 Global Disaster Management and Therapeutic Governance of Communities. In The End of the Development-Security Nexus? The Rise of Global Disaster Management. Jens Stilhoff Sorensen and Frederik Soderbaum, eds. Pp. 81–98. Special Issue of Development Dialogue 58:1–179.
Reid, Anthony, ed.
    2006 Verandah of Violence: The Background to the Aceh Problem. Singapore: Singapore University Press.
Samuels, Annemarie
    2012 After the Tsunami: The Remaking of Everyday Life in Banda Aceh, Indonesia. Ph.D. diss., Leiden University.

Shalev, Arieh Y.

2007 PTSD: A Disorder of Recovery? *In* Understanding Trauma: Biological, Clinical and Cultural Perspectives. Laurence Kirmayer, Robert Lemelson, and Mark Barad, eds. Pp. 207–24. New York: Cambridge University Press.

Summerfield, Derek

1999 A Critique of Seven Assumptions Behind Psychological Trauma Programmes in War-Affected Areas. Social Science and Medicine 48(10):1449–62.

2000 Childhood, War, Refugeedom and "Trauma": Three Core Questions for Mental Health Professionals. Transcultural Psychiatry 37:417–34.

2001 The Invention of Post-Traumatic Stress Disorder and the Social Usefulness of a Psychiatric Category. British Medical Journal 322:95–98.

2004 Cross-Cultural Perspectives on the Medicalization of Human Suffering. *In* Posttraumatic Stress Disorder: Issues and Controversies. Gerald M. Rosen, ed. Pp. 233–45. Chichester, West Sussex, England: John Wiley and Sons.

2008 How Scientifically Valid Is the Base of Global Mental Health? British Medical Journal 336:992–94.

World Health Organization (WHO)

2005 Briefing Note on Psychosocial/Mental Health Assistance to the Tsunami-Affected Region. February 4. WHO Department of Mental Health and Substance Abuse.

Young, Allan

1995 The Harmony of Illusions: Investing Post-Traumatic Stress Disorder. Princeton, N.J.: Princeton University Press.

Zarowsky, Christina, and Duncan Pedersen

2000 Editorial: Rethinking Trauma in a Transnational World. Transcultural Psychiatry 37:291–29.

CONTRIBUTORS

Carmela Alcántara, Ph.D., is an Associate Research Scientist, Center for Behavioral Cardiovascular Health, Department of Medicine, Columbia University Medical Center.

Tom Ball, Ph.D., is an enrolled member of the Klamath Tribes, who received his doctorate in Special Education and Rehabilitation in 1998 from the University of Oregon.

James K. Boehnlein, M.D., is a Professor of Psychiatry at Oregon Health and Science University.

Naomi Breslau, Ph.D., is a Professor of Epidemiology and Biostatistics, Michigan State University.

Whitney L. Duncan, Ph.D., is an Assistant Professor of Anthropology at the University of Northern Colorado.

Byron J. Good, Ph.D., is a Professor in the Department of Global Health and Social Medicine at Harvard Medical School.

Mary-Jo DelVecchio Good, Ph.D., is a Professor in the Department of Global Health and Social Medicine at Harvard Medical School.

Jesse H. Grayman, Ph.D., is an Assistant Professor in the School of Humanities and Social Sciences at Nanyang Technological University, Singapore.

Bridget M. Haas, Ph.D., is an Adjunct Assistant Professor of Anthropology at Case Western Reserve University and a Visiting Scholar at Project Narrative, Ohio State University.

Devon E. Hinton, M.D., Ph.D., is an Associate Professor of Psychiatry at Harvard University and the Director of a Southeast Asian Clinic in Lowell, Massachusetts.

Erica Caple James, Ph.D., is an Associate Professor of Anthropology at the Massachusetts Institute of Technology.

Janis H. Jenkins, Ph.D., is a Professor of Anthropology and Adjunct Professor of Psychiatry at the University of California, San Diego.

Hanna Kienzler, Ph.D., is a Lecturer in the Department of Social Science, Health, and Medicine at King's College London.

Brandon Kohrt, M.D., Ph.D., is an Assistant Professor of Psychiatry and Global Health at Duke University.

Roberto Lewis-Fernández, M.D., is a Professor of Psychiatry at Columbia University.

Richard J. McNally, Ph.D., is a Professor of Psychology at Harvard University.

Theresa D. O'Nell, Ph.D., is an Associate Professor of Anthropology at the University of Oregon.

Duncan Pedersen, M.D., is a Professor at the Department of Psychiatry, Division of Social and Transcultural Psychiatry, McGill University.

Nawaraj Upadhaya, M.A., M.Sc., is with the Transcultural Psychosocial Organization (TPO) Nepal, Kathmandu, Nepal, and HealthNet TPO, Amsterdam, the Netherlands.

Carol M. Worthman, Ph.D., is a Professor of Anthropology at Emory University.

Allan Young, Ph.D., is a Professor of Anthropology at McGill University.

INDEX

CPSIA information can be obtained
at www.ICGtesting.com
Printed in the USA
JSHW012351220922
30887JS00001B/2